Occupation by Design:
Building Therapeutic Power

Occupation by Design: Building Therapeutic Power

Doris Pierce, PhD, OTR/L, FAOTA

Endowed Chair in Occupational Therapy
Eastern Kentucky University
Richmond, Kentucky

 F.A. Davis Company • Philadelphia

F.A. Davis Company
1915 Arch Street
Philadelphia, PA 19103
www.fadavis.com

Printed in the United States of America

Last digit indicates print number: 10 9 8 7

Acquisitions Editor: Margaret Biblis
Developmental Editor: Peg Waltner
Production Editor: Ann McKelvie
Cover Designer: Louis J. Forgione

As new scientific information becomes available through basic and clinical research, recommended treatments and drug therapies undergo changes. The author(s) and publisher have done everything possible to make this book accurate, up to date, and in accord with accepted standards at the time of publication. The author(s), editors, and publisher are not responsible for errors or omissions or for consequences from application of the book, and make no warranty, expressed or implied, in regard to the contents of the book. Any practice described in this book should be applied by the reader in accordance with professional standards of care used in regard to the unique circumstances that may apply in each situation. The reader is advised always to check product information (package inserts) for changes and new information regarding dose and contraindications before administering any drug. Caution is especially urged when using new or infrequently ordered drugs.

Library of Congress Cataloging-in-Publication Data

Pierce, Doris E.
    Occupation by design : building therapeutic power / Doris E. Pierce.
       p. ; cm.
    Includes bibliographical references and index.
    ISBN 10: 0-8036-1048-3   ISBN 13: 978-0-8036-1048-4
    1. Occupational therapy. I. Title.
    [DNLM: 1. Occupational Therapy—methods—Handbooks. WB 39 P615o 2003]
RM735.P546 2003
615.8'515–dc21

                        2003043404

To occupational therapy students, the most remarkable students one can have; to the creativity and love of my family and friends, the source of my own strength; and to the grass that grows in the cracks of the LA freeways.

. . . Foreword

In the mid-1980s a group of University of Southern California (USC) occupational therapy department faculty and graduate assistants met regularly, carrying on an exciting discussion about the major concepts that could be recognized as the core of the academic discipline of occupational science. It was a heady time of divergent definitions, models, diagrams, and relentless drive to express and communicate individual ideas about a topic to which most have devoted their professional lives—understanding occupation.

The process of such academic dialogue has continued and grown, from the classrooms of the first PhD program in occupational science to the research and writings of that program's graduates and those of other occupational scientists attracted by these ideas, which are important to the health of people around the globe. The sharing in occupational science symposia (first at USC, then elsewhere in America, and in Japan, Australia, Great Britain, and Canada) became more formalized with the development of the International Society of Occupational Scientists, the Society for the Study of Occupation: USA, and similar groups in other countries. The research and knowledge began as a trickle; we hope to see it flood the fields of health care and the everyday lives of people everywhere.

But how can we accomplish this task? It is first necessary to understand oneself and others as occupational beings with a biologically innate need for occupational engagement with the world around us. Yet other background remains necessary: understanding the complexity of occupation, those sometime routine engagements in doing and being with which we shape ourselves and our lives, and understanding and developing skill to use occupation therapeutically.

Once occupational therapy students learned biomechanical activity analysis, an extremely limited focus on one aspect of occupation with therapeutic potential. In contrast, the power of the tool that is occupation—appealing, intact, and dead-on accurate for the real goals of people engaged in therapy—is almost overwhelming in its life-transforming potential. To enable occupational therapists to use this tool in the creative ways that have been the hallmark of our profession since its inception, we need to see ourselves as designers of therapeutic occupation and develop design skills focused on the strengths of occupation as a therapeutic tool. This book is written to guide the process of knowledge and skill development for this purpose.

Dr. Doris Pierce has been a part of the process of development of occupational science for use by occupational therapists for most of the last 20 years. I enjoyed her enthusiastic participation in the dialogues of the initial study group as well as in classes in her doctoral studies in occupational science. That dialogue continued for years outside the classroom as we met to discuss definitions, concepts, and ways to apply our knowledge to ourselves through the use of occupational diaries and other self-analytic methods.

Discussions of the issue of balance in occupation have intrigued us for years, and her review of previous concepts and suggestions for a new way of viewing occupational balance is a definite contribution to the field. But most useful to occupational therapists is the expansion, in this book, of ideas that were briefly shared in journal articles emphasizing the unique therapeutic qualities of occupation. One last characteristic that has always been important to me personally and professionally is the idea that learning, working, and living itself can be fun. Dr. Pierce's book clearly approaches the idea of designing therapeutic occupation from a perspective that is not only academically solid and creative but also fun! Ideally, using these materials to guide one's study of occupational design can be not only productive but also pleasurable and restorative, for the individual and for the field of occupational therapy.

Ruth Zemke

... Acknowledgements

I would like to acknowledge, most of all, Ruth Zemke, PhD, OTR, FAOTA, of the University of Southern California. If it had not been for her willingness to engage in discussion and research exploring these broad concepts regarding occupation, *Occupation by Design* would never have been created. We started out to write the book together, but that was not to be. I salute Dr. Zemke's investment in the building of occupational science as a community of scholars.

I would also like to acknowledge the Occupational Therapy faculty of the University of Southern California for their courage, vision, persistence, and leadership in establishing and nurturing the discipline of occupational science. They are a team of stars who have bypassed that stuffy pomposity so endemic to academia, passionately exploring occupation for its applications to their own lives, to their research, and to their overriding commitment to the profession of occupational therapy.

I would especially like to thank the occupational therapy students of Creighton University with whom I explored early drafts of the book through its use in classes. Their input was invaluable to me. Future student readers of the book will not appreciate the degree to which they should be grateful to those students for its organization and style. Also, I am especially grateful to the graduate assistants who have been primarily involved in assisting with the preparation of *Occupation by Design*: Brad Egan of the Omaha Geeks, Michelle Fischer, and Xiaorong Wang.

I would like to express my appreciation to the staff of F. A. Davis for their professionalism and for their investment in the publication of occupational therapy theory, especially Margaret Biblis, Susan Rhyner, and Peg Waltner. Lynn Borders Caldwell shepherded the book gently through its formative stages allowing it to become what it is now, despite a much longer timeline than we originally anticipated. F. A. Davis really knows how to take care of its authors.

I would also like to recognize here the talent of the artist for *Occupation by Design*, Amy Sands. Her ability to take my ideas and convert them into visual form is amazing and adds much to the book.

And a broad thanks to the friends, family, faculty, chairs, deans, and students who have dealt mildly with me in my crankiest moments of writing and been forgiving of the volumes of time it has required to complete this work.

... Preface

Occupation by Design is an occupational scientist's dream. It is a dream of providing powerful interventions based in a sophisticated understanding of our field's primary modality: occupation. Writing this book has provided a 7-year, intellectually exciting struggle to craft an introductory synthesis of this powerful concept for occupational therapy students. It has been rewarding. Still, I will be glad to dance my way back now to the simpler pleasures of conducting research and writing up data.

Occupational therapy students, later occupational therapists, are remarkable people. Occupational therapy is a young profession. We have long operated without a complex understanding of occupation and activity, focusing intensely on treatment and sidestepping our need for a deeper understanding of the phenomenon we apply. We have prepared our students as best we can, with theories from here, there, and everywhere (often incompatible in their underlying assumptions), with practice frameworks, some research on clinical reasoning, a strong valuing of occupation and activity, and field experiences we hope will help them integrate this patchwork into effective interventions. I remember how that felt—overwhelming and difficult. I did not understand, as a new therapist, that this lack of clarity was not necessarily my own fault. It is as if we expect students to forge individually, through experience, the synthesized knowledge of occupation and its therapeutic use that we cannot yet give them in their education. And, remarkably, some do just that. Now our understanding of occupation itself is blossoming. Occupational science publications are increasing. Documents of our association are emphasizing occupation-based practice. Occupational therapy is evolving into a mature profession whose interventions emanate from a unique knowledge base, as in medicine and psychology. To reach its full potential to contribute to the lives of its clients, occupational therapy needs many bridges built between the study of occupation and its use in practice. This book is, I hope, one of those bridges.

Occupation by Design is largely a synthesis of theory and research on occupation and activity. I have learned from my students, however, that one must constantly argue the "why" of studying various aspects of occupation. That is, they want to know how each aspect of occupation might make them better therapists and how they will put such knowledge to work. They are service-driven! So although the primary intent of the book is to provide an introductory exploration of occupation, I have included throughout an explanation of how each described aspect of occupation can be used in practice.

The book follows a strong and simple structure, which I hope will provide readers with a map to hold in mind as they navigate through a concept-rich landscape. The structure is a target divided into thirds, with therapeutic power as the center of the circle. The circle is repeated with sections highlighted, as a signal at the beginning of each chapter that "You are here." The book covers three primary aspects of occupation: its subjective dimensions, contextual dimensions, and therapeutic applications through the occupational design process. What can be learned from each third of the book makes a different contribution to effective occupation-based interventions. Mastered together, they are powerful.

The process of the book, if worked through from beginning to end, unfolds in the following entwined sequences:

- From building insight into one's own occupations, to gaining skills for grasping the occupational patterns of diverse others, to applying occupation as therapy
- From viewing occupation from the perspective of the subjective experience of an individual (very American and historically comfortable), to seeing occupation as having contextual dimensions inseparable from individual experience (less developed in occupational therapy), to using both subjective and contextual dimensions of occupation to build effective interventions
- From an appreciation of the creative design process that lies behind all projects, to designing occupational experiences for oneself, to designing for others, and finally, to designing therapeutic occupations for practice

Each chapter ends with exercises called Power Builders to help actively develop skills for exploring and applying the concepts described. A selection of client cases appears in Appendix A for use with the Power Builders. A recommended list of occupational narratives and narratives of disability to be used with these exercises are provided in Appendixes B and C.

I hope you find the process and the content of *Occupation by Design* as enjoyable, thought-provoking, and creative as I have in its writing. It is the kind of project that never seems quite done, always offering more to think about and explore in occupation. The breadth of the book has been one of its most difficult aspects for me as a scholar, and I hope readers are forgiving for all the important work that surely has been left out. Yet the importance to occupational therapy students and practitioners of a broad overview of occupation seemed pressing. May this effort contribute to your understanding of yourself as an occupational being, and to the power and creativity of your practice.

Doris Pierce, PhD, OTR/L, FAOTA
Endowed Chair in Occupational Therapy
Eastern Kentucky University

.... Contents

Becoming a Designer of Therapeutically Powerful Occupations

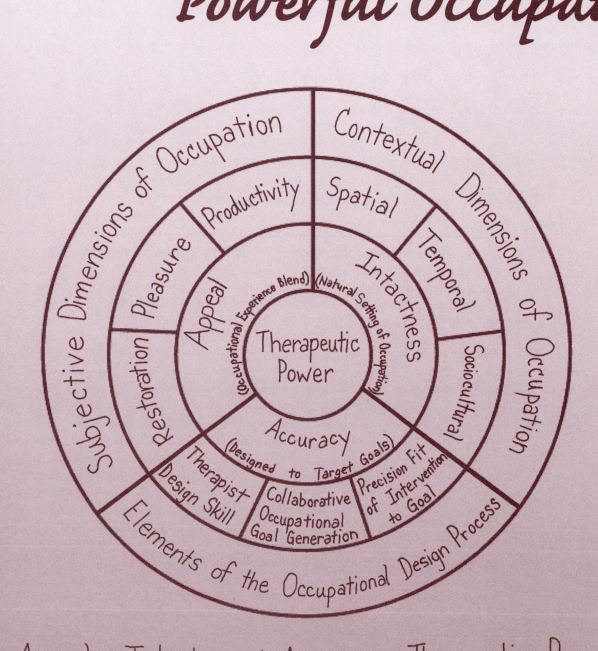

Appeal + Intactness + Accuracy = Therapeutic Power

CHAPTER 1

Welcome to Occupation by Design

What Is an Occupation? An Activity?

A Little Occupational Science History

Understanding Occupations: First in Yourself and Others, Then as Therapy

You Are What You Do: The Occupations of Occupational Therapists

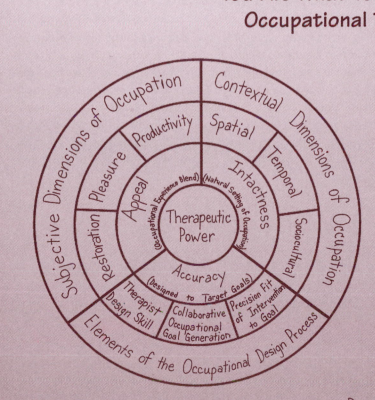

Appeal + Intactness + Accuracy = Therapeutic Power

Welcome to *Occupation by Design*. You must be an occupational therapist. Well, maybe you are just starting out as an occupational therapist, or maybe you are very experienced, but you are still one of those unique individuals who use occupation to facilitate positive changes in people's lives. For me, being an occupational therapist has been exciting, challenging, creative, and sometimes frustrating. It has always been growth provoking. It is a privilege to spend our days helping people reclaim activities that make them who they are. Often, we can see our clients changing before our eyes. We share in their emotional struggles and joy as they work in occupational therapy toward goals important to them. If you imagine the occupational therapy community made up of a large group of individuals all focusing their life work in this way, you can see that you have indeed joined a unique profession.

Helping your clients learn or reclaim occupations is a complex art backed by science. In this book, I have tried to lay out for you the three primary skills that are used by all occupational therapists, regardless of the specialized areas in which they choose to practice: (1) understanding occupation, (2) developing design skills, and (3) applying occupation in practice. As an artist starts out by doing perspective and still-life drawings, you will be asked to appreciate the complexity of occupations in your life and in the lives of everyday people before you try to apply creative occupational interventions to people with disabilities. Here, you will also be encouraged to develop your creativity and problem-solving skills, so essential to becoming an effective therapist. An introduction to treatment through the use of occupation is also provided here. This will give you the foundation on which you can build special expertise for different populations and types of disabilities with which you will work in the future. If I had to choose one focus of this book, I would say it is an introduction to occupation for occupational therapists.

What Is an Occupation? An Activity?

So, before we go any further, let's stop to consider the meanings of the terms *occupation* and *activity*. These are the two central concepts of occupational therapy. They are terms so closely related that they are often used interchangeably. Their meanings have been tangled together since the beginning of the profession (Pierce, 2001a). But they are actually different, and both are important. Because we, as occupational therapists, use human "doing" as both the means and the ends of intervention, it is critical that we fully comprehend the terms occupation and activity (Gray, 1998). That is, doing something is the therapeutic event. Begin able to do something in particular is also the goal toward which the client and therapist work.

Definitions of Occupation and Activity

Activity and occupation are both related to human doing, but in different ways. Here are the definitions of both terms that I proposed recently in the *American Journal of Occupational Therapy* (Pierce, 2001a, p. 139):

> "*An occupation is a specific individual's personally constructed, nonrepeatable experience. That is, an occupation is a subjective event in perceived temporal, spatial, and sociocultural conditions that are unique to that one-time occurrence. An occupation has a shape, a pace, a beginning and an ending, a shared or solitary aspect, a cultural meaning to the person, and an infinite number of other perceived contextual qualities. A person interprets his or her occupations before, during, and after they*

happen. Although an occupation can be observed, interpretation of the meaning or emotional content of an occupation by anyone other than the person experiencing it is necessarily inexact.

An activity is an idea held in the minds of persons and in their shared cultural language. An activity is a culturally defined and general class of human actions. The commonsense meanings of activities, such as play or cooking, enable us to communicate about generalized categories of occupational experiences in a broad, accessible way. An activity is not experienced by a specific person; is not observable as an occurrence; and is not located in fully existent temporal, spatial, and sociocultural context.

Can you see the difference in these two terms? If not, don't be worried. Many highly experienced occupational therapists are just beginning to consider the differences between activity and occupation. This text is just an introduction. As you work your way through the book, you will begin to understand the differences between occupation and activity and why they are important.

Distinguishing between Occupation and Activity during Intervention

Here is a treatment example for you to think about, to illustrate the difference between occupation and activity and why it is important in occupational therapy. I was working once with a 9-year-old boy with autism. Let's call him Tim. He had an aversion to textures that really disorganized his behavior at school, especially during art activities and snack time. He also had cognitive delays, was almost entirely nonverbal, and rarely made eye contact. The activity I thought might be helpful for trying to reduce his sensory defensiveness was sculpting things out of play dough. I had a variety of colors of play dough, and some small plastic tools for shaping, pressing out, cutting, and rolling the dough. We worked at a quiet table, across the room from the other children, who were doing a big history collage project. Tim was clear about not wanting to join in the cutting and pasting of the collage, which did not surprise either his teacher or me, because his cutting skills and sensory defensiveness were a poor fit with the task.

The activity I had in mind for Tim that day was making simple things, like a little ball or a pancake, out of play dough. Once the occupation began, however, I saw something completely different from what I had anticipated when I was thinking at a broad activity level. The experience Tim had and the occupation that occurred were not like the activity idea I had imagined. When Tim opened the cans of play dough, which was a bit of a struggle, the smell of the fresh dough was strong. I could smell it. I thought he was going to gag, but he did not. I helped him to dump out some of the dough. I showed him how to roll it out into a pancake with the rolling pin and then encouraged him to try it. At first he did try, but then, when his palm touched the dough, he drew back. He did not want to do any more. We continued on for a little while. I encouraged him to try, by continuing with my demonstrations. I helped him hold a little plastic knife to cut the play dough without touching it. When I tried to get him to manipulate the play dough directly with his hands, however, he began to scream as soon as he touched it. We then quickly moved outside to the playground to give Tim space to move around and to reduce our disruption of the classroom. Later, I came back and put the play dough away. We had gone a little farther with the play dough texture than Tim could handle.

Can you see how the activity idea I had and Tim's occupational experience were different? The activity of manipulating play dough is thought of as fun, creative, free, spontaneous, and colorful. The occupational experience Tim had was aversive, persuaded, somewhat scary, stinky, and nasty-feeling. That was, obviously, not my best therapy session, but does it show you how important it is to distinguish between occupation and activity? It is critical that we understand that our vague idea about doing something is not necessarily the experience our client is having during intervention.

A Little Occupational Science History

One of the reasons that the meanings of *occupation* and *activity* have been tangled and interchangeable for so long is that they were both incorporated into the field at its inception but from different theory bases (Pierce, 2001a). *Activity* came from theories of industrial efficiency that were being used to design prostheses and adapt work activities for World War II veterans. The activity approaches were focused on getting persons with disabilities up to the performance level of skilled workers by measuring the movements, forces, and grasps used by skilled workers and then adapting them. *Occupation* came from moral treatment and social reform movements that were concerned with the quality of the actual experiences of disadvantaged people such as recent immigrants, factory workers, soldiers, and asylum patients. Occupational approaches focused on changes in time use, habits, skills, and self-organization. But the field was very young in the late 19th and early 20th centuries, just getting organized, and was not yet ready for fine theoretical distinctions between occupation and activity.

Today, occupational therapy has come a long way from its early roots. After many years of practice based on knowledge imported from other disciplines, occupational therapy is now operating increasingly from its own disciplinary knowledge base: occupational science. For a lengthy period of our history, the field emulated medicine and medical thinking. This worked well to gain us access to providing interventions for physically disabled clients in hospital settings, and the field expanded rapidly. Educational programs became more sophisticated, and the knowledge base of the field slowly grew. Although early theorists had remarked on the importance of "work and play and rest and sleep" (Meyer, 1922/1977, p. 640), it is only recently that much research into occupation and activity, separate from their use in therapy, has been done. This book is very much grounded in an occupational science perspective because I am an occupational scientist.

When people ask me what occupational science is, I always wonder what the answer should be. I have three answers. (1) Occupational science is a discipline. (2) Occupational science is a movement. (3) Occupational science is a story.

"Occupational science is an academic discipline, the purpose of which is to generate knowledge about the form, function, and meaning of human occupation" (Zemke & Clark, 1996, p. vii). In the debut article on occupational science in the *American Journal of Occupational Therapy*, we argued that the basic study of occupation would serve occupational therapy by providing knowledge about its primary modality that would not come from any other academic discipline and thus strengthen the efficacy of the applied science of occupational therapy (Clark, Parham, Carlson, Frank, Jackson, Pierce, et al, 1991). The PhD Program in Occupational Science at the University of Southern California accepted its first students in 1989 and graduated its first doctorally prepared occupational scientist in 1994. The *Journal of Occupational Science* is completely dedicated to publishing occupational science research. Occupational science symposia and research societies now exist in many countries.

"The occupational science movement . . . [is a] new discipline, separate from but supporting the applied science of occupational therapy. As a discipline, occupational science would be more like sociology or biology, which are not directly concerned about matters of practical application" (Kielhofner, 1992, p. 327). In this quote I like the term *movement*. Occupational therapy has always had a strong social conscience. In the early days, occupational therapy was allied with the moral treatment and settlement house movements, and it adopted arts and crafts movement concerns about the lives of workers in an industrial age. Later, the field responded with patriotic efforts in the World Wars. In the 60s and 70s, occupational therapy supported civil rights and the independent living movement, and benefited from renewed cultural interests in crafts and consciousness raising by using these approaches in mental-health settings. Today, occupational therapy is moving increasingly into community-based practice and entrepreneurial models. Like occupational therapy, occupational science is also very responsive to social movements. Feminist theory and a concern for the subjective experience of the individual mark a decidedly liberationist and individual rights standpoint in the discipline. Occupational science in Australia is especially marked by a concern for occupational justice, the rights of people to be purposefully engaged in rewarding activity, especially those in institutional settings, such as prisons, orphanages, and other long-term-care settings.

Occupational science is also a story, different every time, depending on who tells it. It is a story of passionate occupational therapists, predominantly female practitioners, pushing forward to create an academic discipline because it would better serve clients if we did so. This is an unusual story in the academic world. Although an interest in occupation has been with us since the creation of the field, it is easiest to trace the story of occupational science from the work of Mary Reilly (1976) in occupational behavior. After Reilly's leadership of the Department of Occupational Therapy at the University of Southern California, Elizabeth Yerxa became department chair. It was Yerxa who made the dream of the basic science of occupation real by mandating that her faculty work together to produce the proposals and curricula that were to become the first doctoral program in occupational science. Yerxa retired just as the program began. Florence Clark, who has been a dynamic leader and highly successful researcher and theorist, replaced her. I have no doubt, however, that she would attribute her success to the strong group of faculty members who surround her, all with active research agendas related to occupational science. Although the University of Southern California has served as the hub of this evolving discipline, there are now occupational scientists on many faculties around the United States and the world, occupational science degree programs at several levels, and active occupational science societies in many countries.

The story of occupational science will continue for many years. In a way, you are now a part of this story, as you take the occupational science offered here and integrate it into your own knowledge base, to support your own excellent practice, exactly as the early visionaries of occupational science dreamed that the story would unfold. Occupation-based practice is a clear revival of our long-held valuing of occupation as a therapeutic modality, yet it bases intervention on occupational science knowledge. This book is my effort to build a bridge for practitioners between occupational science and its applications in occupational therapy. As I have said elsewhere (Pierce, 2001b), the bridge between occupational science research and its applications in occupational therapy will be accomplished in three ways: (1) effective education in understanding occupation and occupation-based approaches, (2) demonstration sites where knowledge of occupation is being effectively applied in practice, and (3) generative discourse regarding how knowledge of occupation is best applied in occupational therapy. This book is presented as a contribution to the effective education of practitioners in strong occupation-based practice. You

Generative Discourse
Demonstration Sites
Effective Education

Knowledge of Occupation   Powerful Occupation-Based Practice are a new generation of therapists whose work will be more scientific, more effective, and more valued by clients than ever before.

Understanding Occupations: First in Yourself and Others, Then as Therapy

To understand occupation as a modality for intervention, you must first study it in typical individuals. That is why this book so emphasizes that you explore occupation in your own life and in the lives of people you know. Developing your insight into typical occupation before you try to examine or treat a disrupted occupational pattern in a person with disabilities is critical to strong clinical skills.

Why Study Occupation? I Just Want to Treat Clients!

Sometimes students say to me, "But why do I need all this occupation theory? Just show me what to do as a therapist." Some are too polite to say this, but they still wonder. They are excited about their new profession and in a hurry to experience helping clients. Perhaps they have seen occupational therapists working with clients who have made it look easy; maybe they were using some play activities, or cooking, or designing a splint.

Think about it this way. Would you want to be treated by a physician who did not want to understand anatomy before treating you? Would you want to drive on a bridge designed by an engineer who did not want to study physics, engineering design, and building materials before supervising the construction of that bridge? Would you want to have a prescription filled by a pharmacist who did not study chemistry? This is the relationship between basic and applied science. The basic sciences study and describe phenomena. The applied sciences develop effective ways of using those phenomena to serve society. Being a competent professional means that you have basic science knowledge on which you base a unique reasoning process. Although what professionals do may look fairly simple from the outside, it is not. In fact, the better the theoretical reasoning of a professional, the easier he or she will make the work appear. Here are some examples of the relationships of basic and applied sciences.

Basic Science	Applied Science
Anatomy, Physiology	Medicine
Physics, Math, Geology	Engineering
Chemistry, Math	Pharmacy
Psychology	Clinical Psychology
Astronomy, Physics	Aeronautics
Earth Science	Meteorology
Biology	Agriculture
Anatomy, Kinesiology	Physical Therapy
Sociology	Social Work
Occupational Science	Occupational Therapy

The Structure of the Book

In the sequence of the book, you will first study an aspect of occupation, and then you will explore how you might use that knowledge in treatment. At the end of the book you will find a whole section on intervention using occupation. Here is a quick tour of the book's contents to get you oriented. It's very easy to understand how it is laid out because it is so structured. The best way to see the structure of the book and how the ideas of the book fit together is to look first at the circular diagram of the therapeutic power of occupation.

The book and the circular diagram are set up to explain the central concern of occupational therapy: the therapeutic power of occupation. See that in the middle? To understand therapeutic power, you need to understand three main concepts of how occupational therapists use occupation as intervention—occupational appeal, intactness, and accuracy. Each of these is based on different aspects of occupation. *Appeal* applies the subjective experience of occupation. *Intactness* applies the contextual dimensions of occupation. *Accuracy* describes how occupation-based interventions occur. To apply your understanding of occupation and occupation-based practice, you also need design skills. All of these topics are woven into the

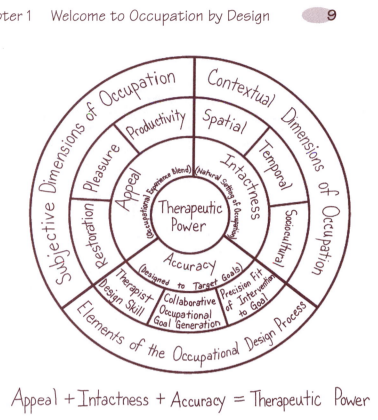

Appeal + Intactness + Accuracy = Therapeutic Power

book, along with lots of fun ways to try them out. Altogether, the approach presented here is called *occupational design process* (Pierce, 2001b). Briefly, here is an overview of each book section.

Section I. Becoming a Designer of Therapeutically Powerful Occupations

The first section of the book (where you are now) prepares you for your explorations of occupation. It includes this introductory chapter and a chapter on design process. *Design process* is the creative thinking used by occupational therapists to problem solve, set goals, and create ideas for intervention and programming. To be an occupational therapist requires highly developed creativity. We do not treat from cookbook protocols. The life challenges of people with disabilities are complex, exist in real-world situations, and emanate from deeply felt desires to create authentic, satisfying lives. Effective use of occupation to meet clients' therapeutic goals requires the therapist to master the convergent and divergent thinking of design process.

In Chapter 2, you will learn the seven phases of design process:

1. Motivation
2. Investigation
3. Definition
4. Ideation
5. Idea selection
6. Implementation
7. Evaluation

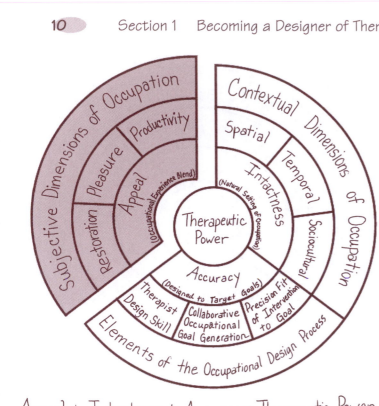

Appeal + Intactness + Accuracy = Therapeutic Power

You will have opportunities to practice these seven skill sets through exercises that I call Power Builders because they will build your ability to provide therapeutically powerful interventions. I encourage you to do as many Power Builders as you feel you will need to get your skills to the level your clients will require of you. When using the Power Builders, you will also have the opportunity to practice your skills through the use of the client cases and narratives provided in the resource appendixes at the back of the book.

Design process works in all areas of life, from planning a party to starting a new occupational therapy program. If you use the Power Builders to practice these skills, you will see a change in your own creative thinking and problem-solving abilities. After Chapter 2, Power Builders at the end of each chapter help you explore a dimension of occupation, apply it to yourself and others, and experiment with using that dimension to design interventions. After you have had many opportunities to practice your design skills in Chapters 3 through 13, you will circle back to specifically consider the use of design process in occupational therapy intervention, in Chapter 14, Therapist Design Skill.

Section II. Designing for Appeal: Pleasure, Productivity, and Restoration in Occupations

The appeal of an occupation to a client will greatly affect the degree to which he or she relates to it as an effective intervention. If you suggest doing something that the person with whom you are working does not find enjoyable, important to reaching his or her goals, or rejuvenating, he or she is likely to reject it or engage in it in only a quick and superficial way. This is the origin of old jokes about "doing basket weaving," when patients in psychiatric settings were often given basket making to do, regardless of how appealing they might or might not find that particular activity. Of course, basketry can be very useful in intervention, but only for someone to whom it appeals.

Appeal results from a combination of the pleasure, productivity, and restoration in an experience. The chapter on pleasure covers play and leisure, sensation, humor, ritual, and addiction. *Productivity* includes the need for challenge and avoidance of boredom, work ethic, work identity, and stress. *Restoration* addresses sleeping, eating and drinking, self-care, and quiet-focus activities such as hobbies and spirituality. The section starts off with a chapter discussing balance between these aspects of the experience of occupation. All chapters have Power Builders at the end that provide ways to apply the ideas from the chapter to increase your understanding of occupation in your own life, in the lives of others, and in your design of interventions. Using this carefully developed understanding of the pleasurable, productive, and

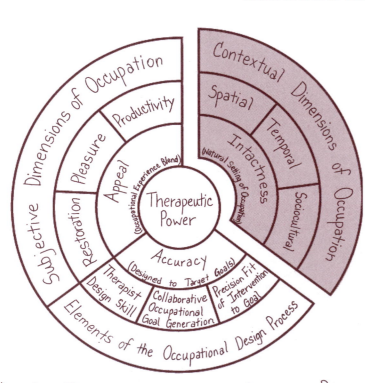

Appeal + Intactness + Accuracy = Therapeutic Power

restorative aspects of occupation, the occupational therapist can design appealing interventions that will motivate and engage clients in working toward treatment goals.

Section III. Designing for Intactness: The Spatial, Temporal, and Sociocultural Dimensions of Occupation

The *intactness* of an occupation is the degree to which an occupation would occur in the usual context for that individual if it were not being used as intervention. For example, results improved when I treated infants and toddlers with feeding problems in their homes, using the preferred ethnic foods of their families, with the mother or other family members working with the children, and at usual mealtimes. *Intactness* is a newer concept for occupational therapy than is appeal. We have understood appeal since the beginning of the profession. It was only in the second half of the 20th century, however, that occupational therapists increasingly began moving out of hospital settings and into community settings. Community-based therapists are seeking greater intervention effectiveness by working in the natural settings of their clients. Another great example of intact intervention is on-site industrial rehabilitation, in which an injured worker receives occupational therapy at his or her job site, working with the usual machines, coworkers, space, and job demands to which he or she will return full time when therapy is complete.

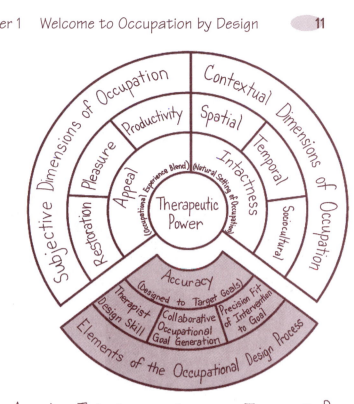

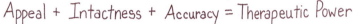

Appeal + Intactness + Accuracy = Therapeutic Power

To design intact interventions, the therapist must understand the temporal, spatial, and sociocultural contexts of an occupational experience. The section on intactness starts out with an evolutionary perspective on human occupation to lay the basis for understanding modern occupational context. *Spatial context* includes the physical body, environmental conditions, object use, and the symbolic meaning of spaces. *Temporal context* addresses circadian rhythms, social schedules and clocks, subjective variations in the experienced speed of time, orchestration of a daily pattern of activities, and typical development of occupational patterns. *Sociocultural context* describes identity, the continuum from solitary to completely interactive occupations, relationships, cultural diversity, gender, and healthcare cultures. Again, all the chapters in this section have Power Builders at the end that provide ways of applying the ideas presented to increase your understanding of occupation in your own life, in the lives of others, and in your design of interventions. Throughout these chapters, the implications for intervention of understanding these dimensions of occupational context are explained. Also a full chapter at the end of the section focuses on using intactness to increase the therapeutic power of occupation-based interventions.

Section IV. Designing for Accuracy: Elements of the Occupational Design Process

After spending time in study of the subjective and contextual dimensions of occupation in Sections II and III, you will reach Section IV, focused completely on intervention. Having developed your basic science knowledge of occupation, you will be ready to consider the applied science of using occupation as intervention. The section on intervention accuracy is the shortest of the three main sections, for two reasons. First, it is meant to serve only as an introduction to occupation-based practice, to complement the book's primary focus on understanding occupation. Second, research on occupation-based practice is, ironically, a rather new area in occupational therapy. I expect that much research on occupation-based practice will be published in the coming years as the field brings the explosion of occupational science knowledge to bear on intervention. This section attempts to gather together an overview of our current understanding of best practice in using occupation in intervention.

To provide Section IV with a base from which to consider the design of occupation-based interventions, a small study of occupation-based program development in an independent and assisted-living center for elders is described in Chapter 13. Then, in the following chapters, the experiences of the therapists in that study are used to illustrate the concepts being presented about intervention. Chapter 14 looks specifically at design process in occupational therapy. Chapter 15 focuses on developing effective collaboration skills to create goals of intervention that truly reflect the life priorities of the client. Chapter 16 is perhaps the most ambitious, asking us to consider not just how, but how well, we are using occupation in treatment. That is, this chapter examines how precisely the intervention fits the goals of the client. Finally, Chapter 17 summarizes accuracy in occupation-based intervention. As in all the other chapters, Power Builders are provided for you, focusing even more in this last section on intervention design and drawing heavily on the cases in Appendix A.

Section V. Conclusion

The last section of the book contains a summary chapter and the resource appendixes. The summary chapter, You Are What You Do, will challenge you to think about what kind of life you wish to lead and what type of therapist you envision becoming. Central questions about your career plans will be posed for you to answer. The appendixes contain the client cases and recommended occupational and disability narratives for your use in the Power Builders throughout the book.

You Are What You Do: The Occupations of Occupational Therapists

Throughout *Occupation by Design,* you will find yourself challenged:

- To become more creative
- To understand the dance you dance in your own daily occupational pattern
- To gain greater insight into the lives of the people around you
- To appreciate the unique perspectives of people with disabilities
- To become the finest occupational therapist you can become

You will be offered occupational appeal, intactness, and accuracy as avenues to potent intervention. Developing in these ways will be completely your choice. Like the students who ask me why they need to learn about occupation, you can choose to quickly forget the concepts presented here and practice largely from the traditional approaches of occupational therapy's past. If you so choose, you will not be alone, and in many ways it will be the easier path. Or you can accept these opportunities to live an occupationally aware and creative life as a therapist, continuing on an ever-rising spiral of mastery to strong therapeutic power in your interventions. This will be the better choice for your clients but will require your commitment and creativity. I wish you joy in the choice you make, and hope that *Occupation by Design* will be of help. You will be what you do.

References

Clark, F., Parham, D., Carlson, M., Frank, G., Jackson, J., Pierce, D., Wolfe, R., & Zemke, R. (1991). Occupational science: Academic innovation in the service of occupational therapy's future. *American Journal of Occupational Therapy, 45,* 300–310.

Gray, J. M. (1998). Putting occupation into practice: Occupation as ends, occupation as means. *American Journal of Occupational Therapy, 52,* 354–364.

Kielhofner, G. (1992). *Conceptual foundations for occupational therapy.* Philadelphia: F. A. Davis.

Meyer, A. (1922/1977). The philosophy of occupational therapy. *American Journal of Occupational Therapy, 31,* 639–642.

Pierce, D. (2001a). Untangling occupation and activity. *American Journal of Occupational Therapy, 55,* 138–146.

Pierce, D. (2001b). Occupation by design: Dimensions, creativity, and therapeutic power. *American Journal of Occupational Therapy, 55,* 249–259.

Reilly, M. (1976). *Play as exploratory learning.* Thousand Oaks, CA: Sage.

Zemke, R., & Clark, F. (1996). Preface. In R. Zemke & F. Clark (Eds.), *Occupational science: The evolving discipline* (pp. vii–xviii). Philadelphia: F. A. Davis.

CHAPTER 2

The Creative Process of Designing Occupations

Design Is a Constant in Life and in Practice

Academic Approaches to the Design Process

Building Your Skills within the Seven General Phases
of the Design Process

You Are a Designer of Occupations

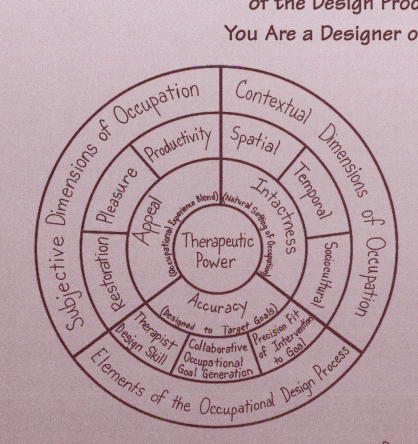

Appeal + Intactness + Accuracy = Therapeutic Power

Design Is a Constant in Life and in Practice

Like beads on a string, the occupations in which we engage over a day, a week, or a year make up the experience we have of our lives. We are what we do. We create ourselves

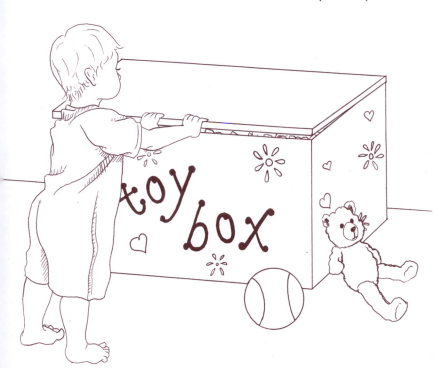

through our actions. For occupational therapists to be the premier experts on human occupation, they must understand the creative design process by which humans plan and implement occupations. Each time we attempt an occupation that is new and challenging for us, we use creativity and design process. For a young child, just figuring out how to open a toy box could be a significant problem-solving challenge. Adults use design process to plan and accomplish projects as large as building homes, writing novels, and launching corporate products. Think about your own life. What have you created lately? A dinner? A trip? A career plan? An event? A new home space? A garden? Our greatest creativity is required in complex tasks with which we are relatively unfamiliar. A. Jean Ayres (1985) called this *praxis*: ideation, planning, and execution of a novel task. Creativity is not an inborn trait, like eye color. Creativity and an understanding of design process are talents that are developed with practice.

More important, occupational therapists must develop sophisticated design skills to create powerful occupational interventions that meet the needs of clients. Design process includes all of the creative thinking from the initial realization of why you want to do something, through considering different ideas, to doing and reflecting on your action. The thinking involved is of many different kinds and tends to alternate between divergent thinking, which opens up and expands an idea, and convergent thinking, which is about narrowing down for precise definitions and choices (Koberg & Bagnall, 1981). For the sake of clarity, in this book we will look at the design process as including seven phases:

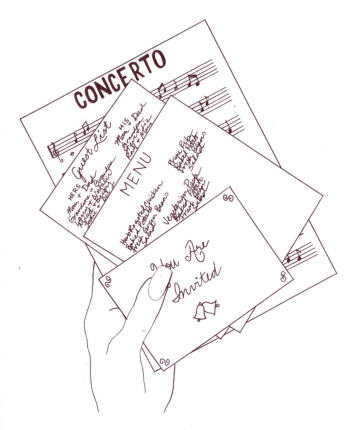

- Motivation
- Investigation
- Definition
- Ideation
- Idea selection
- Implementation
- Evaluation

Creativity in a Typical Therapist's Day

Here is an example of the degree to which occupational therapists require creativity in practice: a typical day for a school-based occupational therapist. Perhaps she will work one-on-one in the classroom with five different children. For each of them, the therapist might bring five different activities that address their goals, trying to insure that most are new to the child and engaging. That makes 25 new ideas in one day. Now, when she is working with each child, many of the activities will have to be adapted quickly to better fit the child's physical or cognitive skills, or they may have to be replaced quickly because the child does not find them interesting. That adds perhaps 25 more ideas during the interventions. Now, the therapist is up to 50 new ideas.

During that day, the therapist also administers a standardized developmental evaluation to a kindergarten child with autism. Because the child is not able to complete the standardized assessment she was planning, the therapist must change quickly to doing clinical observations of the child to complete her evaluation. This requires several problem-solving efforts as she attempts to assess different areas of function using the evaluation room setting and the activities she has available. After doing what she can there, she moves with the child to the playground, which is empty at that time, to do some observations of gross motor skills. How many creative ideas were required in that evaluation? It is difficult to count, but perhaps 10 is a realistic number. So, she has now reached 60 new ideas in 1 day.

Later in the day, the therapist has an hour set aside to work on an intervention program she would like to propose for the emotional and behavioral disorders classroom in her school. She is making a budget, which requires listing supplies for 1 year of intervention. To do this, she must imagine what the areas of intervention would be, and then what activities might work well to address them. A conservative guess of how many ideas she has to come up with for this might be 30. So, that makes 90 ideas.

After school, she joins the parents and teachers of one of the children she sees for his annual Individualized Education Plan meeting. During the meeting, she uses her creative skills to contemplate how best to explain what she sees in this child's progress to his parents and teachers, as well as to participate in a brainstorming session concerning how his need for after-school peer group involvement might be met. How many ideas is that? Well, let us just say she has probably reached 100 in her typical day. And she will need another 100 new ideas and problem solutions the next day, and the next, and the next.

There is nothing sadder to see in practice than a knowledgeable and competent occupational therapist who is bored, burned out, or ineffective because of a lack of creative design skill. Unfortunately, occupational therapy education has tended to focus on teaching content instead of process, taking for granted the creativity of the therapist and spending little time on the novice therapist's creative skills.

Using the Design Chapter as a Reference for the Rest of the Book

This chapter focuses on the basics of design skill: understanding the seven phases of design and learning a few techniques for strong skills within each phase. Unlike most of this book, which centers on building an understanding of different aspects of occupation and occupation-based practice, this chapter on design is very much about the creative process. Here you will learn about design process, and then, in the other chapters of the book, you will develop your design skills by applying them to the concepts presented in those chapters. In many ways, this chapter serves as a reference for working with the concepts in the rest of the book. To begin, we will first look at the design process as it is taught in three very different professional disciplines: architecture, engineering, and medicine. Through the eyes of an occupational therapist, it is easy to see that the students in all three types of training are learning to engage in similar occupations. The primary activities in their professions are lengthy and complex, depend on creative thinking, demand extended planning, and require a specific outcome that must meet the needs of the consumer. The chapter then describes seven phases of the design process and the strategies that can be used within each phase. The chapter concludes with Power Builder exercises for the development of design skills.

Academic Approaches to the Design Process

Helping students to understand and develop their creative thinking and problem-solving skills is especially strong in the professions of architecture, engineering, and most recently, medicine. Although the content of the three disciplines is radically different, the creative thinking required is similar. Before moving into consideration of design phase strategies, let's review how these three applied fields are teaching their students using what they may call design process, problem solving, planning, situation management, or problem-based learning.

Architectural Design: The Studio Method

Architects in training learn the process of designing homes, landscapes, office buildings, industrial complexes, and other structures through the studio method (Duerk, 1993; Jones, 1981; Wade, 1977). In this approach, architects in training are assigned workspace with other students in a large room full of drafting tables. They then spend as many waking hours as possible in this studio, working on design assignments of increasing complexity over the span of the curriculum. The problems with which the students are presented vary from a 1-day "sketch" problem to a "long" problem of up to 8 weeks in length. Always, the produced solutions to these problems are drawn plans. The process of architectural design is generally considered to extend through the phases of programming (data gathering), design development and refinement, construction and ancillary designs (interiors and landscapes), and evaluation and recording of the project (Straub, 1978; Wade, 1977). Students regularly give formal presentations of their thinking and designs to juries of architects, from whom they receive criticism and grades. In the studio, many informal discussions and desk-side critiques of the designs occur. Students are required to give knowledgeable feedback on each other's work and to work in teams on large projects. More traditional classroom instruction in other subjects, such as construction materials and architectural history, is also part of

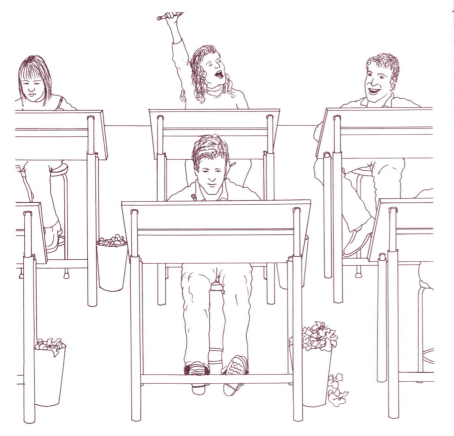

the curriculum. However, it is in the studio that the focus is on the student's development of creative design skills.

One of the unique aspects of architectural design is the degree to which it takes into account the perspective of those who are purchasing or inhabiting the product of their design effort. "An immature architect designs for himself, not his 'users'" (Straub, 1978, p. 3). Consumers often give input on the design in the initial survey stage, at interim presentations of the emerging design, and in formal review of the final design. This is not unlike the occupational therapy process, in which therapists collaborate with their patients to set goals, review progress, and evaluate outcomes of intervention.

Engineering Thinking: Emphasis on Problem Solution

In engineering, the process of creative thinking is viewed as successful problem solving (Cropley & Cropley, 2000; Fogler & LeBlanc, 1995). Historically, the focus in engineering has been more on the product of the work than on the process for getting there. This is in direct contrast to the fine arts orientation of architecture, which attends to the creative process shown in evolving sketches of the designer's conceptualization. Engineering students are generally trained through courses in physics, electrical theory, industrial processes, and other pertinent types of knowledge, and then presented with problems to solve. Engineering schools are well known for the challenging problems with which they confront their students, such as the World Solar Car Race, or team racing to design ways to deliver an egg intact from the top of a building to the ground using only $5.00 worth of materials. In their coursework, different students often use different approaches to the same assigned problem. Some students may band together to create solutions. Others may research previously used solutions. Creative thinking has always been challenged in these engineering problems. However, until recently, the creative process itself received little explicit attention in the engineering curriculum.

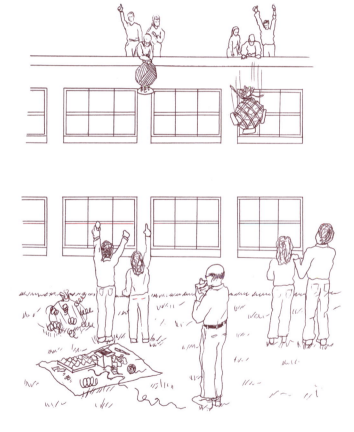

Confronted with fast-paced technological change and increased global competition, engineering schools in the United States are beginning to integrate into their curricula an understanding of the problem-solving process itself. In the early 1990s, the National Science Foundation funded a study by the University of Michigan of engineering problem solving in a group of major American corporations, to produce information that could be used in undergraduate training of engineers (Fogler & LeBlanc, 1995). The teaching materials generated from that study still propose problems and ask for student solutions. However, the problems are identified to the students as they occur in different phases of the problem-solving process. In engineering, the phases of problem solving are called problem definition, generating solutions, deciding on a course of action, implementation, and evaluation (Fogler & LeBlanc, 1995). Engineers are especially strong in their abilities to manage complex project implementations.

Medicine: Problem-Based Learning

In medical education, efforts are being made to provide students with experiences in independently solving the types of problems with which they will be faced in practice. This problem-based learning approach resembles engineering education in its emphasis on solving assigned problems, or cases. Problem-based learning originated in the late 1950s and 1960s, at Case Western Reserve University in the United States and McMaster University in Canada (Boud & Feletti, 1991). By the 1980s, problem-based learning had begun to spread to medical schools all over the world. Occupational therapy programs have also begun to adopt the principles of problem-based learning in the last few years (Royeen, 1994).

Although problem-based learning is implemented in many different ways, some primary characteristics hold true across all settings (Boud & Feletti, 1991). The approach centers on presenting problems for a small group to work on together. It emphasizes

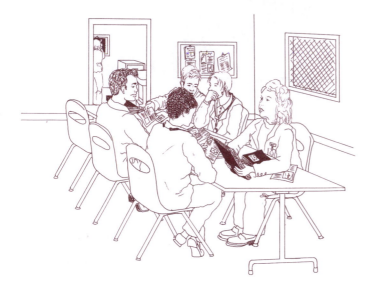

working on the problem in the context in which it usually occurs, usually a medical treatment setting. Instruction is in the form of facilitating the learning process in tutorials, rather than providing information in a more traditional format. Students are expected to seek out the information they require for their work on the case. Often, students focus on a single problem rather than taking multiple simultaneous courses.

The rationale behind problem-based learning is that it strengthens the students' abilities to adapt to changing practice settings, to work within teams, and to address the puzzles of daily practice, which cannot all be covered in detail during the limited time span of the professional curriculum. In problem-based learning, students develop competencies in the areas of problem analysis and definition, group brainstorming, identification of information needs, accessing information resources, and reflection on their own lifelong learning process.

Building Your Skills within the Seven General Phases of the Design Process

All of life, all the decisions and plans that we make, require creativity. That is, we must have the ability to generate new ways of seeing opportunities and new solutions to the challenges presented to us. This is the design process (Koberg & Bagnall, 1981). Design of our occupations and the larger patterns within which they are related is a constant process for each of us. This chapter describes the basics of design process to give you an understanding of the seven general phases of design and some strategies for each phase. The basic phases will be considered in a typical sequence, although the design process does not always adhere so nicely to this stepwise order. The phases include: motivation, investigation, definition, ideation, idea selection, implementation, and evaluation. They alternate between divergent and convergent thinking.

Just as it is true that skills are best developed by clients while they are engaging in therapeutic occupations, your own design skills will develop best by exploring them, using them, and trying them out in different ways. Reading a book chapter will not give you design skills! The best way to develop those is to do design! In this chapter you are provided with strategies to use in each design phase. Read through them now, and consider them a reference for the rest of the book, as you study aspects of occupation and occupation-based practice.

The strategies come from many different disciplines, but have been selected according to their effectiveness in teaching occupational therapy students. At the end of most of the chapters you will find Power Builders, which include opportunities to practice your design skills as you study your own occupations, those of others, and their applications in intervention. Careful reflection on each phase of design within the exercises will make the design process more explicit, allowing you to practice your design skills and reflect on your skill development. With time, these insights will also result in increased abilities to do the fast, on-your-feet creative thinking that is constantly required in daily practice. And remember, design is a playful, open process. Stay loose in your thinking, healthy and rested, and out from under pressure if you wish to be a great designer.

In the following description of the seven phases of design, an example will illustrate the different strategies that can be used to work on a particular challenge. For no particular reason, except that it is fun, I will use here the example of planning a party.

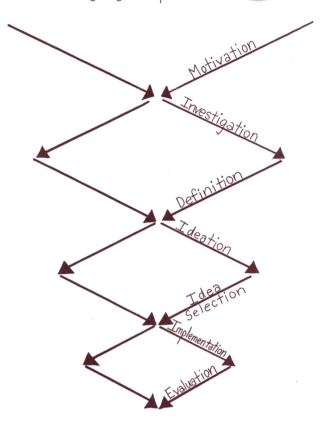

Phase One: Motivation

Recognizing a problem, being irritated by how things are, feeling the need to do something, preparing to jump, getting excited: these are all ways of describing the motivation phase of the design process. It is not a phase filled with detailed actions. Yet it is critical to the success of any undertaking. If you do not take the time to question whether you really want to do something and why, you will not be able to sustain the energy to come up with creative solutions and complete them. The motivation phase is convergent, zeroing in on a commitment to take action, although you may not know at that time exactly how you will accomplish your goal.

The most difficult aspect of motivation is not insight into what needs doing but commitment to take action. Often we already have an idea about some portion of our occupational pattern we want to change, but we have managed to avoid dealing with it, sometimes for years. One of the hardest parts of recognizing a potential change in occupations is being strong enough to break your own habits. Habits are potent organizing forces in our lives, enabling us to go through complex occupational patterns without constant processing and decision making about what to do next in routine activities. Habits are often formed when we are young and unable to discern how they may shape our lives in the long run. In the process of creativity, the most effective way to recognize and accept a change of pattern that might affect familiar habits is to begin slowly. Do not think so far ahead that you become overwhelmed with a feeling of resistance. Do not begin to try to figure out how you will reach your goal. Simply remain in this design phase of recognizing and accepting that the present pattern is not satisfactory, until the desire to avoid dealing with the question you have recognized has lessened. Rushing ahead into action before you have become comfortable with the idea of making a change is a sure way to sabotage a difficult project. Remember, if you are having trouble with any phase of design, just slow down and give it time.

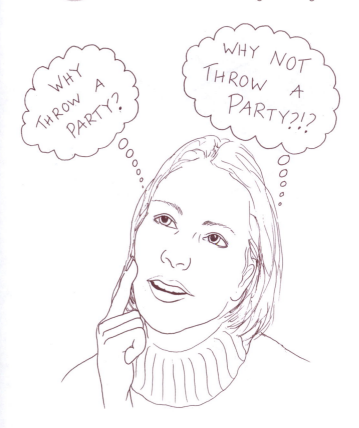

Some people have trouble with being too easily convinced to commit to projects. They say they will do something without really considering whether or not they are sufficiently motivated to carry out the project. This results in completing projects that do not give them much satisfaction, doing things poorly, or just not completing things that they have said they would do. It is as important to stay with the phase of motivation long enough to figure out that you do *not* want to do something as it is to figure out that you do.

Perhaps if you have good pragmatic reasons why you should do something but you are feeling unexcited, you could reflect on why it is important to you long enough to identify the main points that you value about this action. Then you may be able to change the project to accentuate those aspects. For example, an instructor may require a term paper for a class you are taking and you feel completely uninterested in writing it. Still, you do want to pass the class. Upon reflection, you find one aspect of the class that is very interesting to you and begin to imagine what you would like to learn about that topic. You propose to the instructor that your paper focus on that topic. The time flies while you research and write up your paper. The paper turns out to be very original and exciting, and you pass the course.

Strategies for Motivation

Journal. A journal is the ultimate tool for self-reflection. To use your journal to increase your design skill in the preparation phase, write to yourself on the following topics: my style of preparing to begin a task, things I would like to do differently, risks I have taken, what is hard for me about changes, and things I would change if it were easy to do. Ask yourself what you like and dislike about the idea you are contemplating doing. Write a description of what would be the best outcome of this idea.

In the example of planning a party, journaling might include the following sort of entry:

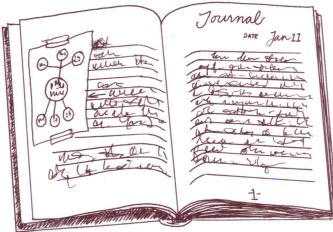

Why do I want to do a party? Well, it would be fun! I like to give parties. Everybody gets together and has a good time, laughing and joking around. Special foods are fun too. It would be nice not to have to invent each party from scratch, though, to be able to go to the garage and pull out the box with all the usual decorations and the list of supplies from the years before. If you gave the same kind of party every year, people would remember it and look forward to it too. And every year, it would probably get better, because you would figure out what worked well and what didn't and change the party a little every year. I wonder what kind of party would be best? Well, what do I want out of the party? I want it to be memorable and unusual, fun, not formal, OK for all ages, and not so much work to put on that I have to keep it small. I want it to include music and dancing and emphasize something seasonal in the theme. It would be OK if it started out small the first year, as long as it was fun, for me as well as for the guests.

Benefits listing. An approach that is effective against that feeling of hesitancy to engage a big challenge is to make a list of all the positive benefits that might result from making changes (Koberg, 1981). Don't forget to include intangibles, like increases in the pleasure you take from your occupations, decreased stress, recognition from others, opportunities that may open up for you from this change, or increased time for other things.

Own the project. If you find yourself avoiding a challenging design task, try asking yourself, "Who is responsible for doing this?" over and over until you see that the answer is "I am." Do this mentally or in writing.

Hang a sign. One way to strengthen your feeling of responsibility for making a change or doing a project is to post notices. There are lots of different ways to do this. Make a big sign naming your new project and hang it in a prominent place. Write it in soap on the bathroom mirror: "I WILL . . .." Tell people about what you are about to do. Cover the refrigerator or a bulletin board with magazine clippings related to your project (Koberg & Bagnall, 1981).

Risk taking. Fear is the greatest barrier to the creative process: fear of failing, of what people might think, of looking silly, of doing something new. You can increase your risk-taking abilities by accomplishing increasingly risky, novel activities. Start very small, by just trying usual things in new ways. Later, you might try a new sport, prepare a new meal, take a different kind of car out for a test drive, learn a dance, or start a new hobby. Envision yourself successfully accomplishing this activity in great style.

Pros and cons. This tried-and-true method is to simply list on two sides of a paper the reasons why you should or should not do something you are considering.

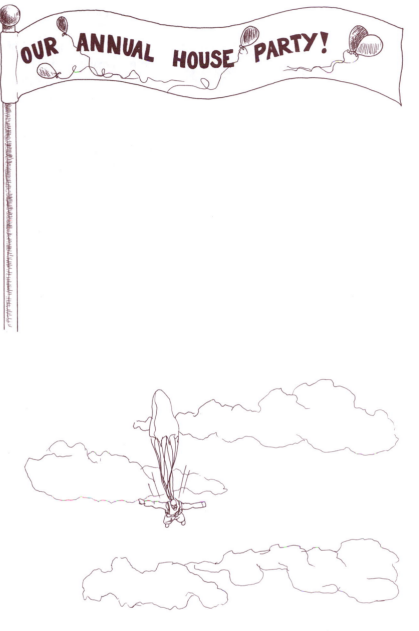

Phase Two: Investigation

Investigation is a divergent phase. Investigating something you are going to do opens up your mind to new possibilities and gives you insight into the primary aspects that may be involved in your project. Information is gathered, and the problem you wish to solve through your actions is explored. Aim for quantity of information, not quality. At this phase, it is counterproductive to get caught up in judgments about how things might best be done or what direction would be better to take. The skilled designer will simply spend time in this phase being exposed to as much information and as many new ways of seeing the challenge as are possible.

Once lots of information is accumulated, it is time to sort through it to identify some of the main themes involved. Investigation depends heavily on flexibility of mind: the ability to question, to turn your idea around 100 different ways and consider its parts. To do this requires some time to sift through your information and reflect on what is there.

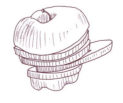
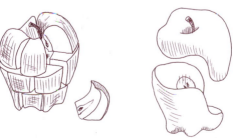

Strategies for Investigation

Journal. Again, as in all of the skills of design, journal writing is a useful way to advance your thinking. Write down everything you know about your question. You will be surprised at how informed you are. Consider what kinds of knowledge are missing from this list and use that to pursue more information. In your journal, try drawing, modeling, or listing the different parts of the question and how they relate to each other. Review the following exercises for potential writing topics. Using a journal is a way of setting aside time for focused thinking. Just keep at it on a regular basis, and you are bound to gain a rich perspective on the actions you are contemplating.

Make an appointment. You can gather and explore information most easily by making appointments with yourself for when you will do so. Set a time each day to seek out information, write in your journal about the idea, or read information you have accumulated. Perhaps just a morning written reflection is all you need. Or, if there is a clear deadline for completion of your project, be sure to schedule blocks of time into your calendar to do your investigating.

Research written information. The most obvious strategy for investigation is to go to the library and search for information. Today we also have great resources on the Internet.

Use human resources. A good way of getting another perspective on the project you are considering is to talk to others about it. Remember, people make good information resources too in any design phase. Talk to people who seem to be doing well at what you are interested in or may even be doing it as part of their jobs. Talk to people who are very different from you in age, culture, or experience. Find books by people who are involved in the activity you are investigating, and see what they have written. Consider whether there may be some type of organization or association that may have useful information for you.

Observe. Put yourself in a place where you can observe something related to your idea. (Get permission if necessary.) Stay there and make notes (if appropriate in that setting) about your idea that are spurred by what you are seeing. Remain there until your observations do not generate new ways of seeing your project.

Ballooning. Explore how far you can develop your idea by ballooning. Write your topic in a circle in the middle of a sheet of paper. Draw lines out to connecting circles, or balloons, that contain parts of this idea or expand the idea in a related direction. Draw lines from these balloons to new balloons too. Continue ballooning outward for as long as you can. (Ballooning is sometimes called mind mapping.)

Classify. Look through your gathered information and try to find any topical groupings. To do this, you can simply take your written materials and sort them by stacking them in different piles, making lists of themes or color-coding by categories with markers. For some people, drawing a visual model of the groupings is useful. By looking for the main ideas in your information, you will clarify your understanding of the project.

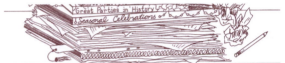

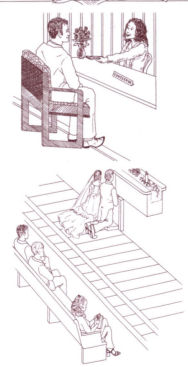

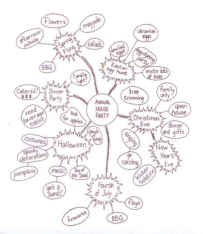

Phase Three: Definition

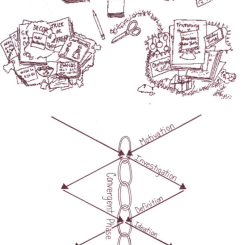

Definition is a convergent phase, bringing your thinking out of the broad exploratory phase of investigation to specify exactly what you wish to accomplish. Many developing designers make the mistake of not spending enough time on reaching a clear definition. This results in a poor design later, with efforts all over the map but few results or little satisfaction. Often, failure to fully clarify the definition of a project will result in having to go back later and redefine.

It is important to realize that the convergent phases are strongly linked in the overall design process. When working on the definition phase, it is good to go back to what you have said in the previous convergent phase, motivation. If you identified a particular characteristic of the project as important to you, you will want to insure that it is included in the definition. For example, in creating an annual house party, I said I wanted it to be fun for me, fun for my guests, informal, memorable/unusual, and seasonal, and to include music and dancing. Also, as I have worked on the idea in the previous phases, I have realized it cannot be overly expensive, so that is an additional criterion.

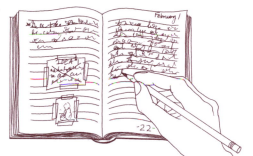

Do not worry too much about how you will do something when you write your definition, or that the definition sounds like too big a project. Figuring out methods or how big a piece of this mission statement you can accomplish will come later. The important thing is just clarifying your definition.

Strategies for Definition

Journal. At this point, write in your journal about the essence of your intent. What exactly are you trying to accomplish and why? What will it look like and feel like if it turns out well? Try some of the following exercises in your journal:

Check on motivation. Compare your definition to what you said in the motivation phase. Make sure everything that motivates you about this project is included in the definition.

Boil down a definition. Write your definition in as few words as possible. Keep rewriting it, eliminating extra words, until you get down to two or three words that express the essence of what you wish to do (Koberg & Bagnall, 1981).

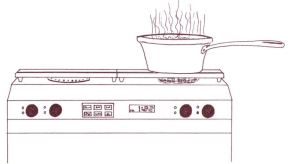

Use battling definitions. Write your definition several different ways. Pit them against each other, choosing the best one. Decide why the winning definition is best. (See the battle on pg 26.)

Create priorities. (See example on pg 26.) For more thorough definition development, use the following steps:

1. List everything you think is important about how your project should turn out.

2. Group the words/phrases in your list.

3. Prioritize the groups according to which is most important.

4. Create a succinct definition that includes all of your main priorities.

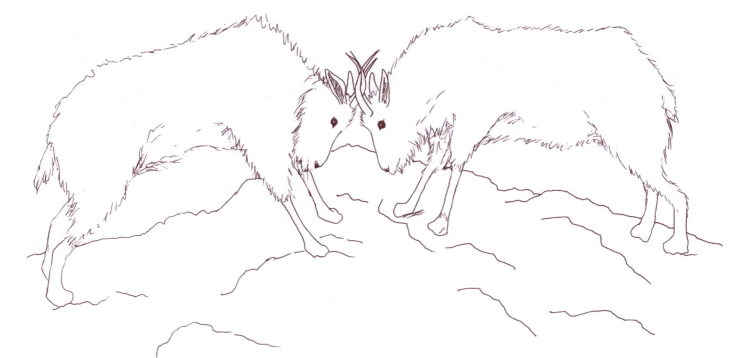

U	original	S = seasonal
A	fun for me	A = activities
A	fun for guests	D = doable
S	seasonal theme	U = unique
S	food of that time of year	
A	fun for kids AND adults	
D	not too much preparation	
A	dancing	
A	music	
D	not too expensive	
U	cool decorations	
A	things to do	
A	not sitting around	
S	food reflects theme	
D	easy to prepare food + drink	
U	different	
S	repeatable every year	

Most important = seasonal
    2nd = activities
    3rd = doable
    4TH = unique

I will create an annual housparty with a seasonal theme that includes lots of fun things to do, and is doable for me.

Phase Four: Ideation

Just as in the previous divergent phase of investigation, it is quantity, not quality, that you seek in the ideation phase. In ideation, you want to generate as many ideas of how to accomplish your definition as possible. Your charge is simply to come up with as many potential plans for enacting the project as you can. They can be impractical, wild, expensive, or time-consuming. The more different ways you can imagine to create change, the more creative will be the action you eventually select. This is not the time to be conservative, careful, or realistic. Remember, divergent phases are about stretching your thinking and opening your mind to new ideas.

It is typical that this design phase requires great mental efforts from the designer. This is where the core conceptualization of the project is born. It requires great energy and can be surprisingly tiring. Anxiety and general feelings of frustration are not unusual. These unpleasant feelings can result in mental blocks and moving too quickly out of this phase. It is important to understand these feelings as "normal" for ideation. Also, remind yourself that, like the punchline at the end of a joke, the release of this emotional tension at a later phase of the creative process will provide you with the pleasurable feelings of solving the puzzle that is your project.

Insure that you have the energy to work creatively through all of the challenges of the design process. First of all, acknowledge that you are making great demands on your creativity. Attend carefully to your physical health during this period. Get plenty of rest. Albert Einstein and Henry Ford took lots of catnaps. Try to do your thinking when you are freshest. Watch out for junk food, caffeine, and alcohol, which can drain your physical energy. Remind yourself constantly that you are in a period of incubation and that creativity takes time. If you are trying hard to generate ideas and they are not coming, take a mini-vacation from it. Take a break, go somewhere, do something else, take a day off, or just get your mind away from the project for a while. You will return refreshed and much more creative.

Strategies for Ideation

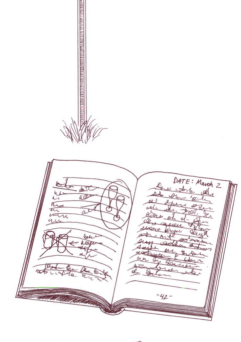

Journal. Look back into the information you have gathered to look for ideas on how to proceed on generating options for action. Ask others how they would do it. How has it been done in the past? How would it be the most fun to do it? List your ideas. Cover a minimum of one page with different ways of getting it done. Concentrate on coming up with the greatest number and variety of ways to accomplish your goal. Do not allow yourself to detour into speculation into the practicality or affordability of one or more of these ideas. That is the surest way to block your creativity. Just focus on filling those pages with possibilities.

Idea dump. Our culture harbors a myth that the great ideas of creative people come to them out of the blue. They shout "Eureka!" and the problem is solved, an important discovery made. This myth wraps the real process of creative thinking in mystery, obscuring our understanding of it. Actually, the biggest roadblock to creativity in the ideation phase is getting stuck on one idea. Sometimes, as we consider a situation and how to address it, a great idea does come to us. It is tempting, at this point, to go straight into implementation. However, you must understand design well enough to simply add this idea to the possibilities you are accumulating and continue with your process. It may turn out to be the best one, but it is unlikely. So, dump that idea right now! Write down the idea that you think may be the best one for how to accomplish your defined project, and deliberately set it aside. Do not let that one idea get you stuck in an uncreative single-mindedness. Be strong! You can do it!

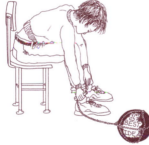

Brainstorm. A brainstorm . . . just what is it anyway? Brainstorming is a powerful strategy for creating a large volume of ideas in a short time. Many people think brainstorming is just getting together and trying to reach a consensus on some question, but they are wrong. If you don't understand the basic rules of brainstorming, a discussion like this often disintegrates into frustrated examinations of only a few possible ideas with uneven participation from different members of the group. However, if you follow the following four simple rules (Koberg & Bagnall, 1981), you should be able to quickly produce lots of different ideas, either in a group or by yourself:

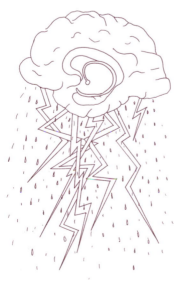

1. No judgment. The point of brainstorming is to produce ideas, not to examine them. No matter how far out they may be, they will contribute in some way to the eventual plan of action. If you begin discussing the feasibility of different suggestions, a less open atmosphere will prevail, and the flow of new ideas will stop. No negative comments allowed!

2. Anything goes. Remember, the crazier the idea sounds, the better. That is how you break through from the few ideas you had at the beginning of the brainstorming session to the wealth of exciting possibilities you will have at the end.

3. Tag on. Feel free to take ideas already mentioned and add onto or adapt them. (Be careful not to detour into justifying an idea or explaining why one way is better than another.) For instance, you might say, "Yes, do what she just said, but how about doing it in this other location?" You can tag on by modifying part of an idea, making a part of it larger or smaller, substituting one thing for another, or rearranging the pattern of how it happens. In this way, ideas get turned around and reshaped.

4. Quantity. Remember, it's quantity that you want, not quality. Just keep the ideas coming. Don't allow quiet to settle over the brainstorming session while you try to think of another great idea. Everyone contributes. Take the ideas you have and play with them. Keep the momentum going.

Good luck with your brainstorming! It is easier to brainstorm in a small group than by yourself, but both work with practice. Remind the group of the rules, and then all dive in. It is helpful to have someone jot down the ideas where everyone can see them as they are generated. Don't go too long in your brainstorming session. A fully creative 5 minutes will produce a remarkable change in the number of creative ideas for a project. When the ideas start to come slower, stop the session. You may want to hold a follow-up session the next day to collect any later thoughts group members have had as they have mulled over the ideas that came up.

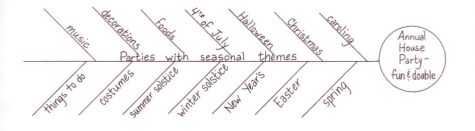

Fishbone diagram. In engineering, a follow-up analysis to brainstorming called a fishbone diagram is used (Fogler & LeBlanc, 1995). This is a type of visual classification of the concepts that were generated in the brainstorming session, so that the variety of possibilities that have been produced can be examined.

Once you have brainstormed, begin your fishbone diagram by drawing the backbone line. Draw a circle at the head end and write inside it the main challenge to the session. The backbone represents the main challenge to the brainstorming session, or the problem that was presented for solutions. Examine the ideas listed in the session and try to identify the primary groupings. For each group, draw a "rib" extending out from the backbone and label it with a group name. Record all the ideas of that group on lines extending out from that rib. Move the ideas around, or even break them down, until they are all recorded along the fish bones. This will give you a new perspective on the primary aspects of the problem you are trying to solve and its potential solutions.

Phase Five: Idea Selection

Once you have generated a creative variety of potential solutions to your challenge, it is time to select the one you will use. This is a critical step. Take your time and think carefully about your choice. Because idea selection is a convergent phase, go back and check what you said was important in motivation and definition. Check to see if you have shifted the intent of your project as you have explored potential plans of action. Does your definition need refining? Once you are clear on your exact objective, examine the options you have generated for the one that is most likely to achieve that end. Continue until you are sure of your choice. Here are some strategies for selecting your idea for action.

Strategies for Idea Selection

Journal. Again, journaling is a good way to work your way through this choice. Describe your intent clearly. Then, write about each potential solution, analyzing its strengths and weaknesses in relation to your objective. Perhaps one of the following investigation strategies would be of use in making a choice. Take your time. Write in your journal on successive days as you decide.

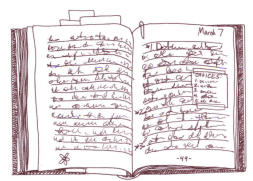

Check convergent phases for criteria for success. Remember, all convergent phases are linked. In a strong design process, the convergent phases should all reflect the same aspects of the project as important. The things you named as motivating you about the project should show up in your definition. In the idea-selection phase, these same characteristics of your project are used as criteria to select the best idea to match your intent. So, to prepare to choose among the ideas you produced in the ideation phase, review the descriptors that you identified as important to the project in the motivation and definition phases.

Plus/minus matrix. Set up a matrix of four criteria for a successful outcome across the top, and the top ideas for your project could be down the side. Award pluses and minuses in the grid boxes for whether each idea meets each criterion. Add them up for each project. Which idea did best? Do the results feel right to you? If not, rethink your criteria, or try a different matrix exercise from among those that follow.

Ranking matrix. Consider the results of your motivation and definition phases. Then, list the criteria by which you will judge whether or not your project was successful. If it was supposed to be fun, then fun is one criterion. Also consider criteria that you may not have mentioned before. Using a short list of criteria, create a matrix where you rank a list of ideas against each other on each criterion. Add the results across the rankings to see which idea leads the others. Check on how you feel once you see the results. If the best-ranked idea does not "feel right," check your criteria. Do they really reflect what is important to you? If necessary, revise the criteria and rank them again. The important part of this process is not the numbers themselves, but the thinking you must go through to create criteria and rank the ideas against each other. If you're doing this activity in a group, share your thoughts about why certain ideas are ranked in the way they are.

Rank and weigh matrix. This strategy expands the ranking strategy by weighting the criteria. The process is otherwise the same. Carefully choose criteria. Set up a grid with the criteria across the top and the ideas down the left side. Weigh the criteria against each other, numbering them according to their value. Rank the ideas against each other, completing the grid. Before adding up the rankings, multiply each number in the grid by the weight of its criteria. Add up for each idea. Check how the results feel to you. Consider whether your rankings and weightings seem right. Redo if necessary. Remember, it is the thought process that is important here, not the numbers.

Combo. Consider whether two of your top-ranked ideas could be combined. (Caution: Do not use a combo just to avoid a difficult decision. You might create a larger project with two competing parts instead of choosing one best idea.)

	fun activities to do	fun to decorate	affordable	good for music and dancing	easy to prepare	informal	good for all ages	TOTAL
Christmas	−	+	−	+	+	−	+	+1
Easter	+	+	+	−	−	−	−	−1
Halloween	+	+	+	+	+	+	+	+7
4th of July	−	−	−	−	+	+	+	−1
New Year's Eve	−	−	−	+	−	−	−	−5

	fun activities	fun to decorate	affordable	good for music & dancing	easy to prepare	informal	good for all ages	TOTAL
Christmas	5	5	4	3	3	4	1	25
Easter	2	2	1	5	5	3	4	22
Halloween	1	1	2	2	2	2	3	13
4th of July	4	4	3	4	1	1	2	19
New Year's Eve	3	3	5	1	4	5	5	26

	x4 fun activities	x1 fun to decorate	x5 affordable	x2 good for music & dancing	x6 easy to prepare	x3 informal	x7 good for all ages	TOTALS
Christmas	5/20	5/5	4/20	3/6	3/18	4/12	1/7	88
Easter	2/8	2/2	1/5	5/10	5/30	3/9	4/28	92
Halloween	1/4	1/1	2/10	2/4	2/12	2/6	3/21	58
4th of July	4/16	4/4	3/15	4/8	1/6	1/3	2/14	66
New Year's Eve	3/12	3/3	5/25	1/2	4/24	5/15	5/35	116

Jury presentation and refinements. In architecture, part of the idea-selection process is a formal presentation of the leading options to a panel for feedback (Jones, 1981; Wade, 1977). This is an especially important strategy if you will have consumers or other participants in the project you are planning. Not only will they have good input for you, but also the jury process will build their support for the plan you choose. A jury presentation is almost a requirement if you must obtain funding from other people to go forward.

Trials. A good way to judge the potential effectiveness of your chosen plan of action is to give it a trial. For instance, if you are planning a new type of service delivery for the occupational therapy department where you work, try it out first with only one or two patients. This will show you the relative chances of success that your chosen plan may have, expose unknown barriers, and give you opportunities to fine-tune your plan.

Phase Six: Implementation

After all the effort you have spent on generating and selecting a creative plan of action, executing it may almost seem simple. But this is not the time to abandon your design skills. Implementation requires a careful plan and attentive execution. Although implementation is much more focused than an early divergent phase, such as investigation, it is still divergent. You may be required to make on-site adjustments as you carry out your design, create ancillary designs for unexpected developments in your plan, or track multiple simultaneously occurring aspects of your project. During implementation, you have to think on your feet!

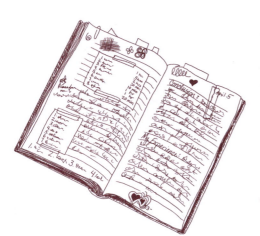

Strategies for Implementation

Journal. As you carry out the idea you have selected, write about your experience. Be sure to include your feelings, unexpected occurrences and how you handled them, how you kept track of what needed to be done, and how you knew that things were going well or poorly at different times. What parts of implementation were hardest and what parts most enjoyable? Did it turn out as you expected? What surprised you the most?

Time/task list. The simplest form of a plan is a time/task list. It is a listing of each task that needs to be done and the estimated time that task will take.

Gantt chart. A Gantt chart is a useful engineering technique for organizing large multipart projects (Fogler & LeBlanc, 1995). It is a grid that shows the different portions of the selected plan and how long they are scheduled to take. Laying out your plan on a Gantt chart can help you to visualize how the implementation fits into the time you have to complete it. The chart is also useful as a tracking device during execution, enabling you to keep tabs on all of the different aspects that may be occurring simultaneously. Be sure to include in your Gantt chart periodic checks on progress, input from participants, and adjustments to the chart.

make scary spider pinata	3 hrs
get cheesecloth for ghost costumes	1 hr
get decorations	1 hr.
put up decorations & pinata	2 hrs.
get dry ice	30 min
get ghost make up	30 min
make punch	30 min
get snacks & drinks & candy	2 hrs
get band	2 hrs.
clean house	2 hrs
set up apple bobbing	30 min
make invitations + mail out	2 hrs.
carve pumpkins	3 hrs.

	September	October							
		week 1	week 2	week 3	week 4	10/27	10/28	10/29	PARTY!
house & decorations			buy decorations				clean house Carve pumpkins	decorate house	
costumes	get cheesecloth at Labor Day Sale				buy make up			put out make up do Family costumes	show guests how to make ghost costumes
food & drink						buy party food & drink	prepare drinks cooler; get dry ice	Make punch Put out chips, etc...	refill bowls
activities		get band		make scary spider pinata		hang pinata	set up apple bobbing tub	show band where to set up	lead bobbing do pinata dance
invitations		make & send out invitations							

Critical path. A critical path chart helps you to think through and depict how different aspects of your plan are related to each other in time; that is, which parts must be done before others, which can hold up the entire process, and which are more flexible in their timing? A critical path chart usually diagrams a flow of events by using arrows from one event to the next. Your project may have several paths. Multiple paths can flow toward a critical event and then continue as a single path. Some paths may be unconnected to any others. The exercise of sketching those relationships will improve the creative execution of your idea. And, like the Gantt chart, a critical path chart can assist you in tracking your implementation.

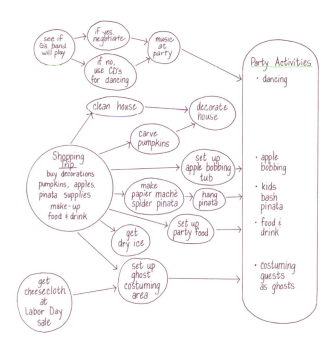

Phase Seven: Evaluation

The most neglected phase of the creative process is evaluation. We can become so caught up in our final product that we forget all about the last phase of the design process. Having accomplished our objective, we stop without examination or closure. Failing to debrief or reflect after a big project happens more often than not. It stunts our own growth as designers. The evaluation phase provides richer opportunities to build design skills than any other phase. At that time, you can examine your outcome and experience, recognizing both your design skill successes and the areas in which you can improve. All of us have definite strengths and weaknesses in specific phases of design, which do not change from one project to the next. If you spend a little time looking back on your design efforts, you can grow from your experience. You may even save yourself from repeating the same mistakes. Furthermore, if the project you have just completed is ongoing or likely to be done again, the information you collect at this phase is invaluable.

When a project is complete, you will also have gained a different perspective on those early phases of motivation, investigation, and definition. Re-examine your journals and reflect on the earlier phases from the viewpoint of the entire project. Ask others who observed your process about your creative design skills in the different phases. For some projects, you may need to submit a formal report, with evidence supporting your accomplishment.

Great occupational therapists do not become so without reflecting on their practices. Reflection is the foundation of professional development. By spending time thinking about how a completed intervention unfolded, you will learn much about that client population, what you would do differently next time, and your own strengths and learning needs as a therapist. In practice settings, it is easy to see which therapists are reflecting on their practice. Over the years, they are the ones who grow, develop expertise on which others depend, and remain excited about working with clients.

Strategies for Evaluation

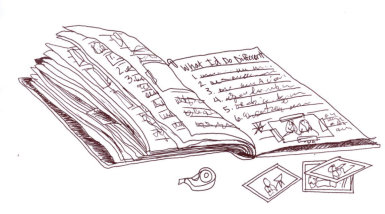

Journal. Now that you have completed your project, what do you think of your outcome? What turned out better than expected, worse, or just about as you anticipated? What did others have to say about it? What would you change if you could? If the project is ongoing, what adjustments will you make now? How have you evaluated your relative success? Look back in your journal where you defined what you were trying to do. Can you present evidence that measures how well you met your objectives? How do you feel about your outcome?

Look at the entire design process. In what design phases were you the most creative? What phases are the most difficult for you? What was the most satisfying part of the whole project? The most stressful? The one from which you learned most? The one you wished you had spent more time on? The one that was the most fun?

This might be a journal entry after a Halloween ghost party:

Wow! It took a long time to figure out what kind of annual house party I wanted to give, but I think this one was the right choice. I am sitting here the day after and I know I should get up and start cleaning up all the decorations and everything, but first I just want to think about this a bit. If I am going to do this every year, I want to make sure I figure out what to do better next year. It was so much fun, hilarious, and what a scene, everyone dancing in their vapors! Things I would change include forgetting the apple-bobbing (too wet and too many things to organize), getting some blacklights for the dancing area, starting the band a little later (after the kids are ready to go home), having the guests help each other to put on the cheesecloth ghost vapors and ghost makeup (too much to greet people coming in as well as costuming people), and separating the cheesecloth area and the makeup area into different places (got too crowded around the mirror). It was great watching people meet each other as they put on their makeup! Everyone had a blast. I am sure it will be even more fun next year, and more people will put on ghost costumes. Seems like some of the guys weren't into costumes. As far as my design process, I think I did best at ideation, because having so many ideas to choose from was how I got to this great party. I think what I did worst was the idea-selection phase. I had so many ideas for fun activities for the party that I picked too many and did not just try to pick the best couple. It was way too much to keep track of during the party and took away from the fun of the party for me. Also, I have to think some more about the seasonal foods idea that I wanted. We did have the spooky punch with the dry ice and Halloween candy, but maybe next year I will make some popcorn balls or something.

Criteria ratings from self or others. You can rate your success against the criteria for success you developed for idea selection or create criteria from your definition. The ratings can be done by you, by users of your project, or by others who observed the project. If you are completing a large project for which you must turn in a final report, you may want to do a more formal evaluation rating.

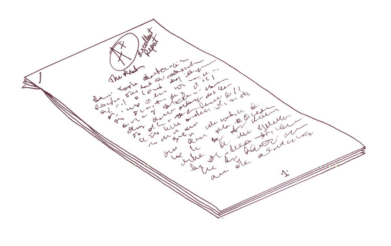

Academic method. If you are having trouble judging your relative success, you can use one method with which all college students should be quite familiar. Give yourself a grade, including credit for all you learned along the way about creativity and your own design process.

Interviews. A good way to get a creative picture of how well you succeeded in accomplishing your objectives is to interview those who have been involved in your project. Describe to them what you intended to do, and then ask how they think you did. After the first interview, adjust your questions to try to get more and better information from your next informant. Remember, you want them to talk, so keep your own comments brief and be a good listener. Count on being surprised and informed by what you hear.

You Are a Designer of Occupations

You are a designer of occupations, in your own life and in your future as an occupational therapist. In this chapter, you have been exposed to the evolving process of creative design. You are now familiar with strategies you can use in each of the design phases. The strength of design process is in its alternations between divergence, which opens and stretches thinking to incorporate new ideas, and convergence, which carefully weighs action choices. How smoothly you can move your thinking from one creative mode to another depends on you. All of us have natural strengths and weaknesses in different phases of design. To be a truly masterful designer, especially in working with clients and their families, requires developing beyond these natural talents to a more articulate perspective on your own design skills. This chapter will serve as a resource to you as you do so.

In the following chapters of this book, you will have many opportunities to use design strategies as you explore occupation and occupation-based practice. In the next section, you will see how we each create our own unique balance of occupations by blending the characteristics of productivity, pleasure, and restoration in the makeup of a day, as well as how this blend can be used in treatment. As you work your way through the section on the spatial, temporal, and sociocultural dimensions of occupation, your insight into how the context of occupation is used to design effective interventions will increase. In the last section of the book, you will focus on occupation-based practice. There, you will also look more specifically at design skills in practice in Chapter 14, Therapist Design Skills.

Just as a trained dancer uniquely appreciates the patterns of his or her own dance, an occupational therapist must be a true connoisseur of the complexity, richness, and beauty of the occupations that surround him or her in daily life and in work with clients. Just like a dancer, to become a skilled designer and an effective therapist, you will need to practice your design skills and reflect on them regularly. Like architects, engineers, and physicians, occupational therapists must be highly sophisticated designers if they are to consistently produce solutions to the difficult challenges presented in practice.

POWER BUILDERS

In the rest of this book, you will have opportunities to use the strategies described in this chapter to do design work related to the unique concepts presented in each chapter. The following Power Builder exercises serve as an introduction to those applications of design process and an opportunity to begin building your design skills.

1. A good way to experience the design process is to use all of the phases from beginning to end on a project. Perhaps you have a project in your life that you wish to accomplish, an assignment to complete, or a new hobby you would like to try out. The type of project that you choose is not important. It can be large or small, but certainly a project larger than can be done in 1 hour is necessary to really dig into the challenge of design. Take time to explore each phase as you progress through the design process. Try different strategies at each phase to see which ones work best for you. Keep records, through either a journal or a file of notes and artifacts. Be sure to spend enough time on reflection once you reach the evaluation phase, especially reflection on your own design skills.

2. A more formal way to do the exercise just described is to complete design reports for each phase as you work your way through a project. Design reports are analyses of your experiences with a selected project, at a specific phase of the design process. Each design report should answer the following questions:

    *   What strategies did you use in this design phase?
    *   What do you see as the primary intent of work at this design phase?
    *   What worked well in this design phase and why?
    *   What were some of the difficulties in this design phase and why?
    *   What are your own strengths and weaknesses in this phase?
    *   How has your conceptualization of your project changed in this phase?

3. Do either of the first two Power Builders as a group working together on one project.

4. For classroom use of design skills to learn about occupation, try this. Create six groups to work on a seven-step design process. Each group will pick one of the subjective or contextual dimensions of occupation: pleasure, productivity, restoration, space, time, or sociocultural context. The objective of this design project will be for each group to create a learning experience about that dimension of occupation for the other five groups to share. In this way, all six groups will have different topics but will be working on approximately the same phase of design process at the same time. Working sessions can begin with orientation to potential strategies to use in each phase, time to use the strategies on the different group projects, and sharing of how the process is going in the different groups at the end of the work time. Hearing about the successes and struggles of other design groups is very helpful in this format because it shows not only what is common

to the experience of design but also how differently projects can turn out, depending on the choices and preferences of the group working on the project.

5. Watch for and identify design process occurring around you and in your own life. What phase of design is occurring? (You may often see mixed phases.) What strategies are being used? How well are they working? Examples can be simply noted and reflected on personally, recorded in a journal, or shared with a partner or a group.

6. Design for yourself the perfect day, using a seven-step design process.

7. Browse through the Power Builder at the ends of the other chapters of this book.

References

Ayres, A. J. (1985). *Developmental dyspraxia and adult onset apraxia.* Torrance, CA: Sensory Integration International.

Boud, D., & Feletti, G. (1991). *The challenge of problem-based learning.* New York: St. Martin's Press.

Cropley, D., & Cropley, A. (2000). Fostering creativity in engineering undergraduates. *High Ability Studies, 11(2),* 207–219.

Duerk, D. (1993). *Architectural programming.* New York: Van Nostrand Reinhold.

Fogler, H. S., & LeBlanc, S. E. (1995). *Strategies for creative problem solving.* Englewood Cliffs, NJ: Prentice Hall.

Jones, J. C. (1981). *Design methods: Seeds of human futures.* New York: John Wiley & Sons.

Koberg, D., & Bagnall, R. (1981). *The all new universal traveler: A soft systems guide to creativity, problem-solving, and the process of reaching goals.* Los Altos, CA: William Kaufmann, Inc.

Royeen, C. B. (1994, December). Problem-based learning in action: Key points for practical use. *AOTA Education Special Interest Section Newsletter, 4,* 1–2.

Straub, C. C. (1978). *Design process and communications: A case study.* Dubuque, IA: Kendall/Hunt Publishing Company.

Wade, J. W. (1977). *Architecture, problems, and purposes.* New York: John Wiley & Sons.

Designing for Appeal:

The Subjective Experience of Pleasure, Productivity, and Restoration in Occupations

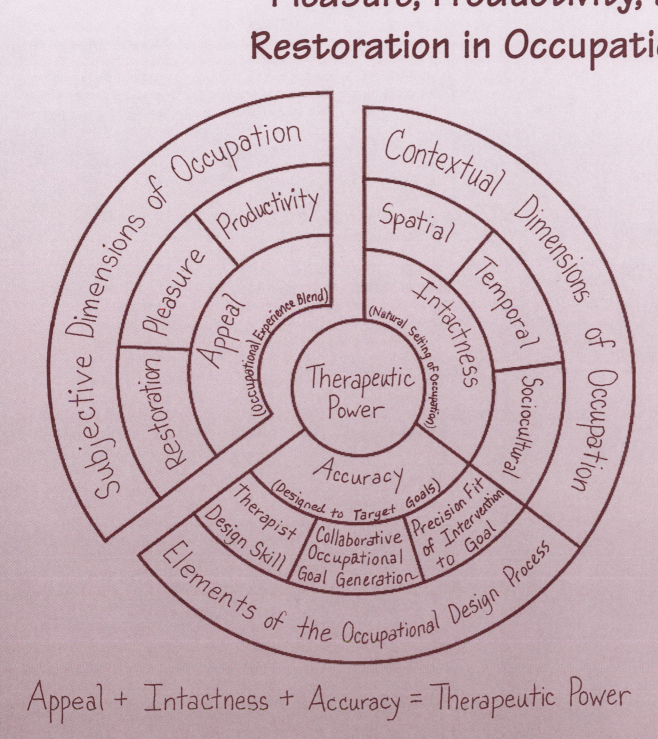

Subjective Dimensions of Occupation

Productivity

Pleasure

Appeal

Restoration

(Occupational Experience Blend)

Contextual Dimensions of Occupation

Spatial

Temporal

Intactness

Sociocultural

(Natural Setting of Occupation)

Therapeutic Power

Accuracy

(Designed to Target Goals)

Therapist Design Skill

Collaborative Occupational Goal Generation

Precision Fit of Intervention to Goal

Elements of the Occupational Design Process

Appeal + Intactness + Accuracy = Therapeutic Power

In Chapter 1, you were introduced to the overall plan of this book. In Chapter 2, you learned about the design process, which you will be using throughout all of the following chapters. Section I is introductory, giving you a view of the landscape before you set out on your expedition into mastery of the central concepts and skills of the occupational therapist.

Now you are ready to begin Section II, which is focused on the subjective experience of occupation. That is, Section II addresses in five chapters the pleasure, productivity, and restoration in occupation; the issues involved in balancing these qualities of daily experience over a day or a lifetime; and the way in which these characteristics of occupational experience can be used to design appealing therapeutic occupation. This section helps you to explore the experience of occupation by seeking to understand your own occupational experiences and patterns first. The last chapter of this section on appeal in occupation-based intervention gives you an opportunity to begin developing some early treatment skills. Also, each of the chapters in this section ends with Power Builders, which you can use to practice your design skills in combination with the concepts presented in the chapter. If you can relax and enjoy your reading, consider how the ideas explain and give you insight into your own life, and try some of the Power Builders at the end. Then, chapter by chapter, you will build toward powerful intervention skills. Occupation is the central concept of occupational therapy. Know it well and you will be a great therapist, no matter what type of patient you see, or what your employment setting may be.

In the section that follows this one, you will explore the contexts in which occupation occurs, and again, you will practice your design skills through the Power Builders at the end of each chapter. Like Section II, Section III ends with a chapter focused on the use of context in intervention design. In Section IV, you will then be ready to look more closely at the skills of the therapist in interaction with the client. Section V provides a summary of the book and some closing thoughts.

So, here you are, ready to begin Section II, with a broad chapter addressing the many questions about striking the right balance of different types of occupational experiences to create a good life. I hope you enjoy this section. In it you will find many clues to great therapy and to what kind of therapist you are destined to be.

CHAPTER 3

The Notion of Balance

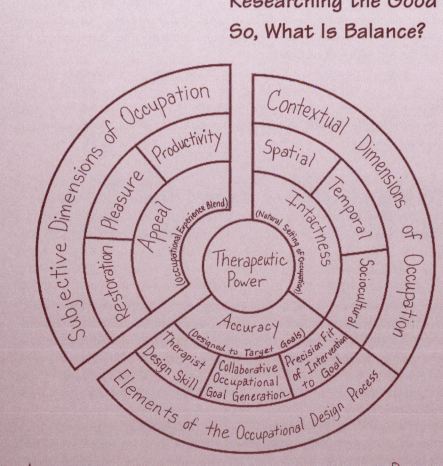

Appeal + Intactness + Accuracy = Therapeutic Power

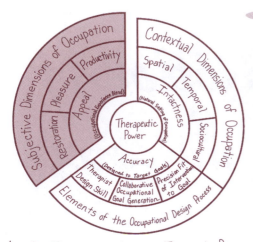

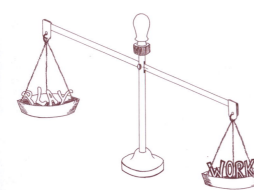

Appeal + Intactness + Accuracy = Therapeutic Power

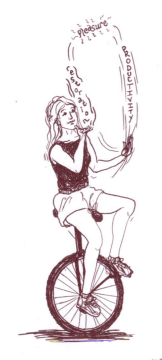

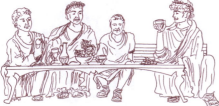

The Notion of Balance

In occupational therapy, we often say a balanced life is important to health and well-being. By this, we usually mean that a relatively equal distribution of time spent in work and in leisure will yield an optimally satisfying life. However, little research has been done on this idea. What is balance exactly? Does it really result in greater quality of life? Most of what we understand about a balance of occupations in our life is cultural wisdom. It is deeply rooted in the history of Western societies, especially in the history of industrialism (Cross, 1990; Gellner, 1988). Striving for balance may be more accurately described as a form of resistance, or adaptation, to the historical changes imposed on our daily occupational patterns by modern forms of paid work. When occupational therapy began, it simply adopted this notion from the surrounding culture that a balance of occupations was healthful.

When we speak of balance in occupational therapy, we are speaking about finding an appropriate division of a person's time between different categories of activity, such as work, play, leisure, and self-care (Reilly, 1974). These commonsense (Geertz, 1983) categories carry great wisdom, tapping essential differences in human activity. However, as occupational scientists have begun to examine these categories more closely, they have found them to be too linear, value laden, decontextualized, and insufficiently descriptive of subjective experience (Pierce, 1997; Primeau, 1996).

In this and the following chapters of this book, you will explore how your own subjective experiences of occupation are made up of a unique mix of pleasure, productivity, *and* restoration. These three characteristics certainly echo the familiar classes of play, work, and rest found in the occupational therapy literature. However, this conceptualization is radically different. Restoration, pleasure, and productivity are not categories between which one must choose to describe an occupation but, rather, three characteristics that are blended within all occupations.

Each occupational experience is a unique blend of the three. After chapters on these three important dimensions of occupational experience, this section ends with a chapter on how you can use pleasure, productivity, and restoration to increase the power of your treatment by designing therapeutic occupations but, with high occupational appeal for each individual you treat.

The Cultural History of the Idea of Balance

Greek Civilization

The notion of a balanced life dates far back in Western history, to the early Greeks, who prized intellectual leisure pursuits above any other form of activity (Primeau, 1996). The Greeks saw work simply as the penalty for natural human sinfulness. Of course, the ability of the Greeks to invest time in leisure pursuits was supported by the labor of slaves.

Agrarian Europe

In European cultures before industrialization, the rhythms of work and leisure were driven primarily by how much daylight there was and what seasonal tasks had to be accomplished. Every day of the week was a work day, all day. Work was primarily produced in households, through agriculture and light cottage industries. All family members partici-pated, regardless of age. People visited while working and supervised children. Lots of breaks were built in for meals and rest. Many holidays broke up the year: saints' days, sea-sonal religious events, market days, carnivals, weddings, funerals, and celebrations of har-vest and planting (Cross, 1990; Primeau, 1996).

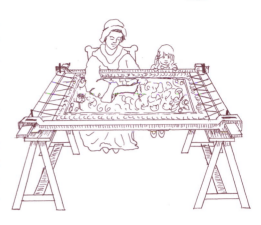

Before the 16th century, individuals constantly negotiated a balanced life by blending the activities of their days to result in a desirable amount of pleasure, a neces-sary amount of productivity, and a healthy amount of rest. The division between work and leisure was not so clear then as it is now, and the notion of children's play was not yet known. Most people believe that the life they lead reflects a typical human pattern. Yet the amount of change that has occurred historically in how we experience our lives is surprising!

The Protestant Reformation

One of the most significant historical forces shaping our daily experience of occupations is the Protestant work ethic. During the Reformation, Protestants split off from the Catholic Church. They asserted that, in contrast to Catholic beliefs, it was a life of hon-est labor, thrift, prosperity, and the production of goods of high quality that marked those who had earned admission to heaven (Gellner, 1988). In the Protestant view, leisure was feared for its potential temptations into sinfulness. This group of radical reformers grew and prospered under their new work ethic. A middle class was created between the elite and the poor, completely changing the structure of European society (Cross, 1990; Primeau, 1996).

The Protestant movement reorganized the calendar and the rhythm of our occupa-tions today. The many religious holidays and festivals in the Catholic calendar were set aside. Instead, a regularly occurring, work-free Sabbath was adopted. The Sabbath day was dedicated to religious life and restoring oneself through healthful leisure, such as walks, hunting, or study. This is how the work week that shapes our lives in Western culture today was born. Can you imagine what life was like before the change to the 7-day work week? How would your life be different without the weekday/weekend rhythm to which you are accustomed?

Today, you can easily observe the Protestant work ethic operating in your own life, regardless of your religious beliefs or ethnic heritage. These ideas permeate modern Western life. Do you value work success over pleasure or rest? Do you sometimes feel guilty when you are enjoying yourself because you are not working? Do you take pride in the craftsmanship of your work, or your fairness in business dealings? Do you config-ure your occupations differently on weekdays from on Sundays? In the next chapter, Productivity in Occupation, you will have an opportunity to examine in greater detail how the Protestant work ethic influences your life and the lives of the clients you will work with as an occupational therapist. The Protestant work ethic pulls our culture toward a heavier emphasis on productive occupations and avoidance of pleasurable occupations.

SUNDAY	MONDAY	TUESDAY	WEDNESDAY	THURSDAY	FRIDAY	SATURDAY

Further, it contributes to the idea of categorizing what kind of occupation one is engaged in according to when it is occurring. During the week, you work, and on the Sabbath, you do not. This strong conceptual split in how most people think about their work and leisure occupations continues today (Primeau, 1996).

Industrialization

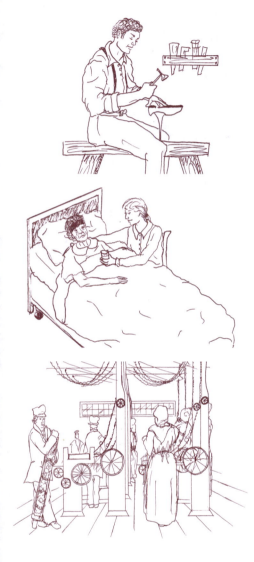

The rise of industrialization and paid employment further emphasized that work and nonwork were opposite and separately occurring occupations. In this period, the two types of activities became defined, according not only to when they occurred but also to where they occurred. What took place in a workplace, such as a factory, was recognized as work and was rewarded with a paycheck. All else was considered nonwork.

By the 1800s, large portions of the population were working outside the home. Many men gave up the independence of the family farm or small industries for the family wage offered by industry. Only the elite and skilled craftsmen were able to resist this pressure to move into the large, synchronized pattern of the factory in which each worker did only a portion of the work leading to the finished product. Work was no longer generally experienced as a series of steps with the resulting satisfaction of a finished product. Through industrialization, work was redefined in spatial and temporal terms. It occurred when the time clock recorded that the worker was within the factory. Our attitudes about work were completely transformed. Work became defined not only by the day of the week but also by its location and what it paid.

During industrialization, the work of those still at home was rendered nearly invisible by these new definitions of work and nonwork. If an activity did not earn money, it was not considered real work. This especially devalued the lives and daily efforts of women, who were actively engaged in many essential unpaid occupations, such as household work and caregiving for children and elderly relatives (Primeau, 1991).

The working conditions in the early factories were terrible. Work hours in the factories were long, with few breaks. Keeping pace with the machines was exhausting. Unsafe conditions regularly caused injuries and deaths. In the mill towns, workers living in dormitories created a new culture far from the behavioral conventions that would have guided them in their smaller hometowns. The incidence of alcoholism and out-of-wedlock births skyrocketed. Adverse health effects on factory workers were also quite clear, especially for women and children.

Reforms

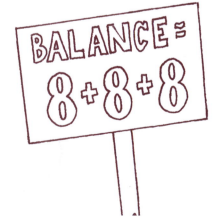

These terrible working conditions created a social reform movement calling for a more balanced, healthy life for workers. This reform movement was a type of organized resistance to the impact that industrialization was having on people's lives. Eight hours of work, 8 hours of leisure, and 8 hours of rest were promoted as a healthier standard. This resulted in the institution of a variety of labor laws, which moved women and children out of factory work, placed some limits on unsafe conditions, and strengthened the ability of male workers to influence their work situations. The notion that a balanced life was something everyone deserved was born out of this societal struggle to adapt to the changes in our lives caused by industrialization, and it is still with us today (Cross, 1990).

Victorian Ideals

Perhaps in reaction to these changes in society, the Victorian era was characterized by a new focus on home and family life (Cross, 1990). Women were encouraged to remain in the home sphere, acting as the coordinators of a balanced family life of engagement in work, recreation, and rest. The idea was discovered that children required play to fully develop, further supporting their exclusion from factories. Play, a new category of activity, was defined as opposite to work. Being the domain of children, unpaid and nonproductive, it was not highly valued. Yet it was romanticized as integral to children's growth and their maturation into successful adults. The toy industry sprang up to support it. By thus placing play in diametric opposition to paid, male, factory-based work, our strong categorization of activity into work and play, or leisure, was engraved in Western thinking for centuries to come (Cross, 1990).

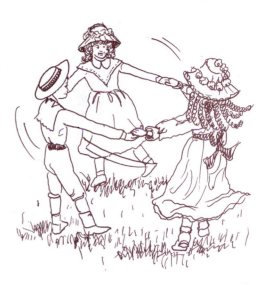

Modern Time Famine

This historically shaped and value-laden thinking regarding our daily activities continues to control how we experience our lives today. Under the influence of the Protestant work ethic, we invest our lives in our paid work, often wondering where the satisfaction in our efforts has gone. We are under a time crunch as we put in increasing numbers of hours on our jobs (Primeau, 1996). Off the job, we engage in a round of leisure activities carefully scheduled for maximum enjoyment. In double-career families, women struggle to complete household work during evenings and weekends, importing the efficiency of the workplace into the home, which used to be a place of relaxation for the family (Hochshield, 1997). Modern culture is experiencing a time famine, largely because of the way in which we categorize our experiences into work and nonwork (Linder, 1970). We work harder and longer to pay for luxury and recreation in our off-the-job time. We constantly seek more pleasure, attempting to balance the high emotional demands of our jobs against the lack of satisfaction they provide. The siren call of a balanced, healthy, and satisfying life pulls strongly at us. However, our attempts to design such a life are usually frustrated by our own historically shaped values regarding our daily activities.

Occupational Therapy: Transcending Cultural Categories for a Deeper Understanding of Occupation

The Founders' Ideas of Balance

True to the culture from which it sprang, occupational therapy adopted at its inception the notion of balance as a valued aim for patients (Christiansen, 1996; Primeau, 1996). The thinking of the founders of occupational therapy was very much rooted in social reforms to improve life conditions for workers, immigrants, and neglected populations of patients (Quiroga, 1995). Adolf Meyer (1922) philosophized about an appropriate balance of work, rest, and leisure. Like others, he fell into the trap of separating work and nonwork,

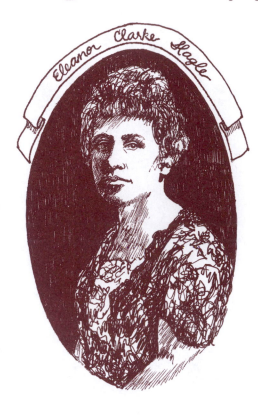

although he did introduce revolutionary concepts regarding how we compose our lives through the time we spend in different occupations. His important ideas about the value of occupations of rest were not much developed in the field, probably because of our cultural overemphasis on productivity. Eleanor Clarke Slagle (1922) used habit training to institute a curative balanced round of activities in the lives of asylum patients. Later, Mary Reilly (1974) used work, play, leisure, and self-care to describe the categories of human occupation that should be kept in healthy balance.

The Problems of Cultural Categories

As a field, occupational therapy operates primarily out of the cultural ideas about occupation that have been handed down to us and shaped by history. Unfortunately, the cultural categories are value laden in ways that do not serve us, or our clients, very well. They devalue the lives of women, children, and others who are not engaged in paid employment. Even for those of our clients who are well matched to the demands of the Protestant work ethic, the categories are not particularly useful in strategizing how to design a truly balanced, satisfying life from available resources.

In the more recent history of occupational therapy, occupational scientists have begun to examine occupation in greater depth than ever before. Research has begun to explore occupation's history, the way in which an occupation is experienced by an individual, the contexts in which occupations occur, and the ways in which occupational experiences create meaning in our lives. The rationale for studying occupation is that the better we understand it, the more powerful will be our use of occupation in treatment. As occupational scientists delve deeper into occupation, the weaknesses of our historically shaped categories become more evident, and we are challenged to move on to more useful descriptors (Pierce, 1997; Primeau, 1996). To do so, we must set aside work, play, and leisure and develop a new language for talking about occupational experience.

It is likely that broad cultural categories of human action, such as work, play, rest, self-care, and leisure, will best serve the field by being used as activity descriptors. Activities differ from occupations in that they are general cultural ideas of human action. Activities are not experienced by a particular individual and do not occur in a real place and time. They are shared cultural ideas about what people can choose to do. Occupations, on the other hand, are one-time experiences of a particular person, who constructs the occupation and its meaning, and interprets the surrounding context of that occupational experience. Occupations are authored by individuals. Occupations are experiences of doing (Pierce, 2001).

A pattern is a design that is discernible across multiple occurrences. It is an observable or reportable shape in the way events, objects, or people are related to each other, across space, time, or relationships. Much of science is the discovery and description of patterns. The way that occupations occur over someone's day, or how they occur in differently situated individuals, is an occupational pattern (Pierce, 1996, p.17).

Creating Balanced Occupational Patterns

When we wonder how it is that one creates a balanced life, the question we are really asking is this: "How can our occupational pattern be constructed in a way that is optimal in providing all that we desire from our lives?" This potent, age-old question must be entered into by first examining what an occupational pattern is.

In occupational therapy, we often speak of simple types of activities, such as Reilly's (1974) typology of work, play, self-care, and rest. However, real-time experiences of occupation are not easily classified in this way. What we call play, because it is the activity of a child, can be experienced by that child in a way very similar to work: as a serious task directed toward creation of a specific product. We might feel confident calling an engineer's paid activities *work* and then hear him describe getting lost in the fun of a challenging new project. And who has not heard someone say, after a busy weekend, that he or she is going off to work to get some rest?

The problem of using commonsense categories in the search for patterns of occupation is this: to be effectively operationalized, concepts must be grounded in and identify distinctly different and clearly bounded conditions (Reynolds, 1971). That is, the categories, or types, must be mutually exclusive. Apples and oranges are the classic example of mutually exclusive types. The historical origins of our cultural categories have not provided us with descriptions of clearly different types of occupations. The field's traditional classifications require us to choose from among a limited set of relatively vague and overlapping categories. If, as occupational therapists, we are to be the premier experts on occupation, we must move to deeper and more accurately descriptive concepts than those offered by the commonsense language of our culture. For this reason, it is important to recognize when and why we are using broad cultural activity categories and when we need to move to more accurate description of the blending of productivity, pleasure, and restoration within the unique, one-time occupational experience of a specific individual.

Another problem in trying to apply traditional categories, such as work and play, is that an observer will always know less about the personal experience of an occupation than will the individual engaged in it. What looks to us like serious, goal-oriented effort may be experienced by that person as deeply enjoyable. Occupational therapy has always valued highly the subjective experience of the individual (Yerxa, 1983). For this reason, the descriptors that we use in our search for optimal, or balanced, patterns of occupation must emphasize the preeminence of the individual's perspective on his or her occupation. At this point, we must limit our use of broad categories, such as work and play, in which the culture or the person observing defines the essential character of the occupation at hand, to the times when we are speaking only in generalities. To accurately address the real experience of the occupations of individuals, we must move to subjective descriptions. That is, we must depend on the individual experiencing the occupation to inform us, rather than make assumptions about that person's experiences from cultural categories. Individuals experience each engagement in occupation as a variable and irreplicable blend of three characteristics—productivity, pleasure, and restoration.

The Three Subjective Characteristics of Occupational Experience

At first, the idea of an occupation described by the individual experiencing it as pleasurable, productive, and restorative does not seem so different from our field's adopted cultural categories, such as work, play, leisure, and rest. But look more closely. The radical difference in this approach is in the little word *and*. By saying that humans experience each engagement in occupation to some degree as pleasurable, productive, *and* restorative, we are freed from difficult forced choices—between work and

a choice:

WORK or PLAY or LEISURE or SELF-CARE

OR

PLEASURE AND PRODUCTIVITY AND RESTORATION

play, for example. A person's real experience of an occupation can simply be seen as a unique, irreplicable blend of these three characteristics. Assessing the degree to which each of these characteristics was experienced provides a more accurate description of an individual's engagement in occupation. By adopting this blended description, we have dramatically increased our potential for examining what a balanced life may be!

We have begun to study how an occupation is experienced by an individual in terms of the degree of productivity, pleasure, and restoration he or she feels during engagement in that occupation (Zemke & Pierce, 1994). In this way, many more aspects of occupational experience are opened to investigation, and our field's valuing of the perspective of the individual is honored. Within this approach to research on occupation, a wealth of questions can now be undertaken that would not previously have been possible. Interesting questions abound regarding the blend of the three characteristics within occupation and how they might produce balance.

- How do people bring pleasure into being productive?
- What do we get out of apparently nonpurposeful activities like watching television?
- Are the rich really enjoying themselves more than are the poor?
- How does occupational experience vary between individuals? Between cultures?
- Under what conditions are two, or even three, of the characteristics at a high level within a single occupational experience?
- Do the characteristics tend to display a general pattern over a day, a week, a year?
- Is there a pattern across development?
- Can balance be identified, assessed, and perhaps even prescribed through the three characteristics?
- Does the pattern that produces balance differ from one individual to the next, or is there a general occupational pattern that tends to yield a feeling of balance?
- Is balance really related to health?

There seem to be trends in relationships between the characteristics of restoration, pleasure, and productivity (Zemke & Pierce, 1994). For instance, pleasure can reach high levels in conjunction with high levels of productivity or restoration, but restoration and productivity rarely reach high levels within the same occupation. As might be expected, both productivity and restoration show strongly repeating circadian rhythms. This is only the beginning of mapping occupational patterns through the use of these three characteristics.

Researching the Good Life

A variety of research approaches have been used to examine that elusive and perfect occupational pattern that we call the "good life." A well-designed, balanced, and personally successful life is a difficult thing to quantify or assess. Several different but closely related concepts have been studied in this area—happiness, subjective well-being, quality of life, and life satisfaction. Happiness has most often been operationalized in research as subjective well-being, or the measure of how happy individuals perceive themselves to be. The terms *life satisfaction* and *quality of life* tend to be used in research on individuals who may be seeking the good life under difficult circumstances, such as aging or disability. These two terms do not seem focused on assessing an optimal life. Rather, they are meant to examine what might be an adequate life given certain limitations.

Happiness, Subjective Well-Being, Quality of Life, and Life Satisfaction in Typical Individuals

A variety of factors have been linked with subjective well-being. Interestingly, 6 out of 10 people rate themselves as "pretty happy," and 3 out of 10 as "very happy." Only 1 in 10 rates himself or herself as "not too happy" (Myers, 2000, p. 56). So the natural setpoint for perceived happiness is not in the middle, but on the high end. This high average supports an optimistic and sociable approach to life that is functional and effective for most people.

The ability of humans to adapt fairly rapidly to changes in life circumstances is central to understanding subjective well-being (Diener, 2000). Sudden changes, such as being diagnosed with a disease or winning the lottery, are accommodated to within a few days, and levels of happiness move back toward their previous levels. This explains why wealth is not highly correlated with happiness, except for those living in or near poverty levels (Furnham & Argyle, 1998). We accommodate to a certain lifestyle, and it no longer makes us dramatically happy or unhappy. It is just our usual life. Similarly, physical attractiveness in college students and physical health in elderly people show only slight correlations with subjective well-being (Diener, 2000).

Popular culture would have us believe that possessions, fame, beauty, wealth, or a life of ease is what make us happy. However, research shows specific factors are correlated with subjective well-being. Strongest among those factors are social support and friendships, marriage, employment, and leisure satisfaction (Argyle, 1999; Myers, 2000).

Involvement in valued occupations has shown a high correlation with subjective well-being in the few studies that have looked at this factor. Leisure satisfaction is one of the strongest overall predictors of life satisfaction (Furnham & Argyle, 1998). Engaging in personal projects that beneficially affect life, allow self-expression, and are socially valued increases subjective well-being (Christiansen, 2000). The work of Csikszentmihalyi (1991) on flow, or optimal experience, clearly demonstrates this tie between doing and happiness. (Flow is discussed more fully in the next chapter.) And again, in the tie between task experiences and subjective well-being, adaptation is an important factor because the novelty, age appropriateness, participation opportunities, and situational meaning of particular life tasks are constantly changing and being re-evaluated within the life view of each person (Cantor & Sanderson, 1999).

Life Satisfaction of Elders

Occupational therapists often work with elderly individuals who have just suffered a traumatic disability, are managing a chronic illness, are in the process of a planned or unexpected retirement, or are living in nursing homes. By understanding life satisfaction in elders, therapists are better equipped to identify threats to quality of life and to design more effective interventions that use valued and life-enhancing activities. Research on subjective well-being in elders shows findings similar to those in the broader population, except that health and leisure satisfaction weigh more strongly for elders. In one study of male elders, engagement in purposeful activity correlated positively with life satisfaction (Madigan, Mise, & Maynard, 1996). In an independently living group of elders of both genders, it was found that although the amount of engagement might decrease with age, changes in activity expectations and continued participation in valued activities contributed to high levels of life satisfaction (Griffin & McKenna, 1998). In another study of elders in nursing homes, engagement in self-generated, rather than prescribed, activities contributed to life satisfaction (McGuinn & Mosher-Ashley, 2000). In a study of retirees, self-determination and the seeking of leisure occupations that were novel and challenging increased life satisfaction (Guinn, 1999). Understanding life satisfaction in the elderly population also requires grappling with the question of how wisdom—that "integration of cognitive, reflective, and affective elements" (Ardelt, 1997, p. 15) with age—supports life satisfaction.

Living Well with Disability

As is true in working with the elderly population, understanding how the life satisfaction of persons with disabilities is threatened and supported by specific factors makes the occupational therapist's interventions more effective. Research on the quality of life of those living with disability shows that engagement in activity plays a central role in satisfaction. In research on individuals with spinal cord injury, the factors of marriage, noninstitutional residence, access to the environment, satisfactory paid or unpaid employment, social and psychological functioning, and time since injury supported increased life satisfaction (Dijkers, 1999; Post, de Witte, van Asbeck, van Dijk, & Schrijvers, 1998; Richards, Bombardier, Tate, Dijkers, Gordon, Shewchuk, et al., 1999). In personal accounts, people with Alzheimer's disease emphasized the importance of engaging in valued activities as central to their quality-of-life experiences (Snyder, 2001). For patients with rheumatoid arthritis, giving up two-thirds of their leisure activities since disease onset had a primary negative impact on their feelings of well-being (Wikstrom, Isaacson, & Jacobsson, 2001). In a study of adults with mental retardation living in different settings, those in sheltered apartments expressed the highest levels of life satisfaction—in comparison with those in residential institutions and in parents' homes—especially in the areas of access to friends, free time, and total lifestyle satisfaction (Schwartz & Ben-Menachem, 1999). In individuals with multiple sclerosis, life satisfaction was closely tied to energy level, independence in self-care, leisure activities, and housekeeping ability (Lundmark & Branholm, 1996). Although these studies of life satisfaction in people with disabilities differ widely in methods and factors examined, it is clear in the overview that engagement in occupation is central to life satisfaction in persons with all types of disabilities. This strong relationship between life satisfaction and occupation makes it all the more clear how important occupation is in both intervention design and collaborative goal setting with clients.

Depression: High Risk for Low Quality of Life

Depression is the greatest risk factor for low quality of life. It can occur in those who are otherwise healthy or in those who are disabled, and in both the young and the old. In the United States, approximately 3 percent of men and 9 percent of women are experiencing the symptoms of major depression at any one time (Downing-Orr, 1998). Depression is quite common in elderly people (Dorfman & Lubben, 1995). Although pharmaceutical treatment of depression is widely accepted, only about 20 percent of persons with depression receive treatment. Often, persons with depression go undiagnosed. Those who do enter treatment are stigmatized, suffer side effects of antidepressants, and are at high risk for suicide. Healthcare providers tend to treat a person with depression as if he or she were weak, exhibiting a character flaw, and to blame for his or her own problems. Occupational therapists who are alert to the common symptoms of both primary depression and depression in reaction to life events can better serve their clients. Clients with depression can be referred to additional services. Negative quality-of-life issues exacerbated by depression may need to be addressed differently. Additional support and problem solving may also be required to assist clients with depression in resolving factors that are negatively affecting quality of life.

A Key to the Good Life: Occupation

Whether we are speaking about typical individuals, elders, those with disabilities, or those with depression, it is clear in this research overview that engagement in valued activities is a key to life satisfaction. For occupational therapists, a basic understanding of life satisfaction is important to grasp that being "pretty happy" is fairly typical, and that adaptation to changes in wealth, physical attractiveness, and even health can be realistically expected without severe long-term impacts on subjective feelings of well-being. The great impact on a person's happiness of broad factors such as marriage, friendships, employment, and leisure (even in comparison with degree of disablement in individuals with disabilities) places the goal setting we do with clients within a whole different set of priorities. Aim to improve these factors in the lives of your clients, and you will probably enhance their overall happiness. Working with elders and those living with disabilities is an especially rich area in which to apply these discoveries in designing effective interventions. As occupational therapists, understanding the good life equips us to live more satisfying lives ourselves, as well as to better assist our clients to live the "good life."

So, What Is Balance?

The study of occupational experience has not yet reached the point at which a balanced life can be adequately described, prescribed, or precisely facilitated through intervention. However, we are making progress in this direction.

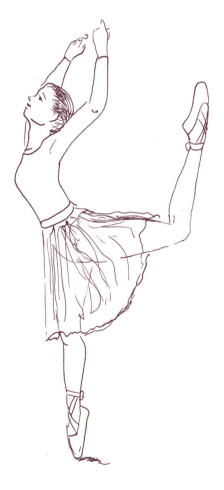

As a student of occupation, you have accomplished several things in this exploration of the complex idea of balance. You have reviewed the historical forces that shaped current cultural categories of activity and notions of healthful occupational balance. You can now recognize how the founders of occupational therapy unquestioningly adopted cultural categories of activity, as well as the belief that a balance of different types of occupations is the healthiest occupational pattern.

By understanding the subjective experience of occupation as a variable blend of productivity, pleasure, and restoration, you can step away from the traditional commonsense categories of activity, yet retain their inherent wisdom. Thus you gain three advantages: (1) You leave behind the many problematic, historically acquired meanings of the cultural categories of occupation; (2) you move from a forced choice between relatively few categories to use a three-dimensional description that is grounded in the perspective of the individual involved; and (3) your thinking in this way opens the potential for better understanding occupation in your own life, in the lives of your clients, and as you will use it in treatment.

Reviewing the research on happiness, life satisfaction, and quality of life gives you a sense of what is typical in well-adjusted individuals and what factors are especially critical in the creation of a good life. The fact that engagement in valued activities is so central to this end provides us with strong evidence of the key role that occupation and occupational therapy has to play in insuring quality of life for individuals who are aging, living with disabilities, or experiencing depression. Keeping in mind the factors that had the greatest impacts on life satisfaction in these studies will help you to insure that you are protecting and targeting the most critical aspects of occupational experience in the collaborative construction of new occupational patterns with your clients.

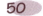

To become a skilled designer of therapeutic occupations, you must become a connoisseur of human occupation. To do so, set aside any concerns with treatment design for a while. In the next three chapters, focus on developing your insight into the patterns of pleasure, productivity, and restoration in your own occupations. It will be an enjoyable and eye-opening experience!

Key Concepts for Strengthening Insight into Balance in Occupations

- Protestant work ethic
- Industrialization
- Work
- Play
- Categories of activity versus blended occupations
- Pleasure, productivity, and restoration
- Happiness, subjective well-being, life satisfaction, and quality of life
- Depression

Building Insight into Your Personal Occupational Experience of Balance

1. Reflect on the following, in discussion with others, as a journal entry, or as a more formal paper or poster presentation:

- What commonly occurring occupations in your life are highly pleasurable for you? Which are high in satisfaction derived from the productivity of reaching goals? Which do most to restore your energy level? Make a list of each.

- Regarding the lists made above, answer one or more of the following: Which list is longest? Why? Are you OK with the life balance that the lists reflect? Does reflection on the lists suggest shifts you might want to make?

- Is there a way to bring more pleasure into your high-productivity occupations? Have you made enough time for highly pleasurable experiences?

- Have you made enough time for highly restorative occupations?

- Think about your occupational pattern this past week. When did you experience the highest feelings of productivity? Of pleasure? Of restoration?

- If you were entering treatment for a recently acquired disability, how would you want the levels of productivity, pleasure, and restoration blended in your experience of intervention? What would most motivate you to remain involved in your occupational therapy?

- Consider these factors that research has shown to have a strong correlation with a high level of subjective well-being: social support and friendships, marriage, employment, and leisure satisfaction. Pick one of these and argue why you think that factor has had the greatest impact on your own well-being.

2. Within a group, have each person write down the activity he or she thinks is most highly pleasurable, most highly productive, and most highly restorative. Share the results. How alike or different were the answers? Why is this?

3. Although you may or may not be Protestant, you are likely to have incorporated in your attitudes some of the Protestant work ethic that is so common to modern Western culture. Reflect, in writing or in discussion with others, on the following questions:

   • Do you ever feel guilty for not being involved in productive occupations? When do you feel this?

   • Have you ever felt that you have worked so hard that it is hurting your health and life balance? If so, why did you do it?

   • Has anyone ever viewed you as "driven?" When and why?

   • In what areas do you, or have you, experienced the pride in craftsmanship that marks the Protestant work ethic?

   • Have you ever experienced a situation in which the golden rule of "do unto others as you would have them do unto you" has been broken? How did that feel? How did your values differ from those of the other person in regard to your understanding of what was "fair?"

4. Brian Little (Christiansen, Little, Backman, & Nguyen, 1999) describes the "life projects" that provide overarching guides to the patterns of our occupations. For you, a life project may be to get your degree as an occupational therapist. What are some of your other life projects? How do they shape your occupational patterns? How do they influence your balance?

5. Ask someone to observe you doing something that is obviously not high level, either in pleasure, productivity, or restoration. Then, have him or her describe to you how much you are experiencing each of these characteristics. How well was he or she able to discern your actual experience? What can you add to his or her understanding of your experience in each of the three dimensions? What does this make you think about our ability to understand the experiences of others? Do you think this ability can be developed? Will this be an important ability for you as a therapist?

Building Insight into Balance in the Occupational Experiences of Others

1. Observe someone you believe to be engaged in a highly productive occupational experience. Can you discern where this individual may also find some pleasure or some restoration in this experience?

2. We often think of children's play as highly joyful and active, the ultimate in pleasurable activity. Observe a child or a group of children at play. Can you identify times when a child is experiencing productivity, the feeling of working toward goals? Can you identify when a child is experiencing restoration (refilling energy reserves) as he or she plays?

3. Have you ever had the opportunity to observe someone who is going through a divorce or unexpected unemployment? How was his or her balance and life quality affected by this?

4. Have you experienced, or known someone who has experienced, depression? In which of the three subjective characteristics of occupational experience did depression have the greatest negative impact: pleasure, productivity, or restoration?

5. Select one of the cases in Appendix A and reflect on the following questions, either in writing or through discussion.

   - What levels of pleasure, productivity, and restoration do you think this person is experiencing in his or her occupational pattern in comparison with a typical individual?

   - If you could affect the level of only one of the dimensions in this person's occupational pattern through intervention, which one do you think it would be most important to target? Why?

   - Which of the dimensions of pleasure, productivity, or restoration has changed the most for this person because of the impact of his or her disability?

   - If you were designing intervention that would be the most appealing to this individual, how would you blend the levels of productivity, pleasure, and restoration to make engagement in treatment as compelling as possible?

   - Of the factors shown by research to have the greatest impact on life satisfaction and happiness, which is most problematic in this case?

Building Design Skills Using Balance

1. Brainstorm for yourself as many highly pleasurable occupational experiences as possible. (See Chap. 2 for rules of brainstorming.)

2. Brainstorm for yourself as many highly productive occupations as possible.

3. Brainstorm for yourself as many highly restorative occupations as possible.

4. Use your understanding of the primary factors supporting life satisfaction to brainstorm as many ideas as you can about how to improve your own quality of life.

5. Use a seven-step design process to design for yourself a 24-hour day that is balanced perfectly in terms of levels of productivity, pleasure, and restoration.

6. If you could only change one thing about the balance of productivity, pleasure, and restoration in your present occupational pattern, what would it be? Use an ideation strategy from the design chapter to generate a list of potential changes; then choose and use an idea selection strategy to pick the best one.

7. Continue Power Builder 6 by completing the implementation and evaluation phases.

References

Ardelt, M. (1997). Wisdom and life satisfaction in old age. *Journal of Gerontology: Psychological Sciences, 52B*, P15–P27.

Argyle, M. (1999). Causes and correlates of happiness. In D. Kahneman, E. Deiner, & N. Schwarz (Eds.), *Well-Being: The foundations of hedonic psychology* (pp. 353–373). New York: Russell Sage Foundation.

Cantor, N., & Sanderson, C. (1999). Life task participation and well-being: The importance of taking part in daily life. In D. Kahneman, E. Deiner, & N. Schwarz (Eds.), *Well-Being: The foundations of hedonic psychology* (pp. 230–243). New York: Russell Sage Foundation.

Christiansen, C. (1996). Three perspectives on balance in occupation. In R. Zemke & F. Clark (Eds.), *Occupational science: The evolving discipline* (pp. 431–451). Philadelphia: F. A. Davis.

Christiansen, C. (2000). Identity, personal projects, and happiness: Self construction in everyday action. *Journal of Occupational Science, 7*, 98–107.

Christiansen, C., Backman, C., Little, B., & Nguyen, A. (1999). Occupations and well-being: A study of personal projects. *American Journal of Occupational Therapy, 53*, 91–100.

Cross, G. (1990). *A social history of leisure since 1600.* State College, PA: Venture Publishing.

Diener, E. (2000). Subjective well-being. *American Psychologist, 55*, 34–43.

Dijkers, M. (1999). Correlates of life satisfaction among persons with spinal cord injury. *Archives of Physical Medicine and Rehabilitation, 80*, 867–876.

Dorfman, R., & Lubben, J. (1995). Screening for depression among a well elderly population. *Social Work, 40*, 295-305.

Downing-Orr, K. (1998). *Rethinking depression.* New York: Plenum Press.

Furnham, A., & Argyle, M. (1998). *The psychology of money.* New York: Routledge.

Geertz, C. (1983). *Local knowledge.* New York: Basic Books.

Gellner, E. (1988). *Plough, sword, and book: The structure of human history.* Chicago: University of Chicago Press.

Griffin, J., & McKenna, K. (1998). Influences on leisure and life satisfaction of elderly people. *Physical and Occupational therapy in Geriatrics, 15*, 1–16.

Guinn, B. (1999). Leisure motivation and the life satisfaction of retired persons. *Activities, Adaptation, and Aging, 23*, 13–20.

Hochshield, A. (1997). *The time bind: When work becomes home and home becomes work.* New York : Henry Holt and Company.

Linder, S. (1970). *The harried leisure class.* New York: Columbia University Press.

Lundmark, P., & Branholm, I. (1996). Relationship between occupation and life satisfaction in people with multiple sclerosis. *Disability and Rehabilitation, 18*, 449–453.

Madigan, J., Mise, D., & Maynard, M. (1996). Life satisfaction and level of activity of male elderly in institutional and community settings. *Activities, Adaptation, and Aging, 21*, 21–36.

McGuinn, K., & Mosher-Ashley, P. (2000). Activity engagement and life satisfaction in elders. *Activities, Adaptation, and Aging, 25*, 77–86.

Meyer, A. (1922). The philosophy of occupation therapy. *Archives of Occupational Therapy, 1*, 1–10.

Myers, D. (2000). The funds, friends, and faith of happy people. *American Psychologist, 55*, 56–67.

Pierce, D. (1996). The brain and occupational patterns. In C. B. Royeen (Ed.), *AOTA Clinical Course: Neuroscience Foundations of Occupation.* Bethesda, MD: American Occupational Therapy Association.

Post, M., de Witte, L., van Asbeck, F., van Dijk, A., & Schrijvers, A. (1998). Predictors of health status and life satisfaction in spinal cord injury. *Archives of Physical Medicine and Rehabilitation, 79*, 395–401.

Primeau, L. (1996). Work and leisure: Transcending the dichotomy. *American Journal of Occupational Therapy, 50*, 569–577.

Primeau, L. (1991). A woman's place: Unpaid work in the home. *American Journal of Occupational Therapy, 46*, 981–988.

Quiroga, V. A. M. (1995). *Occupational therapy: The first 30 years.* Bethesda, MD: American Occupational Therapy Association.

Reilly, M. (1974). *Play as exploratory learning: Studies of curiosity behavior.* Beverly Hills, CA: Sage Publications.

Reynolds, P. (1971). *A primer in theory construction.* Indianapolis, IN: Babbs-Merrill Educational Publishing.

Richards, J., Bombardier, C., Tate, D., Dijkers, M., Gordon, W., Shewchuk, R., et al. (1999). Access to the environment and life satisfaction after spinal cord injury. *Archives of Physical Medicine and Rehabilitation, 80,* 1501–1506.

Schwartz, C., & Ben-Menachem, Y. (1999). Assessing quality of life among adults with mental retardation living in various settings. *International Journal of Rehabilitation Research, 22,* 123–130.

Slagle, E. C. (1922). Training aids for mental patients. *Occupational Therapy and Rehabilitation, 1,* 11–14.

Snyder, L. (2001). The lived experience of Alzheimer's: Understanding the feelings and subjective accounts of persons with the disease. *Alzheimer's Care Quarterly, 2*(2), 8–22.

Wikstrom, I., Isaacson, A., & Jacobsson, L. (2001). Leisure activities in rheumatoid arthritis: Change after disease onset and associated factors. *British Journal of Occupational Therapy, 64,* 87–92.

Yerxa, E. J. (1983). Audacious values: the energy source for occupational therapy practice. In G. Kielhofner (Ed.), *Health through occupation: Theory and practice in occupational therapy* (pp. 149–162). Philadelphia: F. A. Davis.

Zemke, R., & Pierce, D. (1994). [Data set on occupational event log: Student sample.] Unpublished raw data.

CHAPTER 4

Productivity in Occupations

- Productivity Inborn
- Productivity as a Moral Imperative: The Protestant Work Ethic
- Work Identity
- Productivity Stress
- Productivity as a Key Dynamic in Powerful Occupational Therapy

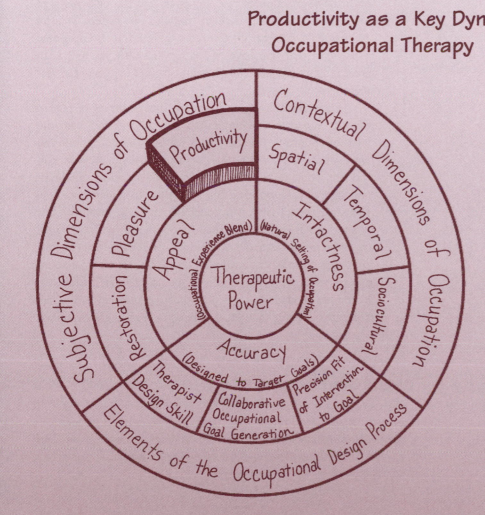

Humans love to be productive. Sure, we moan and groan when we have to leave our fun and go off to work, but striving toward goals is deep in our nature. People get great satisfaction from the challenges that they set for themselves, and our nervous systems crave the stimulation. Our culture values, even overvalues, productivity. The work we do makes us who we are. Building a house, baking a cake, completing a degree, getting a baby to sleep—all of these are satisfying because we are accomplishing a desired goal.

The satisfaction of working toward and reaching goals is different from the enjoyment we receive from purely pleasurable activities. Engaging in occupations that are highly productive means that the activity is experienced as being done for the sake of its outcome. It is goal driven. There are many different types of activities that are usually thought of as high in productivity—paid employment, self-employment, housework, caregiving, studying, and volunteer work. The ability to be productive is essential to who we are as people, as occupational beings.

Occupations that are strongly pleasurable are more oriented to the process, or the moment-to-moment experience, of engaging in that activity. Of course, this does not mean that an occupation must be either enjoyable or productive. Given the right conditions, we can experience both high productivity and high pleasure in an occupation. Such activities that tend to focus on both the satisfaction of reaching goals and the enjoyment of the process involved, such as hobbies or sports, will be addressed in Chapter 5. Can you think of an occupational experience that you have had lately in which you felt both great satisfaction in reaching a goal and great enjoyment in getting there?

In this chapter, you will explore many aspects of human productivity, from the physical to the cultural and from the highs of optimal flow experiences to the lows of burnout. You will question the overemphasis on productivity in Western culture and examine its costs in stress, work addiction, and devaluation of unpaid workers. You will come to understand how this strong emphasis on productivity can also produce such phenomena as pride in craftsmanship, personal growth through career experiences, and even wisdom. As you explore the concept of productivity as a primary characteristic of occupational experience, be sure to consider your own values, beliefs, and history of productivity. It is only through knowledge of yourself as an occupational being that you can become a truly great occupational therapist in your work with others.

Productivity Inborn

Productivity is an inborn human trait. Through evolutionary adaptation, the search for stimulation for our complex human nervous system, and the pursuit of flow experiences, productivity has become increasingly a key factor in what it means to be human.

Productivity as an Evolutionary Adaptation

The human tendency to engage in productive occupations is a survival strategy. The drive to strive toward a goal may even be programmed into our nervous systems through the evolutionary development of the human neocortex. Certainly, the ability to anticipate threats to survival, to plan for physiological needs, and to use strategy to reach goals was enhanced by the sophisticated processing made possible by the addition of the neocortex to the more primitive structures of the human brain. Throughout evolution, individuals who were more productive and goal oriented would have been more likely to survive and pass on their genetic endowments as well as their cultural traditions (Zemke & Horger, 1995).

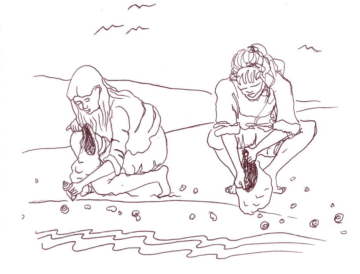

The desire for productivity has evolved into an essential aspect of human nature. For example, have you ever gone to the beach for a relaxing day and spent time there gathering seashells? It is not, for most of us, that the seashells are especially valuable. We haul them home and then don't quite know what to do with them. Yet, in scanning the sands and pouncing on each newly discovered shell with excitement, there is something that drives us on, some satisfaction in simply searching for and gathering shells. Each found shell is a simple goal met, and from that we derive great satisfaction. As in putting together a puzzle or doing a crossword, there is a little thrill of satisfaction in putting each piece or word in its place. In evolution, this drive to scan for pattern and recognize desired objects supported food and materials gathering, tracking prey, monitoring children, and keeping vigilant watch for various threats to survival.

Let's head back to the beach for another example. Did you ever spend time building a sand castle? Through hours of working alone or with others, we build these structures. What are they for? It's obvious that they are not particularly useful. Yet, we work hard at digging, molding sand, assessing our progress, and defending the growing structure from the depredations of waves and toddlers. We take great satisfaction in our own abilities to produce the sand castle out of nothing more than wet sand and our own creative drives. Maybe someone even has the brilliant idea of using some of those seashells to decorate the castle! Building a sand castle is similar to many unpaid activities in which we engage simply for the sake of enjoying our creative productivity—climbing mountains, sewing, bicycling cross country, cooking gourmet meals, gardening, or writing a book. We do not work so hard at these occupations because we await a paycheck, or because we need the product for survival.

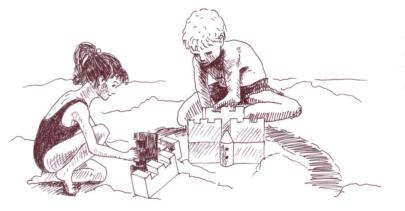

Rather, we gain satisfaction from working toward and reaching a personal goal. In evolution, this type of satisfaction in creative accomplishment supported our invention of new methods for obtaining and storing food, constructing clothing, building shelters, and performing other basic daily activities of human life.

Human Need for Arousal and Challenge

Human productivity is also driven by an almost physiological need for challenge. Even the smallest infant shows a determined intentionality, striving at the edge of skill to

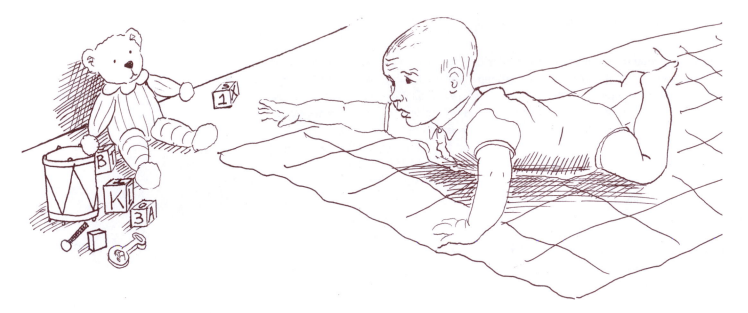

accomplish the next most difficult undertaking (Pierce, 1996). The goals of newborns are simple—keeping a moving object in gaze or hanging onto a nipple until finished feeding. For a slightly older infant, an excited crawling pursuit and grasp of an attractive object yield the greatest accomplishment of the day. By 1 year of age, the toddler can strategize enough to pull a box next to a cupboard to climb up to a counter in pursuit of a cookie. Like an adult testing work skills to his or her limit in a big project, the typically developing child seems driven to set goals just at the far edge of ability. For older children, the drive toward goals is often experienced in games and sports. You will see it in your clients as they strive to reach personal goals of recovery. What is behind this human impulse to strive to the next harder goal?

In the 1960s and 1970s, researchers in the areas of attention, vigilance, and sensory deprivation became intrigued with the degree to which humans seek out conditions of novelty, complexity, and variability. Such *collative variables,* as they called them, resulted in increased arousal (Berlyne, 1960). From infancy to old age, humans tend to seek out challenges in objects or experiences that are novel, developmentally complex, or unpredictable in their responses. These "pacers" result in increased arousal, as we deal with the cognitive uncertainty they provide (Ellis, 1973). A mild level of arousal contributes to attention, interest, and high energy levels. Once the novelty, complexity, or surprise element is habituated to, tension abruptly decreases. As with reaching the punch line of a long joke, this quick drop in tension with resolution of the pacer's uncertainty feels good. By engaging in occupations that are productive and goal oriented, we enter into this cycle of arousal and resolution. When a meaningful goal is reached, the satisfaction can be great. Humans need this constant seeking of the next challenge to maintain arousal and fend off boredom. Can you think of times when you have set goals for yourself just for the challenge of reaching them? Just to make things more interesting and arousing?

Flow Theory

Flow is a state of consciousness in which one is so involved in an occupation that nothing else is noticed. The activity is autotelic, or intrinsically rewarding. Flow theory offers an especially useful perspective on productivity. Flow is so involving and satisfying that it contributes much enjoyment to our experience of occupations that are highly productive and goal oriented. Csikszentmihalyi's (1988, 1991) research on flow, or optimal experience, is based on multiple studies of workers reporting on their subjective experiences of goal-oriented actions. His research groups have included surgeons, artists, burglars, musicians, Jesuits, factory workers, mountain climbers, gamblers, teenagers, writers, and many others.

Occupational therapists use the concept of flow to design appealing therapeutic occupations for their patients. Flow results from a perfect match between perceived skills and perceived challenge. Less skill than is required to meet a challenge results in the uncomfortable overarousal of anxiety. The opposite mismatch of greater skills than are required for a task will result in the equally aversive underarousal of boredom. As each new challenge is mastered and skills increase, greater challenges are required to return to the flow state.

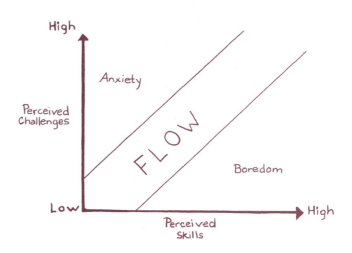

Flow is most likely to occur when the occupation provides clear goals and feedback about relative success and focuses attention on a limited stimulus field. As people focus attention on a task at hand, their awareness merges with the activity, and they feel in control. Their sense of passing time is distorted, and they lose themselves and their awareness of everyday problems. If you think of how a potter feels, completely caught up in throwing a pot on a turning potter's wheel, you can imagine the flow state. Finding flow in our work gives us a unique sense of enjoyment and satisfaction that we cannot enjoy without striving toward goals. Where do you experience this feeling in your life? How you could increase the amount of flow experience in your life by using these ideas about the conditions that produce flow?

The Problem of Boredom

In German, the word for boredom is *langeweile,* meaning a long time. When we are bored, time seems to move very slowly. We feel restless, dissatisfied, and uninterested in what we are doing. The activity in which we are engaged holds no meaning, or value, for us (Barbelet, 1999). Karl Marx (1967/1844) described boredom as the result of a worker's alienation from the experience of work. Alienation results from the meaninglessness of industrialized labor. Jobs that are broken down into small tasks provide no satisfying feeling of accomplishment or completion of a product. Workers have no control over or ownership of the tools and processes of industrial work.

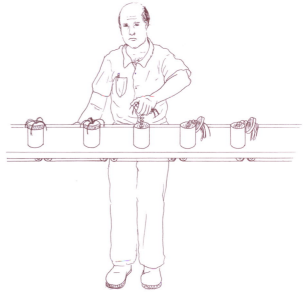

Research has shown that the most boring experiences are those that require attention yet do not provide challenge (Barbelet, 1999). In repetitive work, boredom can be avoided by creating meaning and interest through daydreaming, establishing social relationships in the work setting, devising output goals to challenge oneself, or identifying the importance of the work within some larger framework. There is a negative correlation between boredom and flow: they are nearly opposites (Harris, 2000).

Studies of adults who are chronically bored demonstrate that this condition is the result of compromises they have made in pursuing life goals (Bargdill, 2000a, 2000b). Often they have made life decisions on the advice or at the request of others, modifying their life directions significantly. Habitually bored adults usually do not know how to extricate themselves from these situations and continue in their boring occupational patterns, feeling ambivalent about their lives. They feel stuck, empty, goalless, and apathetic. Often, such feelings lead to increased use of drugs and alcohol or to suicidal ideation. Sometimes life events, such as a divorce or job loss, require new goals to be set to dissipate boredom.

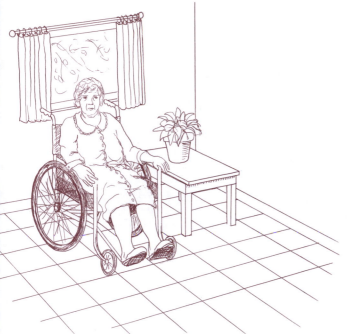

Many of the populations to whom occupational therapists provide service are at high risk for boredom. Elders in nursing homes are at high risk for the "troubling triangle" (Slama & Bergman-Evans, 2000, p. 36) of boredom, loneliness, and helplessness. Although medication is often used to control these feelings, participation in an active daily life that includes engaging goals, social relationships, and opportunities to help others more fully combats such feelings (Ejaz, Schur, & Noelker, 1997). Newberry and Duncan (2001) found a strong relationship between boredom and delinquency. Adolescents who have difficulty imagining possible futures for themselves and are bored in school have a greater tendency to engage in truancy, drug use, and crime. Feeling void of goals, they seek new challenges and escape from boredom through deviant acts. The U.S. Department of Education (1999) estimates that 24 to 45 percent of youths in juvenile justice settings have learning disabilities or emotional and behavioral disorders. Challenged with the difficulty of setting goals for themselves and trying to find satisfaction in the activities of school, community, and family life, they seek to escape boredom and meaninglessness through the excitement and peer network of juvenile crime.

To see an occupational therapy client who is bored during intervention is a very discouraging thing, but it does happen. Therapists who do not use a collaborative, occupation-based approach, in which the client selects the goals, influences the choice of activity for intervention, and envisions the outcomes of treatment, often find themselves faced with bored clients. Out of kindness and faith in the expertise of the therapist, the client may persevere for some time; but without an understanding of why he or she is involved in a particular activity, the client's boredom will soon push him or her to look for something else to do. The classic example of a boring intervention is cone stacking, often used for upper extremity strengthening and coordination. It is not that cone stacking is an inherently boring activity in itself, although it is certainly limited in the challenges it can provide. It is just that clients are often found stacking cones without having an investment in the goal of doing so.

Productivity as a Moral Imperative: The Protestant Work Ethic

The Protestant Reformation

The survival need for productive occupations is undeniable. However, it was not until the Enlightenment that productivity began to be viewed as an indication of moral goodness. In the Reformation movement, radical Protestants declared that morality was not what the Catholic Church declared it to be, but instead included thrift, productivity, craftsmanship, and fairness. They professed the golden rule: "Do unto others as you would have others do unto you." Protestants who prospered under this ethic, but who modestly did not flaunt their wealth, were considered to be "chosen" people and destined for heavenly eternal life. The ultimate importance of leading a productive life, rooted in this movement that so dramatically reorganized European culture, is a strongly embedded value in Western culture (Gellner, 1988). It is a historically shaped value that, regardless of religion, reigns in Western culture. How have you seen the Protestant work ethic operate in your own life?

Industrialization

The rise of industrialization has also exerted a historical shaping force on our attitudes toward work. Before the Industrial Revolution, productive occupations were mostly home-based activities—caring for crops, animals, house, and children. Light cottage industries, such as weaving, were common. These home-produced goods were sold or bartered for things families did not produce themselves. This picture of adult productivity changed dramatically with industrialization.

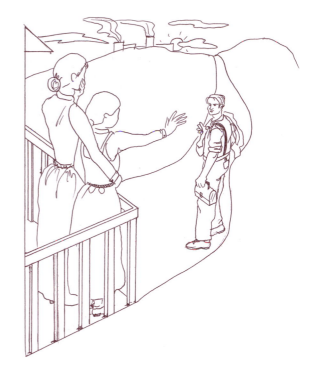

In the 1800s, large portions of the population began working outside the home for pay. Many men moved into factory work, receiving a "family wage," thus shifting the way people valued different forms of productivity. Instead of recognizing the efforts and products of all adults, we, as a nation, began to judge the value of productivity by the wages it produced. Men left their homes, spent less time with their families, gave up the independence of the family farm, and entered the demanding work environments of early factories. Many children and unmarried women worked too. Conditions were unsafe. Hours were long, with few breaks. Keeping pace with the machines was exhausting. Workers had very little influence over their situations.

Craftsmanship

Have you ever been involved in paid work or a hobby that was demanding, highly skilled, and emphasized the quality of the finished piece? Pride in such craftsmanship is rooted in the Protestant work ethic. Examples of this abound in woodworking, model building, cake decorating, needleworking, or motorcycle customizing. The sign of an occupation emphasizing an attitude of craftsmanship is the way in which the product is carefully displayed for the appreciation of others. When you are treating a client using an occupation that offers opportunities for craftsmanship, you can enhance your client's involvement, motivation, pride, and satisfaction in the project by commenting on his or her high-quality workmanship. By doing so, you will also enhance treatment gains from the activity.

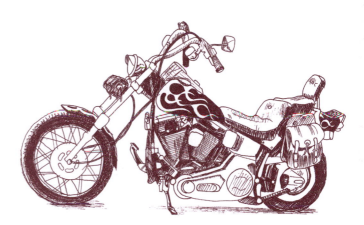

The Cinderella Complex

Sometimes we believe that, if we work hard enough, someone will recognize our hard work and reward us. This is called the *Cinderella complex* (Dowling, 1981). Unfortunately, real life is not filled with princes and fairy godmothers waiting to reward us for our hard work. This feels unfair because we truly believe that hard work proves that we deserve worldly goods and recognition of our moral character. Again, this is the Protestant work ethic shaping our beliefs. Many of the adult patients we serve may feel frustrated by working so hard in exchange for little reward or recognition for their efforts to rebuild lives that have been disrupted by traumatic illness.

Work Identity

Another result of our culture's strong orientation toward productivity is the degree to which we define ourselves through our work. Adults are very much "what we do."

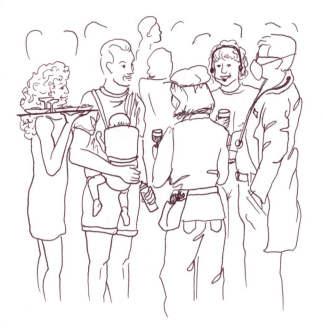

Imagine, for example, that you are at a party where you do not know many people. You begin to chat with someone. One of the most likely questions to arise will be "What do you do?" Perhaps you answer that you are an occupational therapy student. The other person gains insight by imagining your daily occupational pattern of studying, attending classes, maybe holding a part-time job. He or she believes that you have a future in health care. The conversation is likely to continue along this track, exploring where you go to school, how you like it, and so on. You will probably reciprocate by inquiring about the other person's work. You may discover some common ground for further discussion. Or perhaps you won't, and the two of you will drift off to talk in the same way to others. By talking about our work, we are explaining who we are. We are displaying our identities as occupational beings within the larger society.

Types of Workers

The types of paid (and self-employed) workers are nearly innumerable. Here, however, is a very general listing:

- Farmers, fishermen, forestry workers, animal husbandry workers, hunters, miners, and other harvesters of nature
- Manufacturers, crafters
- Construction workers, plumbers, electricians, and other technical service and repair workers
- Salespeople, grocers, butchers, other retailers
- Personal service vendors, such as hairdressers
- Housekeepers, garbage collectors, and other household service providers
- Clergy, doctors, lawyers, nurses, social workers, therapists, and other professionals with specific helping expertise
- Teachers, researchers, writers, editors, publishers
- Office workers, bankers, managers
- Waiters, waitresses, cooks, bakers
- Soldiers, law enforcement officers, fire and emergency workers
- Sailors, pilots, truck drivers
- Prostitutes, drug dealers, and other illegal workers
- Professional athletes, dancers, musicians, artists, actors, media workers

In addition to those who work for financial rewards, there are also unpaid workers, as in the following general listing:

- Caregivers of children and of ill and elderly people
- Providers of unpaid household work
- Students
- Volunteers

Work as Personal Growth

Self-identification through our work can be a powerful avenue for growth. As we go through the phases of our careers, new challenges are offered and met. Often the career path we see in more experienced workers around us can serve as a guide to self-development within our own work. In many lines of work, distinct markers of skills highlight advancement over time and workers are expected to attempt to acquire them. As an occupational therapist, you may move from student to new therapist to expert in special areas. From there, you may go into supervision and administration or open your own practice. Maybe you will become an educator! At each stage of your career as a therapist, different personal strengths and weaknesses will be discovered, and new skills and wisdom acquired. Of course, you will still be just as much yourself in occupations that are less productive and more highly pleasurable or restorative. However, it is likely that you will more strongly associate your unique identity as a person with the occupations that you view as your work. The opportunities that work offers us to grow and change over time contribute to our evolving identities as adults, create a social world within which we define ourselves, and shape the image of us that others hold.

Unpaid Work

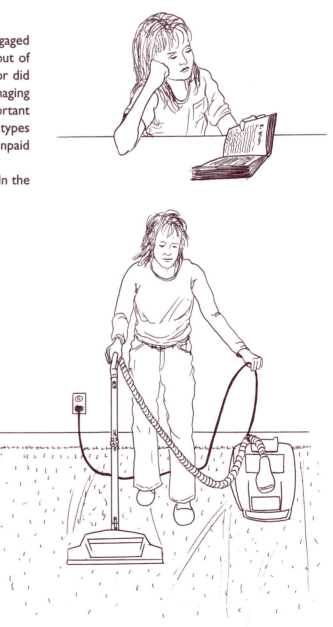

The downside of work-based identity is experienced by those who are engaged in unpaid work (Primeau, 1991). Not only did industrialization take men out of their homes, but it made the work of those who remained in the home or did not receive a paycheck almost invisible (Gellner, 1988). This has been damaging to the self-esteem of these individuals and to their abilities to make important unpaid work contributions to society. Attitudes of disrespect for certain types of work have resulted in a decreased willingness of individuals to assume unpaid work.

Student work is intended to transition a child into a productive adult. In the Western world, this generally entails fulltime elementary, middle, and high school study. For some, student work also includes time in trade school, college, or graduate school. The work of students is as effortful and dedicated as that of other workers, and more demanding of conceptual growth than most adult work, yet it is generally dismissed by adults of the culture as not being part of the "real world." Families and significant others vary greatly in making students feel valued for their daily, fulltime work. Adolescents and young adults often feel pressured to move quickly into paid work. Students intent on finishing high school or college often drop out when faced with these messages about the lack of value of their work.

For hard-working homemakers, it can be embarrassing to be identified as unpaid workers in a modern culture that values paid workers. Yet society could not continue without their work, which provides adequate shelter, food, and clothing for families. Most families in which an unpaid homemaker works do not have enough income to pay someone to do these services, even if the homemaker took employment outside the home. Without this unpaid household work, those in the home who were employed would not be able to continue arriving at their jobs fed, rested, and dressed in clean clothes unless they sacrificed their leisure time to do those unpaid tasks.

Community volunteer work was once a large part of the unpaid work of women, especially upper-class, educated women. There are also charitable and service organizations that are largely composed of male members. The work volunteers do supports many of the community social services traditionally offered in the Western world. Often this work is provided through churches or civic associations. As increasing numbers of women have entered the workforce in recent years, however, fewer women are making fulltime careers of active volunteering (Daniels, 1988).

For occupational therapists, it is critical to have a solid understanding of the work being performed by the unpaid caregivers of clients. In many cases, we rely on the caregiver for support of the home program and for information on daily progress. This is especially true in working with elderly clients or with children, when intervention must occur out of a family-centered approach. Caregivers of elders most often tend to be a spouse, a daughter, or a daughter-in-law, in that order (Olshevski, Katz, & Knight, 1999). Caregivers of children, of course, tend to be mothers, although the incidence of child-rearing by grandparents is increasing.

Caregivers deserve all the support that occupational therapists can provide. In one study of the caregivers of spouses with spinal cord injuries, the degree to which the newly injured individual and the spouse were experiencing stress as a consequence of the injury was approximately the same (Chan, 2000). An especially at-risk group of caregivers are HIV-positive mothers, who must provide care for their children while seeking services and care for themselves (Marcenko, & Samost, 1999). In studies of caregiving work, several strategies have been found to reduce the stress and burden of caregiving: delegating care work, developing competence in care work, understanding and monitoring stress, insuring time for relaxation, including pleasant events in the caregiver's day, increasing social support, and taking a positive perspective on problems (Olshevski, Katz, & Knight, 1999; Van Ess Coeling & Biordi, 2000).

Work Addiction

Have you ever worked extremely hard to accomplish something, in spite of a desire to sleep or to stop working to have some fun? Such determination and sacrifice of other potential occupations in which we might engage is a strategy we all use to reach our goals. However, it works better in smaller projects than it does as a permanent lifestyle. People who let productivity overpower their lives, damaging their health, relationships, and quality of life, are called *workaholics,* or work addicts.

In many ways, work addiction is the "pretty addiction" (Robinson, 1998, p. 170). The Protestant work ethic is so strong in our culture that we value highly productive occupations over all others, in spite of the damage they may do to the individual. Consider, for example, who the people are whom you have been taught to admire. For what are they known? Are any of your heroes famous for their outstandingly pleasurable or restful occupations? Probably not. The people who serve as role models in our culture are those who are highly productive—inventors, corporate tycoons, presidents, missionaries, scientists. We admire those who accomplish grand goals. To be well regarded, people let others know how hard they work and how dedicated to the point of personal sacrifice they are. Unfortunately, the story behind some of these highly productive people is often one of extreme focus to the point of poor health, social isolation, and lack of pleasure and rest in their lives. It is likely that these high achievers did get great satisfaction from their work. But at what cost? These heroes of our culture are living up to the values of the Protestant work ethic to an extreme degree.

Of course, there is a difference between the work addict and those who are simply hard workers or find themselves in a situation that requires them to work long hours. In work addiction, the individual is often depressed, anxious, and chronically tired and engages in a cycle of prolonged work highs followed by crashing lows. Warning signs of work addiction include:

- Constant busyness
- Need for control
- Perfectionism
- Crumbling family relationships and friendships
- Binges of late work on many projects
- Inability to have fun and grumpiness
- Poor driving record (inattention caused by preoccupation with work)
- Impatience
- Poor self-care habits (nutrition, exercise, and rest)
- Overuse of caffeine and nicotine
- Stress symptoms (ulcers, headaches, and high blood pressure) (Porter, 2001; Robinson, 1998; Robinson & Post, 1997)

Although we tend to think of work addiction as a problem of only corporate executives, it can be seen in all walks of life. The key to work addiction is that people view their own self-worth as primarily reflected in their current productivity levels. In Japan, a society that strongly values productivity, the deaths of approximately 10,000 middle-aged workers per year from heart attack and stroke are called *karoshi,* or suicide by work (Robinson, 1998). Other examples of work addicts with which most of us are acquainted are supermoms, superstudents, and healthcare professionals who burn out from not being able to set limits on their efforts to help others.

Loss of Work Identity

In a culture that so highly values productivity, the unexpected loss of identity that accompanies the end of a particular type of work can be agonizing. In addition to suddenly questioning one's identity, one also loses the daily routine of using occupational skills. Networks of social relations that have been created through years of shared work are often lost. Regardless of the type of paid or unpaid work with which one identified or the cause of the cessation of that work, transitions in work identity require an effort to reconstruct one's personal identity around new activities. An occupational therapist can be an effective facilitator in this effort by drawing on his or her wealth of knowledge regarding occupations and activities to discuss, suggest, and assist in experimenting with new occupational patterns.

In paid work, loss of work identity can occur through layoff, termination, retirement, or disability. For those who find themselves suddenly unemployed, there is not usually a need for a significant change in work identity. Rather, such people will probably focus on finding paid employment that uses their current skills. At times, unemployment may trigger consideration of a change in work life, such as when an entire industry is in a downturn. If that is the case, it will be important to spend time in reflecting on the selection of a new work identity. The individual will need to seek educational or training experiences with which to gain necessary competencies for employment, or find an entry-level paid position that will allow development of additional skills in that type of work.

Retirement can pose a serious threat to work identity, raise awareness of mortality, and bring into question the value of one's contribution to society outside of paid employment. A large body of literature addresses the importance of retirement planning for successfully moving from one life pattern to another (Schaie & Schooler, 1998). Short-term retirement adjustment is best when physical health is good, income is adequate to retirement needs, and retirement is the worker's decision rather than a mandate (Gall, Evans,

& Howard, 1997). In recent years, as large numbers of baby boomers reach retirement age, there has been an increase in the use of *bridge employment,* or employment that takes place after the person officially retires from a full-time position (Kim & Feldman, 2000). Often, bridge employment is part-time or temporary employment in the same area of work. In addition to paid work, retirees can supplement bridge employment with personally valued volunteer and leisure activities that they were not able to enjoy during full-time employment. Occupational therapists, with their unique perspectives on human productivity, can be excellent allies in an older worker's reconceptualization of sources of productivity in daily life.

For unpaid workers, loss of work identity occurs when those for whom they provide care move on. The empty nest syndrome, for example, is the loss parents feel when their children leave home to establish themselves as adults in the world. Death of a spouse can similarly result in a widow's or widower's loss of pattern in daily activities, especially if the spouse was ill and required much caregiving work.

Cessation of paid or unpaid work through the onset of disability is likely to generate more serious threats to work identity than does unemployment, retirement, or loss of those for whom one is providing care. In the case of illness and disease processes that lessen or abruptly curtail participation in everyday work, there usually has been little planning done for the transition. Returning to the same type of work may not be possible. Other life issues brought on by the disability, such as economic concerns, disruption of major life plans, and emotional reactions of family and friends, must be dealt with simultaneously. Issues of work identity may seem to be long-term treatment considerations in comparison with more immediate difficulties in learning self-care or adjusting to mobility limitations. Yet the impact of disabling conditions on an individual's work identity can lie at the very heart of self-concept, goals for rebuilding a life, and motivation to participate in occupational therapy.

Productivity Stress

Not all highly productive occupations are experienced as satisfying. When the focus on productivity is allowed to outweigh the well-being of workers, fatigue, stress, impaired health, and burnout can easily result. Stress can also result from major life transitions, such as immigration, marriage or divorce, childbearing, death, or illness. By *productivity stress,* I refer to stress that results from an overemphasis on goal-driven experiences in everyday life.

Sources of Productivity Stress

Stress in highly productive occupations can arise in several different ways. Goals can be set unreasonably high so that it is not possible to gain satisfaction from reaching them. In such cases, called *work overload,* there are two possible responses—(1) reduce standards for productivity to decrease fatigue or (2) maintain efforts to reach goals while experiencing continuing stress.

Environmental factors in work settings that produce constant anxiety, such as noise levels, crowding, or sense of risk, can also rob workers of satisfaction in their work. Examples of work that is inherently stressful because of high demand for attention to safety include operating nuclear power plants, controlling air traffic, and fighting fires.

Some people find their goal-driven occupations boring and lacking in personal significance. Others feel that they work simply out of a lack of choice. For many, the continuously repetitive nature of their paid employment removes the novelty and challenge from the experience. For others, the relative lack of clarity of the goal robs them of the satisfaction of attaining it. Bosma and Peter (1998) found that perceptions of low control over job outcomes and rewards, despite high efforts, were associated with a high incidence of coronary heart disease. A study of stress in nurses (Cheng, Kawachi, Coakley, Schwartz, & Colditz, 2000) found a relationship between declines in health status and the factors of low job control, high job demands, and low work-related social support. All of these situations, in which workers have no hope of attaining flow or experiencing satisfaction in accomplishments, place them under unremitting stress.

In a study of stress and coping in occupational therapy students (Everly, Poff, Lamport, Hamant, & Alvey, 1994), a questionnaire was used to survey the top sources of stress. "At least 86 percent of the subjects reported their top stressors to be examinations, amount of class work, lack of free time, long hours of study, and grades" (p. 1022). Does this sound familiar? Although the students were stressed, many of them reported that this stress strengthened their commitment to their career goals.

Stress, Distress, Coping, and Health

Stress has broad negative effects on health and immunity. An increasing number of studies on stress and immunity have been done in the new field of psychoneuroimmunology (Baum & Singer, 1987; Evans, 1984; Keller, Shiflett, & Bartlett, 1994; Plotnikoff, Murgo, Faith, & Wybran, 1992). Current research posits a model of relationships between stress, distress, immunity, and health. Stressors can be internal physiological events, social conditions, or traumatic experiences. They can be chronic or acute. Distress and coping are the ways in which a person handles the stressor, including his or her coping style, attitude, self-esteem, feelings of being more in or out of control of the situation, social supports, and emotions. Distress and coping serve as filters that can, if effective, decrease the impacts of stressors on health. *Hardiness* refers to the ability to handle stress well, and thus reduce illness, by approaching stressful conditions with attitudes of commitment to the problem, control, and desire for challenge (Maddi, Kahn, & Maddi, 1998).

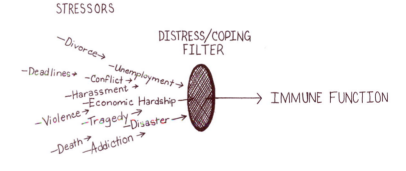

Immune function is deeply impacted by stress and thus impacts health. For example, a study of AIDS patients found that friend support was effective in reducing distress under lower-stress conditions, but family support was effective in reducing distress in higher-stress conditions, and the availability of both types of support impacts health status (Crystal & Kersting, 1998).

By understanding the influence of stress on health, we can recognize stress-related health risks in our clients. Interventions to reduce chronic stress can target clarification of valued and reachable challenges, changes in environmental conditions of work, facilitation of flow, decisions to cease stressful occupations, or changes in the way that a person responds to stressors. In a society that so strongly emphasizes productivity, it is not surprising that the stress of striving toward goals has resulted in a high prevalence of stress-related illnesses.

Burnout

Many studies have documented burnout in various groups of workers. Burnout is the result, after extended work stress, of a complete lack of motivation to continue work.

Here are some examples of different types of workers and other populations and some of the stressors that are causing their burnout:

- Women firefighters: sexual harassment, performance pressure, self-doubt, ill-fitting equipment (Shuster, 2000)

- Refugee children in schoolwork: traumatic stress during immigration experiences (Driver & Beltran, 1998)

- Homeless mothers: lack of services, unsafe shelter environments (Kissman, 1999)

- Middle-school students: economic hardship, family discord, academic problems, schoolwork demands (De Anda & Bradley, 1997)

- Caregivers of elderly people: initial recognition of elder's deterioration, periods of behavioral disturbance in the elder (Olshevski, Katz, & Knight, 1999)

- Prostitutes: poor mental health, drug and alcohol dependence (El-Bassel & Schilling, 1997)

- Cambodian refugees: number of war traumas, resettlement stressors, financial problems (Blair, 2000)

- Social workers: role conflict, role ambiguity, lack of social support (Um & Harrison, 1998)

- Police officers: organizational stressors, lack of reciprocity from citizens and colleagues for efforts, use of violence (Kop, Euwema, & Schaufeli, 1999)

- Nurses: length of career, low levels of education, work on psychiatric wards (Koivula, Paunonen, & Laippala, 2000)

- Nurses: role conflict, role overload, lack of social support (Baba, Galperin, & Lituchy, 1999)

- Nurses: demanding contacts with patients, time pressure, poor rewards, lack of participation in decision making (Demerouti, Bakker, Nachreiner, & Schaufeli, 2000)

- Clergy: bureaucracy, poor administrative support, difficult work conditions (Grosch & Olsen, 2000)

The issue of burnout is especially important for occupational therapists in their own careers. A special category of workaholics, called *careaholics,* are individuals who are not able to say no to those who could benefit from their help. Many of those in the helping professions fall prey to this syndrome, failing to set limits on their work and gradually burning out as competent, creative, and energetic care providers. The work of therapists can also be emotionally demanding because they work with people who are immersed in processes of rapid adjustment and change. When you factor into this picture the productivity pressures in most healthcare settings today, the risk of stress and burnout in occupational therapists is high. Understanding stress, burnout, and their prevention can be important for working with clients and their caregivers, but it can also assist you in supporting your own therapeutic effectiveness by preventing stress and burnout in your own daily occupational patterns as a therapist.

Post-Traumatic Growth

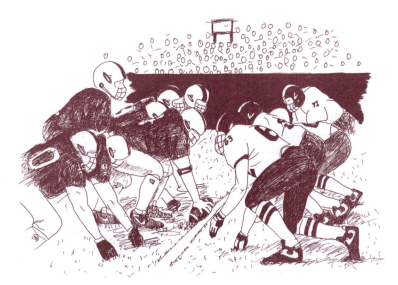

All of us have met persons who seem to seek out stress—professional athletes, executives, or perhaps our own coworkers.

Some seem to be experiencing satisfaction from striving toward their goals. Others do not. Still, they seem drawn to place themselves in demanding situations. Part of the explanation for this behavior may be that the brain produces endogenous opiates under stress. In extreme challenges, epinephrine (adrenaline) is generated as well. If a person enjoys the "high" produced by these brain chemicals more than he or she dislikes the emotional pressure of the stress, he or she will continue to seek out such stressful situations. Corporations sometimes use high-stress, high-productivity occupational experiences, such as mountain climbing, to teach team skills and promote strong goal orientations in upper-level administrators.

Often, as occupational therapists, we are privileged to witness the surge of personal growth experienced by clients after traumatic illnesses or suddenly acquired disabilities. In my work with children on a burn unit, I was always struck by the gusto with which the children would return to their play after having been deprived of it for an extended time. Perhaps you yourself have experienced post-traumatic growth (Aldwin & Levinson, 2001) after personal tragedy, emotional trauma, or illness. Although we would like to avoid such stressful experiences in life, the natural outcomes of such experiences are often increased maturity and wisdom on our parts. As the old saying goes, "What doesn't kill you just makes you stronger."

Productivity as a Key Dynamic in Powerful Occupational Therapy

The better you understand productivity and why humans seek it out, the more powerful you will be as a therapist. Reaching a certain functional level of performance returning to previous levels of productivity is often the sole reason why a patient is referred to occupational therapy. As you work with your patients, you will recognize their problems and strengths in the different areas of productivity described in this chapter. Reflecting on such questions as whether a client suffers a disruption of work identity or how you can create flow conditions during intervention will support the excellence of your interventions. These strategies of treatment provision will be more fully discussed in the final chapter of this section, which addresses the blending of productive, pleasurable, and restorative characteristics in therapeutic occupation to create high appeal for each individual client. Productivity is also an important component in the collaborative goal-setting process, as described in Chapter 15. For now, continue your study of the three primary subjective characteristics of occupation through the following Power Builders on productivity and the subsequent chapters on pleasure and restoration. Suffice it to say that, in regard to intervention, your foundational understanding of productivity will equip you to assist your clients in resolving productivity problems and creating new occupational patterns in their lives that feel satisfying and productive.

POWER BUILDERS

Key Concepts for Strengthening Insight into Productivity in Occupations

- Being productive as an evolutionary advantage
- Need for arousal and challenge
- Flow
- Boredom
- The Protestant work ethic
- Craftsmanship
- Work identity
- Types of workers
- Unpaid work
- Work addiction
- Productivity stress
- Stress, distress, coping, and health
- Burnout
- Post-traumatic growth

Building Insight into Your Personal Occupational Experience of Productivity

1. Reflect on the following by discussing with others, writing a journal entry, or writing a more formal paper or poster presentation.

- Make a list of your goals for today. What do your goals for today tell about who you are in terms of your long-range life goals?

- Whom do you admire? Why? How much of what you respect about this person is because of his or her goal-oriented accomplishments?

- Look around your home. Do you see any objects, handmade by yourself or by others, that you appreciate for their beauty? Can you tell the difference between a well-made object of this kind and one that is poorly made? What does this tell you about your own values regarding craftsmanship? Do you take pride in the quality of some particular type of work that you do often?

- In what occupations have you experienced flow most frequently? Analyze one of these, in terms of the degree to which it provides the conditions of flow: clear goals and feedback on reaching them, focused attention, limited stimulus field, merging of action and awareness, loss of sense of time, and removal from everyday awareness of self and current life problems.

- Describe the most boring experience you can think of. How is boredom related to the lack of a valued goal in this scenario?

- Have you ever felt guilty because you were not being productive? Describe this occasion. How was this feeling based in the Protestant work ethic?

- Have you ever experienced a personal change in work identity? How did the change affect you? What were some of the issues you had to resolve?

- Among those you know personally, who is doing the greatest amount of unpaid work? Does this person feel valued for his or her work?

- When have you experienced your greatest productivity stress? What were the effects?

- Have you ever worked so hard that the ongoing stress degraded your health?

- Have you ever experienced personal growth from loss? If so, how did this occur?

2. *Flow: The psychology of optimal experience*, by M. Csikszentmihalyi (1991), is a must read for any occupational therapist! Available in paperback, this slim volume has the capacity to enhance your enjoyment of all of your productive occupations. Also, facilitating a flow state in your clients will increase the power and generalizability of your treatment exponentially.

3. Do an activity that usually provides flow for you.

Building Insight into Productivity in the Occupational Experiences of Others

1. The next time you are at a social gathering at which you meet new people, listen to the conversation for indicators of the way we define our identities through our work. How did people say who they were? How did you do so? How were these statements related to an assumed set of productive occupations? Reflect on this in your journal or in conversation with someone.

2. Chart your family tree in terms of primary types of work of those to whom you are related. Are there particular types of work that run in the family?

3. Go on a boredom expedition, looking for someone who appears to be bored. Once you find a bored person, observe him or her in a focused way for 10 minutes. What did you see? Why was the person bored? How did it feel to watch a bored person?

4. Select an occupational narrative, disability narrative, or case from Appendix A. How is productivity expressed and experienced in this person's life? Are there productivity problems and issues?

5. Cut out magazine advertisements that show people engaged in highly productive occupations. What do you assume about their lives and what they are like as individuals by seeing them at work in this way? Make a collage to share or reflect on, or, with others, tape all the clippings to a wall in groupings and discuss how the experiences of productivity might be alike and different in the different examples.

6. Interview a person about the productivity in his or her work, using

POWER BUILDERS

questions that elicit information about the following aspects of productivity: arousal levels, goals, satisfaction, flow, self-esteem through work, craftsmanship, work identity, personal growth through work, career progressions within the work, work stress, and burnout. (See Chapter 15 for more background on interview skills.) Select a person who is as different from you as possible, in terms of experience with the work, age, gender, ethnicity, ability/disability. Share your observations afterwards, either through discussion or in written form.

7. With another person or a group of people, conduct interviews concerning productivity, as described above, but with each of you interviewing different types of workers. Compare your conclusions afterward, either in discussion or in writing.

8. Go to a work site and observe productivity, looking for evidence of the following phenomena: arousal levels, goals, flow, craftsmanship, different types of workers and career progressions within the work, and work stress. (See Chapter 16 for more background on observation skills.) Select a person who is as different from you as possible in terms of experience with the work, age, gender, ethnicity, ability/disability. Share your observations afterwards, either through discussion, or in written form.

9. Do the observations described for exercise 8 with another person or person. Make your observations separately and compare notes in discussion afterward.

10. With another person or a group of people, make observations of productivity, as for exercise 8, but with each of you observing different types of workers. Compare observations afterward, either in discussion or in writing.

11. Spend time in a place where you feel others are displaying their craftsmanship and pride in their work. How is craftsmanship defined in this setting? How is the finished product carefully displayed? Share your observations with others.

12. Interview someone you know well concerning post-traumatic growth or the lessons and wisdom the person has gained from a significant negative experiences or events in his or her life. (See Chapter 15 for more background on interview skills.)

13. Interview a primary caregiver for a person with a disability or illness about the experience of productivity in his or her work. (See Chapter 15 for more background on interview skills.) Be sure to ask the caregiver about the following concepts: arousal levels, goals, satisfaction, flow, self-esteem through work, craftsmanship, work identity, personal growth through work, work stress, and burnout.

14. Interview an occupational therapist concerning the experience of productivity in his or her work. (See Chapter 15 for more background on interview skills.) Be sure to ask the person about the following concepts: arousal levels, goals, satisfaction, flow, self-esteem through work, craftsmanship, work identity, personal growth through work, work stress, and burnout.

POWER BUILDERS

Building Design Skills Using Productivity

1. Pick one occupational experience that you expect to be having within the next week that you think will be dull or boring. Brainstorm at least 15 ways in which you could make it more stimulating by using productivity concepts. Select one of these strategies using a simple ranking against three criteria. Try the strategy. Analyze in discussion or writing how well your strategy worked in making your experience less boring.

2. Use a seven-step design process to create an experience for a group of people that helps them learn about some aspect of productivity. This can be done on your own, in a dyad, or in a group.

3. In a group or on your own, select a case from the appendix that shows some productivity problems. Design some interventions to respond to those needs. Try brainstorming to get started, and then simply rank the interventions to decide which you would try first.

4. Imagine that you are working with a 60-year-old male executive who is recovering from a stroke that has left him with some mild speech problems and left-side incoordination. In a group or on your own, brainstorm as many ways as you can think of to use concepts of productivity in working with this client.

References

Aldwin, C., & Levenson, M. (2001). Stress, coping, and health at midlife: A developmental perspective. In M. Lachman (Ed.), *Handbook of midlife development* (pp. 188–215). New York: John Wiley & Sons.

Baba, V., Galperin, B., & Lituchy, T. (1999). Occupational mental health: A study of work-related depression among nurses in the Caribbean. *International Journal of Nursing Studies, 36*, 163–169.

Barbalet, J. (1999). Boredom and social meaning. *British Journal of Sociology, 50*, 631–647.

Bargdill, R. (2000a). A phenomenological investigation of being bored with life. *Psychological Reports, 86*, 493–494.

Bargdill, R. (2000b). The study of life boredom. *Journal of Phenomenological Psychology, 31*, 188–219.

Bum, A., & Singer, J. (1987). *Handbook of psychology and health. Vol. 5, Stress.* Hillsdale, NJ: Lawrence Erlbaum Associates, Publishers.

Berlyne, D. (1960). *Conflict, arousal, and curiosity.* New York: McGraw-Hill.

Blair, R. (2000). Risk factors associated with PTSD and major depression among Cambodian refugees in Utah. *Health & Social Work, 25*, 23–31.

Bosma, H., & Peter, R. (1998). Two alternative job stress models and the risk of coronary heart disease. *American Journal of Public Health, 88*, 68–83.

Chan, R. (2000). Stress and coping in spouses of persons living with spinal cord injuries. *Clinical Rehabilitation, 14*, 137–145.

Cheng, Y., Kawachi, I., Coakley, E., Schwartz, J., & Colditz, G. (2000). Association between psychosocial work characteristics and health functioning in American women: prospective study. *British Medical Journal, 320*, 1432–1436.

Crystal, S., & Kersting, R. (1998). Stress, social support, and distress in a statewide population of persons with AIDS in New Jersey. *Social Work in Health Care, 28*, 41–60.

Csikszentmihalyi, M. (1988). *Optimal experience.* New York: Cambridge University Press.

Csikszentmihalyi, M. (1991). *Flow: The psychology of optimal experience.* New York: Harper Collins.

Daniels, A. (1988). *Invisible careers: Women civic leaders from the volunteer world.* Chicago: University of Chicago Press.

De Anda, D., & Bradley, M. (1997). A study of stress, stressors, and coping strategies among middle school adolescents. *Social Work in Education, 19,* 87–99.

Demerouti, E., Bakker, A., Nachreiner, F., & Schaufeli, W. (2000). A model of burnout and life satisfaction amongst nurses. *Journal of Advanced Nursing, 32,* 454–464.

Dickerson, A. (2000). The power and flow of occupation illustrated through scrapbooking. *Occupational Therapy in Health Care, 12,* 127–140.

Dowling, C. (1981). *The Cinderella complex: Women's hidden fear of independence.* New York: Pocket Books.

Driver, C., & Beltran, R. (1998). Impact of refugee trauma on children's occupational role as students. *Australian Occupational Therapy Journal, 45,* 23–38.

El-Bassel, N., & Schilling, R. (1997). Sex trading and psychological distress among women recruited from the streets of Harlem. *American Journal of Public Health, 87,* 66–71.

Ejaz, F., Schur, D., & Noelker, L. (1997). The effect of activity involvement and social relationships on boredom among nursing home residents. *Activities, Adaptation, and Aging, 21,* 53–66.

Ellis, M. (1973). *Why people play.* Englewood Cliffs, NJ: Prentice-Hall.

Evans, G. (1984). *Environmental stress.* New York: Cambridge University Press.

Everly, J., Poff, D., Lamport, N., Hamant, C., & Alvey, G. (1994). Perceived stressors and coping strategies occupational therapy students. *American Journal of Occupational Therapy, 48,* 1022–1028.

Gall, T., Evans, D., & Howard, J. (1997). The retirement adjustment process: Changes in the well-being of male retirees across time. *Journal of Gerontology: Psychological Sciences, 52B,* P110–P117.

Gellner, E. (1988). *Plough, sword, and book: The structure of human history.* Chicago: University of Chicago Press.

Grosch, W., & Olsen, D. (2000). Clergy burnout: An integrative approach. *Psychotherapy in practice, 56,* 619–632.

Harris, M. (2000). Correlates of boredom proneness and boredom. *Journal of Applied Social Psychology, 30,* 576–598.

Keller, S., Shiflett, S., & Bartlett, J. (1994). Stress, immunity, and health. In R. Glaser & J. Kielcolt-Glaser (Eds.), *Handbook of human stress and immunity,* pp. 217–244. New York: Academic Press.

Kim, S., & Feldman, D. (2000). Working in retirement: The antecedents of bridge employment and its consequences for quality of life in retirement. *Academy of Management Journal, 43,* 1195–1210.

Kissman, K. (1999). Respite from stress and other service needs of homeless families. *Community Mental Health Journal, 35,* 241–249.

Koivula, M., Paunonen, M., & Laippala, P. (2000). Burnout among nursing staff in two Finnish hospitals. *Journal of Nursing Management, 8,* 149–158.

Kop, N., Euwema, M., & Schaufeli, W. (1999). Burnout, job stress, and violent behavior among Dutch police officers. *Work & Stress, 13,* 326–340.

Maddi, S., Kahn, S., & Maddi, K. (1998). The effectiveness of hardiness training. *Consulting Psychology Journal, 50,* 78–86.

Marcenko, M., & Samost, L. (1999). Living with HIV/AIDS: The voices of HIV-positive mothers. *Social Work, 44,* 36–46.

Marx, K. (1967/1844). *Economic and philosophical manuscripts.* Moscow: Progress Publishers.

Newberry, A., & Duncan, R. (2001). Roles of boredom and life goals in juvenile delinquency. *Journal of Applied Social Psychology, 31,* 527–541.

Olshevski, J., Katz, A., & Knight, B. (1999). *Stress reduction for caregivers.* Philadelphia: Brunner/Mazel.

Pierce, D. E. (1996). Infant space, infant time: Development of infant interactions with the physical environment, from 1 to 18 months. *Dissertation Abstracts International.*

Plotnikoff, N., Murgo, A., Faith, R., & Wybran, J. (1992). *Stress and immunity.* Ann Arbor, MI: CRC Press.

Porter, G. (2001). Workaholic tendencies and the high potential for stress among co-workers. *International Journal of Stress Management, 8,* 147–164.

Primeau, L. (1991). A woman's place: Unpaid work in the home. *American Journal of Occupational Therapy, 46*, 981–988.

Robinson, B. (1998). *Chained to the desk: A guidebook for workaholics, their partners and children, and the therapists who treat them.* New York: New York University Press.

Robinson, B., & Post, P. (1997). Risk of addiction to work and family functioning. *Psychological Reports, 81*, 91–95.

Schaie, K., & Schooler, C. (Eds.) (1998). *Impact of work on older adults.* New York: Springer Publishing.

Shuster, M. (2000). The physical and psychological stresses of women in firefighting. *Work, 15*, 77–82.

Slama, C., & Bergman-Evans, B. (2000). A troubling triangle: An exploration of loneliness, helplessness, and boredom of residents of a veterans home. *Journal of Psychosocial Nursing, 38*, 36–43.

Um, M., & Harrison, D. (1998). Role stressors, burnout, mediators, and job satisfaction: A stress-strain-outcome model and an empirical test. *Social Work Research, 22*, 100–116.

U.S. Department of Education (1999). Special Education in Correctional Facilities. In *Twenty-First Annual Report to Congress on the Implementation of the Individuals with Disabilities Education Act* (II-1–II-22).

Van Ess Coeling, H., & Biordi, D. (2000). The relationship between work strategies used by informal caregivers and care receivers and clinical outcomes. *Journal of Applied Gerontology, 19*, 264–284.

Zemke, R., & Horger, M. (1995). Hands: Tools for crafting human adaptation. In C. Royeen (Ed.), *Hands on: Practical interventions for the hand* (pp. 85–103). Bethesda, MD: American Occupational Therapy Association.

CHAPTER 5

Pleasure in Occupations

The Activities of Play and Leisure

Simple Sensory Pleasures

Complex Cerebral Pleasures

Taking Pleasure Too Far: Chemical and Activity
  Addictions

Designing Pleasure into Life

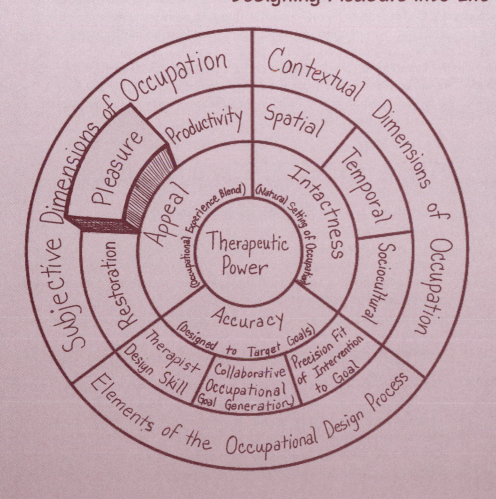

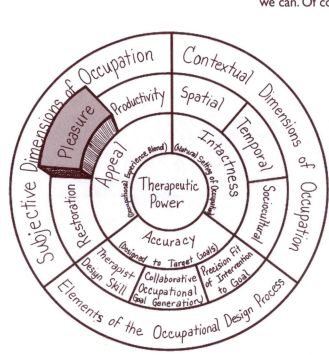

As we design our days of activities, we try to fit in as much pleasure for ourselves as we can. Of course, our enjoyment has to be balanced against our desire to be productive and remain healthy. Did you ever wonder what you would do if you won the lottery? If you had nearly unlimited financial resources, you would probably select an occupation high in pleasure. Until we do win the lottery, however, we must design a pattern of occupations that gives us the enjoyment we desire, still moves us toward our life goals, and takes care of our needs for rest and nutrition.

What activities give you pleasure? Stop and think about this for a moment. Make a short mental list. Some of the pleasurable occupations you chose were almost completely hedonistic, weren't they? If you look closely at your choices, you will also realize that many of the occupations you chose were characterized by high degrees of either productivity or restoration. For instance, if you imagined lying on a tropical beach in the sun with a cold beverage beside you, you're bound to feel a high degree of restfulness associated with this quite pleasurable experience. If you chose a project you always wanted to do, such as remodeling an old barn into a wonderful studio home, you've realized that a lot of productivity is included in your pleasurable occupation. This is the nature of occupation. It contains degrees of all three characteristics: pleasure, restoration, and productivity. Pleasure can be found together with high restoration or high productivity, but rarely with both at once.

In this chapter, we will explore how we design pleasure into occupations. Wouldn't you like to raise your pleasure levels and still accomplish your goals? In occupational therapy, we often design treatments that use pleasurable occupations. Clients tend to be more motivated to engage in therapeutic activities that are enjoyable. That's why occupational therapists need to learn so much about crafts and hobbies. Skillfully designing pleasurable occupations requires a deep understanding of pleasure in human life. To gain perspective on how pleasure operates in our daily occupations, we will consider in this chapter the historical meanings of play and leisure, the role of the limbic system in purely sensory pleasures, and some of the more complex aspects of human pleasure.

The Activities of Play and Leisure

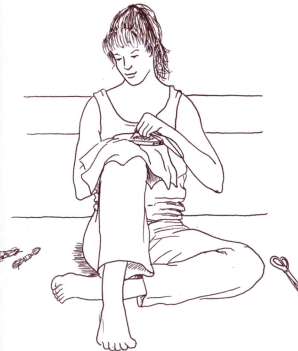

In Chapters 3 and 4, we examined how occupational therapy has long used our culture's commonsense language to describe occupation in terms such as work, play, and leisure. The advantage of using everyday words is that our clients, and others, understand us. The disadvantages are that the meanings are vague and embody all sorts of historical baggage concerning the greater value of some activities in comparison to others.

Leisure

The Protestant work ethic clearly makes work the opposite of play and leisure. The Reformation devalued activities sought out for pleasure's sake and valued leisure only as a reward for good, honest work (Gellner, 1988). Leisure was seen primarily as a way to keep an adult refreshed for productive activities. Often we call the pleasurable occupations of adults *leisure*. Like work and play, the common meaning of leisure is historically rooted in the Victorian idea that the most important aspect of adult occupations is productivity. Any adult occupations that were not work were lumped under the term *leisure*. The term seems to connote both restfulness and pleasure, and refers to all waking activities in which adults engage outside of work hours. Leisure activities today include hobbies, sports, arts, crafts, dance, music, entertainment, travel, and others (Cross, 1990). What are your leisure activities?

Play

According to the Protestant work ethic, play is the less productive and therefore the less important activity of children. Even today, the value of play is often argued by saying it is the work of the child, important for development of skills for adult productivity. Piaget (1962) described three types of play: (1) practice games from birth to 2 years of age, (2) symbolic games using imagination from 3 to 6 years, and (3) games with rules, such as sports, from 7 to 11 years. Reilly (1974), who advocated occupational therapy's increased focus on occupation in the 1960s, described *play* as an occupation that was intrinsically motivated. By this, she meant that it is engaged in for its own sake. It is done for the pleasure of doing it, rather than for the sake of its outcome. Play is a predominance of process over product. It is being in the moment. She described the child's learning of rules of motion, objects, and people through play, as well as the child's developmental progression through stages of exploration, competency, and achievement in play. Too often, we think of play as anything a child does. Actually, that is a misleading definition. Children also work quite hard at reaching their goals. Also, adults play. In the midst of a serious day in the clinic, therapists may joke with each other, or enjoy doing an activity along with a client. The essence of play is pleasure. What are some of the most pleasurable memories of play in your childhood? How do you play now?

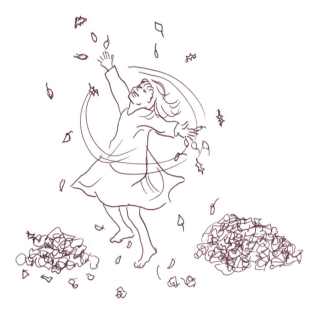

Simple Sensory Pleasures

The Limbic System

Understanding how the limbic system works helps us understand how sensations and memory contribute to the pleasure we find in our occupations. The limbic system is an old, primitive area of the human brain. If our forebears did emerge from the sea, it was the limbic system that assumed regulation of body temperature, heart rate, blood sugar, and other systems necessary to a warm-blooded animal in the cold, unwelcoming air. For this reason, the limbic system is sometimes called the "visceral brain" (McKeough, 1995, p. 126). The limbic system also processes emotional expression and memory (Martin, 1996). It contains the brain's pleasure centers. Generally, the limbic system includes the amygdala, the hippocampus and fornix, the hypothalamus, and the limbic association cortex (Martin, 1996). These structures fit into the underside of the cortex, curving in C shapes just at the top of the midbrain.

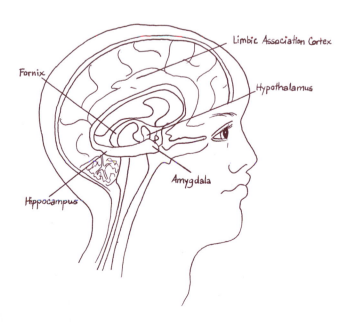

The *amygdala* (Greek for almond) participates in the sense of smell, memory, emotion, and appetitive behaviors, such as eating and sex (Martin, 1996). The amygdala links associations of pleasurable or painful experience to specific stimuli, so that when those stimuli recur, they are more likely to be attended to and taken into long-term memory. The amygdala influences changes in nervous system excitation and ability to respond. The fact that the amygdala projects directly to the dorsal motor nucleus of the vagus nerve, which controls the facial muscles, explains why humans can read feelings so well in one another's faces (Martin, 1996).

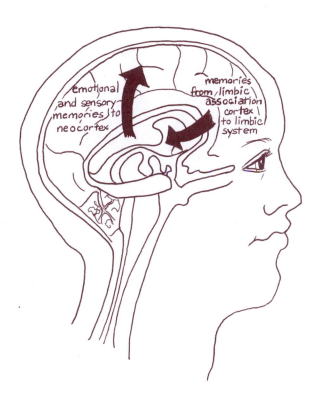

The hippocampus and its efferent pathway, the fornix, play an important part in short-term memory. Nearly all incoming sensation is entered into short-term memory at the hippocampus. However, it is only through attention to those sensations that memories are refreshed and stored in long-term memory. Edelman (1989) calls the hippocampus the "organ of succession" (p. 119) because of its role in perceiving sequence (Martin, 1996). Understanding event sequence is particularly important for formulating quick responses to sensory input.

The hypothalamus is about the size of a pea. It mediates production of reproductive hormones and sensations of sex, pain, hunger, and thirst. One of the main functions of the hypothalamus is to regulate the autonomic nervous system. The hypothalamus contains 40 times more opioid receptors than in other parts of the brain (Martin, 1996; Rose, 1976). These receptor sites attach neuropeptides, producing pleasure or analgesia of pain. Most well known of the neuropeptides are the endorphins (short for endogenous morphine) and enkephalins. They modulate pain and contribute to immune function (Rogawski & Barker, 1985).

The limbic association cortex is on the underside of the frontal, parietal, and temporal lobes. It receives all sensory information except olfaction from higher areas of the cortex, where it has already been partially integrated. The connections of the limbic system through the limbic association cortex to the greater neocortex are responsible for the affective aspects of remembered experience.

The Pleasures of Sensation

Much of what we consider to be pleasurable in occupation is because of our simple animal enjoyment of our senses. As sensation is processed through the limbic system, it is colored with pleasure. Pleasure is highlighted, enhancing the likelihood that information so critical to our survival, such as the taste of food or the texture of a tool, will receive adequate prompt attention and uptake into memory. The hypothalamus responds by affecting the autonomic system through relaxation or increased arousal. Some people seem more sensuous and attuned to sensory input than others. People also seem to differ in terms of which sensory experiences bring them pleasure. There are individual differences in the degree to which different types of sensation impact a person's limbic system. Of the senses of smell, taste, touch, movement, vision, and hearing, which gives you the most pleasure? What sensory deficit do you think would have the greatest negative impact on the amount of pleasure in your occupational pattern?

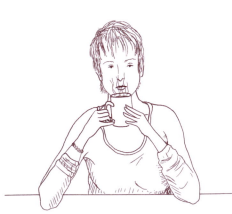

Taste and smell are the simplest forms of sensation, operating on a more transitory chemical level than other types of sensation. Although taste and smell sensations certainly become associated with visual, spatial, or textural memories, they do not form the types of complex, multisensory, and sequential memories that other kinds of sensory experiences provoke (Rose, 1976).

Smell is the most primitive of our senses, and the one least cortically processed. The limbic system has also been called the *rhinencephalon,* or nose brain. Some theorists propose that the limbic system evolved from the sense of smell.

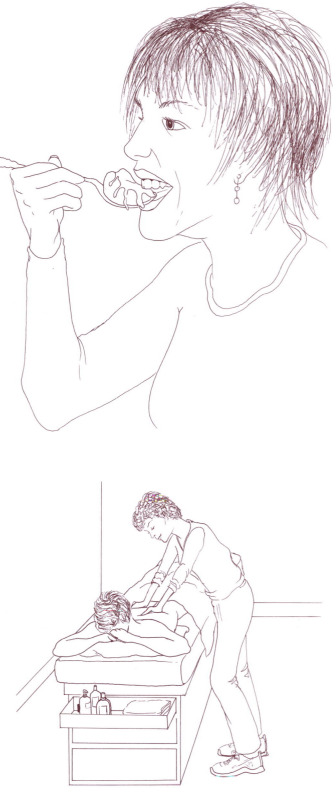

Smell is processed through the paired olfactory bulbs, called cranial nerve I, which lie along the underside of the brain, extending from the central limbic structures to the nose. There are three primary sensory tracts for smell. The very oldest of these leads to the hypothalamus and triggers olfactory reflexes. A not-quite-so-old tract also leads to the hypothalamus, and plays a part in learned associations to smells. The newest tract leads by way of the thalamus to the cortex. Even in the cortex, the olfactory areas are phylogenetically older than other portions of the sensory cortex (Guyton, 1991). In mammals, behavioral responses are often triggered by olfactory cues. Have you ever had an unexpected occurrence of an emotional memory from an olfactory cue? Such a memory is caused by the limbic system's overlapping functions of olfaction, emotion, and memory.

The sense of taste is as poorly understood as smell. It appears that there are four primary taste sensations: (1) bitter, (2) sweet, (3) salt, and (4) sour. Each of these is sensed by specialized taste buds, located in specific quadrants of the tongue, mouth, and throat. Taste is the only sensory input that does not cross to the contralateral side of the nervous system in processing. Our mental representations of taste are highly integrated with smell, texture, and visual aspects of the taste experience. As is also true in the sense of smell, individuals can have "blindness" for particular aspects of taste, such as sour sensation.

Input from several types of receptors yields different types of sensation regarding touch and body position, depending on the receptor's location. Information can be exteroceptive (from the skin surface), proprioceptive (from muscles and joints), visceral (from internal organs), or deep (from deep pressure). Imagine someone giving you a massage—you may feel the softness of velvet or feel like you are floating in water. Although information regarding touch, texture, and pressure can give great pleasure, the pathways carrying this information are not as directly connected to the limbic system as are those for taste and smell (Guyton, 1991). The influence of these sensations on the reticular activating system that influences arousal levels may be the link that gives us pleasure from tactile sensation.

The sense of touch also seems to be closely connected to our experience of sexuality. Orgasm has been shown by electroencephalography (EEG) to be correlated with intense neuronal firing in the septum. Like a mini-seizure, the firing spreads throughout the limbic system, but never enters cortical areas. Following orgasm, our endorphin levels rise, producing a feeling of well-being and relaxation (Changeux, 1985).

Vestibular information from the inner ear about movement, position, gravity, and balance receives constant monitoring at the limbic level. Young children sometimes spin in circles for the sheer joy of it. Few adults break into this type of spontaneous vestibular pleasure seeking. The connections of the vestibular system to brainstem structures and the limbic system affect arousal, emotion, posture, muscle tone, and integration of sensory information (Ayres, 1972).

The visual and auditory senses are processed at a more cortical level than that noted for other sensory modalities. Their connections to the limbic system are the

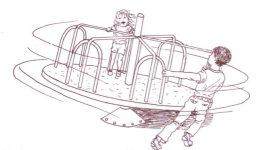

least direct. Perhaps this is why we rarely hear of people driven to overindulge in sight or sound to the point of endangering their health.

Visual perception is highly developed in humans. Seventy percent of human sensory receptors are found in the retina. The more primitive visual tracts lead to the midbrain and thalamus, influencing basic behavioral reactions to the environment. Newer tracts lead to the visual cortex in the occipital lobe. Auditory input ascends to the auditory cortex in the temporal lobe, as well as directly to the reticular activating system to enable quick reactions to auditory stimuli.

The Pleasure of Being Physically Active

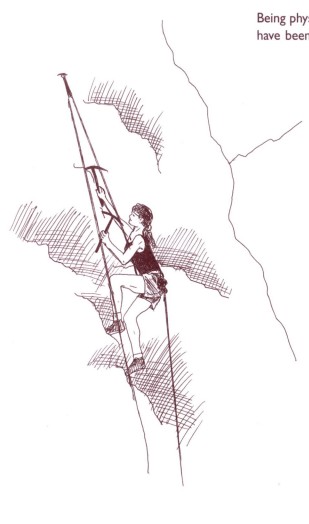

Being physically active and moving through the world can be pleasurable, especially if you have been deprived of this experience for any length of time. Have you ever gotten up from sitting for a long time and just enjoyed stretching your legs and walking, even though you really had no destination in mind? Sensations flow, endogenous opiates are released, and the body provides the mind with a welcome flow of input. Have you heard of a "runner's high"?

Many people in Western culture have dangerously low levels of physical activity. Research shows that complete physical inactivity, such as is experienced during bed rest, has negative impacts on immunity, perception, cognition, and mood (Sandler & Vernikos, 1986). Among older adults living in U.S. retirement communities, only about 15 percent are meeting objectives set by the Public Health Service of 30 minutes of physical activity per day (Pollard, Taylor, & Smith, 2000). It is not inability that stops them, but a lack of belief in their ability to exercise and in the value of doing so. Adults who exercise for health and fitness reasons feel greater self-esteem than those who do not (Tiggemann & Williamson, 2000). In a study of children ages 8 to 16, approximately 80 percent reported 3 or more bouts of vigorous physical activity per week (Anderson, Crespo, & Bartlett, 1998). Twenty-six percent of U.S. children watch 4 or more hours of television per day (McMurray, Harrell, Deng, Bradley, Cox, & Bangdiwala, 2000). Do you get enough physical activity in your own life?

In the case of the pleasure we derive from being active, it may be true that the more we enjoy this particular pleasure, the healthier we will be! In many of the client populations occupational therapists serve, physical activity is a critical factor for maintaining health. If we can make better use of the pleasure of physical activity in occupational therapy, we may be able to kill two birds with one stone—address patient goals through pleasurable and active interventions and also enhance their physical states of health.

Dealing with Pain

In many of the people with whom occupational therapists work, pain reduces the pleasure they experience in their occupations. Chronic pain is especially problematic because it requires ongoing coping, management, and preventive strategies. Persons especially at risk for chronic pain include those with diagnoses of arthritis, fibromyalgia, back injury, cerebral palsy, spinal cord injury, amputation, multiple sclerosis, traumatic brain injury, and stroke (Benrud-Larson & Wegener, 2000). In these diagnostic categories, interventions are focused on the primary diagnosis, and the problem of pain is left largely unaddressed. Ongoing pain can result in depression as well as difficulties with employment, family life, and functional status (Averill, Novy, Nelson, & Berry, 1996; Hunfield, Perquin, Duivenvoorden, Hazebroek-Kampschreur, Passchier, Suijlekom-Smit, & van der Wouden, 2001). Occupational therapists can play an important role in enhancing the quality of life of their patients by advocating that healthcare teams use a broad approach that includes an emphasis on pain management, stress management and coping, and a full return to a satisfying occupational pattern.

Complex Cerebral Pleasures

Many human pleasures are more complex than the simple enjoyment of sensation. Understanding how these more cerebral human pleasures operate is more challenging than comprehending the functioning of the limbic and sensory systems. Indeed, it does not seem that science has come quite so far as to even put much research into this area. There are, however, a few clues.

Thrill Seeking

Bombarding the body with high levels of different types of sensory input can produce pleasure by triggering an adrenaline response. This is one reason why play is so closely associated with fun and pleasure. Children do not hesitate to seek highly arousing sensory experiences, just spontaneously doing something for the thrill of it. Sledding and watersliding are good examples. Many adults also engage in thrill-oriented sports such as skiing, racing, bungee-jumping, rock-climbing, and whitewater rafting. Some people enjoy the thrill of being frightened by movies that are suspenseful, fast paced, violent, or shocking. What are some of your most thrilling occupations? Do they have strong sensory components?

Humor

Think of someone telling a long, detailed joke. Your attention is held, your mind puzzles out where the joke is going, and your arousal increases as it is told. You lean forward slightly, still, eyes on the person telling the joke. The punch line comes, with some unexpected twist, and you laugh, relaxing your position and moving your body. This quick drop in arousal is experienced as pleasurable. When we laugh at slapstick humor that is full of pratfalls and silly-looking accidents, we are experiencing the combination of arousal at what looks like a painful injury and relief at seeing that the individual is unhurt. Sometimes, just being around people who are laughing seems contagious. That's the secret behind television laugh tracks. Research has shown that humor is good for us and supports immune function (Ornstein & Sobel, 1989). When was the last time you had a good laugh?

In recent years, many healthcare settings and professions have begun to recognize the value and importance of humor. Wooten (1996), a specialist in humor in nursing practice, calls humor the "canary of health care" (Uren, 1998, p. 1). This analogy refers to the historical use of canaries in mines to alert miners to declining levels of oxygen. In today's increasingly productivity-driven healthcare workplace, losing your sense of humor

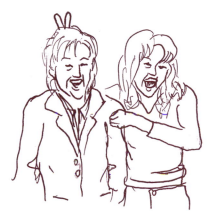

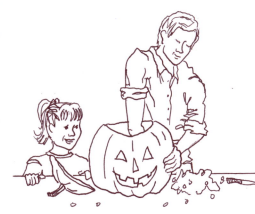

can be an indicator of dangerously high levels of stress and potential for burnout. Norman Cousins (1979) was one of the first to raise the consciousness of healthcare providers regarding the importance of humor in his book *Anatomy of an Illness*, the famous account of his use of humor to cure himself of ankylosing spondylitis. The reasoning behind this remarkable approach is that humor reduces stress and improves immune function.

Humor as a therapeutic approach is now being deliberately applied in many types of settings: intensive care (Thornton & White, 1999), hospice (Showalter & Skobel, 1996), midwifery (Davison & O'Brien, 1997), rehabilitation (Basmajian, 1998), emergency rooms (van Wormer & Boes, 1997), and home care for Alzheimer's patients (Buffum & Brod, 1998). Humor serves both provider and client by reducing stress and increasing trust and communication (Schultes, 1997). Patch Adams, a physician, has led the movement to include clowns on the healthcare team, claiming that the old adage "laughter is the best medicine" is true (Clayton, 1997). There is even a nursing journal devoted entirely to humor, *Journal of Nurse Jocularity*, filled with hilarious perspectives on the work life of nurses.

In a study of the use of humor in occupational therapy, Vergeer and MacRae (1993) uncovered several themes that reveal how humor is best used in practice. Humor can be used either spontaneously or deliberately. Care must be taken not to use humor that may be offensive, or to use abstract humor that excludes patients with cognitive impairments. Laughing at yourself can equalize power relations between client and therapist, and emphasize that you prefer a person-centered approach over a more distant professionalism. Humor creates a more positive work environment and helps staff achieve balance and reduce stress. By understanding humor, one of the pleasurable aspects of occupation, you can enhance the power of your interventions and your own enjoyment of your profession.

The Pleasure of Meaningful Ritual

Performing a deeply meaningful action or ritual can give pleasure beyond what can be accounted for in sensations. Part of this is because of the way the limbic system colors the experience with previous memories and the emotions with which they were associated. A deeply meaningful act is always grounded in a wealth of memories. If a ritual has been repeatedly performed during generally pleasant times, such as at special holidays, it will be strongly associated with previous positive feelings. As you move through the loosely scripted action of a ritual, you relive those pleasant memories. You enjoy a sense of timelessness. Completion of the action can release a flood of emotions. Can you recall ritual events in your life that were highly pleasurable?

Mixing Pleasure and Productivity: Creative Arts, Crafts, Hobbies, Sports, and Fun Jobs

Many of the creative activities that we associate with high levels of pleasure are actually blends of high pleasure and high productivity. The essential difference between productivity and pleasure in occupation is that productivity is experience focused on the product or goal and produces satisfaction in that outcome, and pleasure is the experience of the moment-to-moment process of doing and results in enjoyment. Some of the things adults do during their leisure time are creative activities that include both a goal, or valued outcome, and a pleasurable process. Sometimes our paid work provides us with this mix of pleasure and productivity, if we are lucky enough to do something in which we truly do enjoy the process. These are what Csikszentmihalyi (1988, 1991) calls flow, or optimal experiences. Activities that tend to be thought of as high in both productivity and pleasure are those in which we engage in the pleasurable creation of a product. Here is a list of just a few of these high-pleasure, high-productivity, creative activities:

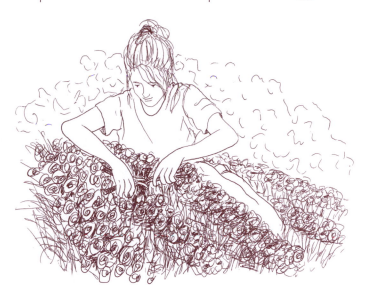

- Art
- Sewing and needlework
- Crafts
- Woodworking
- Sports
- Creative paid work
- Cooking
- Decorating
- Gardening
- Playing music

Taking Pleasure Too Far: Chemical and Activity Addictions

To discuss the pleasurable dimension of occupation without acknowledging the darker side of pleasure that emerges as addiction would be to treat occupation too lightly. Unfortunately, the power of occupation in our lives is not always positive. There are two types of addictions that can be destructive to the occupational pattern desired by an individual—chemical addictions and activity addictions. Chemical addictions are fairly straightforward; they are physiological needs for a particular substance, such as nicotine, alcohol, or drugs. Activity addiction is an involvement with a particular activity to such a degree that it has destructive consequences for a person's life. Addictions are usually destructive to the occupational pattern to which we aspire because of our involvement in actions that isolate us from others and prevent engagement in other activities. The line must be drawn, of course, between a sudden and consuming interest in doing a particular activity and the point at which this passion becomes dangerous. That line must be drawn by each individual, within his or her judgment of what is and is not a satisfying and appropriate occupational pattern. Have you ever gotten completely caught up in reading a book or a series of books by the same author? Perhaps you stayed up late at night reading and were tired and impaired at work the next day. Is this an activity addiction? Probably not. An activity addiction is ongoing, results in disrupted social relations, and impairs the quality of the occupational pattern over a longer period than just 1 day.

Substance Abuse and Addiction

Substance abuse is the overuse of legal substances or the use of illegal substances. Addictions are physiological cravings for legal or illegal substances. The substances to

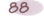

which Americans are most often addicted include nicotine, alcohol, and illegal drugs. Consider the following facts from the 1999 National Household Survey on Drug Abuse (www.health.org/govstudy):

- Approximately 14.8 million Americans used illicit drugs.

- Eleven percent of children ages 12 to 17 used illicit drugs, primarily marijuana.

- Thirty percent of Americans used tobacco: 15 percent of those ages 12 to 17, 40 percent of young adults ages 18 to 25, and 25 percent of adults ages 26 and older.

- About half of the 1.6 million new smokers in a year were younger than 18 years of age.

- Approximately 45 million Americans were binge drinkers (5 or more drinks once in 1 month).

- Approximately 12.4 million Americans were heavy drinkers (5 or more drinks on 5 or more occasions in 1 month).

- Peak age for binge and heavy drinking was 21.

Given the size of these problems in Western culture, any occupational therapist will be dealing with clients who are abusing or addicted to tobacco, alcohol, and/or drugs, regardless of area of practice or the degree to which clients may be disclosing such issues. In some intervention populations, such as persons with spinal cord, head injury, or heart attack, involvement with such substances often precipitates the trauma that results in the need for occupational therapy. Often, difficulty in carrying out recommended and agreed-on interventions results from substance use. In some cases, the life losses and long-term consequences of disablement can push clients who were not previously at risk into substance use and abuse.

Many myths and cultural stereotypes exist regarding involvement with these dangerous substances that can obscure the therapist's perception of lifestyle factors in treatment. For example, although we may think of a drug user as a penniless, skinny junky, hanging out in some fleabag room in a ghetto, this is inaccurate. One of every 10 people who use illegal drugs has a full-time job and is not poor (*New York Times,* 1999). Another example of the way in which culture can cloud our ability to see what is right in front of us is the way in which heavy drinking and binge drinking are accepted as a humorous rite of passage for college students, despite the fact that the combination of driving and drinking is the number one killer of young adults.

The pleasure that individuals gain through the use or abuse of these substances is real. But is it worth the cost? Why do people seek pleasure in this way, rather than in another, less risky way? There are many answers to such a question: the strength of physiological addictions, the need for consolation and release from discouraging circumstances, poor judgment, peer pressure, the denial of potential harm, family patterns, or the lack of experience with other pleasurable activities that might serve the same need. Regardless of the individual situation of each client with whom you work, it is important that you, as a therapist, look at the abuse or addiction as a part of the whole occupational pattern of the person, and ask yourself what this person is seeking through this behavior and how that pleasure might be found elsewhere.

Obesity and Bulimia

For some, the pleasure of food becomes a problem. Obsessions with eating or not eating can have dramatic negative effects on health. In Chapter 6, the role of food and drink in restoring us is fully discussed. Also in Chapter 6 is a description of obesity, bulimia, and anorexia, the disorders of eating. Obesity is continued overeating to the point of impaired health, and is on an epidemic increase in the United States. Anorexia is starving oneself. Bulimia is an out-of-control binge-and-purge cycle of eating. Obesity, anorexia, and bulimia are not substance addictions, but activity addictions or maladaptive occupational patterns. Although we require food, water, and air to survive, we do not say we are addicted to these substances.

Pathological Gambling

One type of thrill seeking that can evolve into a disorder is gambling (McCown & Chamberlain, 2000). Although most people are able to control the impulse to gamble, 3 to 5 percent become pathological gamblers. Pathological gamblers can suffer financial devastation, become involved in illegal activities to pay off debts, and lose important relationships. Similar to those with a drug addiction, pathological gamblers are preoccupied with plans for and stories about gambling, require increasing levels of gambling risk to get the same thrill, are unable to quit despite repeated attempts, and are restless and irritable when not gambling. The prevalence of gambling problems is increasing in the United States, aggravated by escalating opportunities to gamble through state lotteries, casinos, and the Internet. Growing gambling problems in youth, college-age adults, and older people are evident (Curry & Gershensen, 1998; McNeilly & Burke, 2000). Pathological gambling was declared a disorder of impulse control in 1980 in *Diagnostic and Statistical Manual of Mental Disorders (DSM)*, but insurance companies do not cover treatment for pathological gambling. Many individuals participate in Gamblers Anonymous, a 12-step recovery program. Regardless of how it is treated, pathological gambling is a disorder of occupational pattern—a pattern of continuing engagement in activities despite the evident dangers inherent in doing so. Intervention requires a family-centered approach that focuses on constructing a life that is satisfying to the recovering gambler to replace the important role that gambling has played in his or her life.

Technology Addictions

The explosion of technology into our lives has changed our occupational patterns considerably. First radio, and then television, joined the list of typical activities that we fit into our days. Later, we had the advent of video games. Even more recently, Internet addiction has entered the conversation about the pros and cons of technology-based activities in our lives. Are these real addictions? Or are they just new occupational patterns to which we have not yet adjusted and begun to value? To call something an activity addiction means that we believe the degree to which the person is involved in that activity is seriously affecting his or her health and/or quality of life.

The advent of television has inserted a new category of activity into our lives. Where there once existed more physically active choices in the typical occupational pattern, many adults and children today are spending hours passively seated in front of the television. In the United States, more than half of children ages 8 to 16 years watch more than 2 hours of television per day (Crespo, Smit, Troiano, Bartlett, Macera, & Anderson, 2001). High frequency of television watching is correlated with obesity, putting the health of large numbers of children and adults at risk. Do you consider your own pattern of watching television to be your desired level and healthy for you?

In a study of nearly 18,000 Internet users, Greenfield (1999) used an adaptation of the DSM criteria for compulsive gambling and estimated that approximately 6 percent of those on-line are "virtual addicts." That is, their Internet use has resulted in social isolation, depression, and dramatic alterations in lifestyle, or has impaired work performance because of Internet surfing on the job. Those who claim to be addicted to the Internet report feelings of powerlessness and being out of control. Thirty-seven percent of those in the addicted sample of Greenfield's study were involved regularly in cybersex, or Internet-based pornography, chat rooms, or relationships. Internet relationships are quite different from face-to-face relationships. There is anonymity, allowing a person to assume a new identity and hide undesirable physical features. People conversing on-line are dis-inhibited. That is, because of the anonymity, they are far more open and intimate in their communications. As an experience, surfing the Internet is remarkably similar to entering a gambling casino; that is, there are high visual stimulation, time distortion, and specialized areas to enter for certain interactive experiences. Clicking on an Internet site opens a whole new set of possibilities. Just like rolling the dice or dropping a quarter in a slot machine, there is a sense of venturing into the unknown. In a study of 277 undergraduate college students, Morahan-Martin and Schumacher (2000) found that pathological Internet users were more likely to be males, use on-line games and technologically sophisticated sites, and score significantly higher on loneliness scales. Do you know anyone who may be at risk for Internet addiction?

Video games are becoming an increasingly typical activity of children and young adults. In one study (Phillips, Rolls, Rouse, & Griffiths, 1995), 77 percent of the children questioned played video games. Some scholars argue that playing video games greatly resembles gambling and gambling addiction (Fisher, 1994), but is an earlier childhood form of the addiction. Certainly much concern has been expressed about the effects of the violence in video games on the behavior of children. In children counseled to decrease the amount of time spent watching television and playing video games, aggressive behavior was significantly reduced (Robinson, Wilde, Navracruz, Haydel, & Varady, 2001).

As technology introduces new activities into our lives, we seem to have few societal mechanisms for critically considering the loss or damage that may be done through changes in occupational patterns that these new, technology-based activities create. Whether it is watching television, using the Internet, gambling, or playing video games, it is important that we consider the impact on health and quality of life that incorporating, or overusing, these activities has on our own lives and those of our clients.

Designing Pleasure into Life

In Western culture, we have strong values that emphasize productivity in our lives. Sometimes we even feel guilty if we are enjoying ourselves too much. Yet it is possible to have high levels of both pleasure and productivity in the same occupation. It is not necessary for our work to be no fun! As you are learning about pleasure in occupations, you have an opportunity to rethink the design of your occupational pattern to include more occupations that are highly pleasurable, or to include elements of pleasure in your highly productive or highly restorative occupations. Why not? It's enjoyable, it's healthy, and it may even boost your productivity!

Understanding your own pleasures in daily activities will also help you to be a more creative, empathic, and powerful occupational therapist. Sophisticated practice theories, such as sensory integration (Ayres, 1972), activity analysis and use of crafts (Crepeau, 1998; Fidler & Velde, 1999) incorporate an understanding of the processes behind pleasure in occupation to strengthen intervention. Combining your creative skills with your understanding of the limbic system and sensory processing, as well as the more complex pleasures of occupation, gives you powerful access to strategies to improve the life designs of your clients. Never underestimate the power of pleasure in treatment!

POWER BUILDERS

Key Concepts for Strengthening Insight into Pleasure in Occupations

- Play
- Leisure
- Sensory pleasure
- Physical activity
- Pain
- Thrill seeking
- Humor
- Ritual
- Activities that mix high levels of pleasure and high levels of productivity
- Chemical addictions
- Gambling
- Technology addictions

Building Insight into Your Personal Occupational Experience of Pleasure

1. Reflect on the following in discussion with others, as a journal entry, or as a more formal paper or poster presentation:

- What were your favorite childhood play activities?
- What is your favorite type of leisure activity?
- What type of sensory experience gives you the greatest enjoyment?
- What types of physical activities give you the most pleasure, and why?
- When have you had the most physical pain in your life?
- What is the most thrilling experience you have ever had?
- Do you consider yourself a thrill seeker? Do you know anyone who is?
- What is the funniest thing that ever happened to you? Why was it funny?
- What are some highly pleasurable rituals in your life?
- What is the most highly restorative occupation from which you receive a high level of pleasure? What type of pleasure is it?
- What is the most highly productive occupation from which you receive a high level of pleasure? What type of pleasure is it?
- How can you increase the pleasure levels in your highly restorative occupations?
- How can you increase the pleasure levels in your highly productive occupations?
- What would you change about your life if you won the lottery? What type of pleasure are you envisioning in these changes? How can you bring

POWER BUILDERS

that type of pleasure more strongly into your life until you win the lottery?

2. Do something highly pleasurable based on sensory input. Concentrate fully on the sensations for at least 10 minutes. How did you feel afterwards?

3. Rent a comedy video and watch it at a time when you are usually tired from productive activities. Notice how different you feel after laughing at the video.

4. Learn a new joke and tell it to someone.

Building Insight into Pleasure in the Occupational Experiences of Others

1. Do a 2-hour observation of children at play. (More information on observation skills is in Chapter 16. Be sure you have appropriate permissions to observe.) Create an observation scheme of at least 10 points, to prompt your full attention to all that is going on before you. Record all that you see.

2. Do a 2-hour observation of adults engaged in leisure. (Be sure you have appropriate permissions to observe.) Create an observation scheme of at least 10 points to prompt your full attention to all that is going on before you. Record all that you see.

3. Interview an amateur athlete about the pleasures of practicing his or her sport. (More information on interview skills is in Chapter 15.) Create a brief interview schedule before you do the interview. Record responses either in writing or on audiotape. Review the responses after the interview and write a summary (one to two pages) of the main points the athlete made about what the pleasures were in doing this sport.

4. Go to a place where you can watch other people laughing, such as a funny movie or a comedy club. Watch a couple of people from beginning to end of your time there. How did their moods, expressions, body postures, arousal levels, and amounts of eye contact with others change from beginning to end?

5. Ask people to tell you the jokes they know.

6. Observe a group of people participating in a common holiday ritual or conduct an interview of an individual about such an experience. (Use information on interview and observation skills from Chapters 15 and 16.) Write a brief summary of what gives the person or group pleasure in this ritual event.

7. Interview an occupational therapist concerning the experience of pleasure in his or her work.

8. Cut out magazine advertisements that show people engaged in highly pleasurable occupations. What do you assume about their lives and what they are like as individuals by seeing them in this way? Make a collage to share or reflect on, or, with others, tape all the clippings to

a wall in groupings and discuss how the experience of pleasure might be alike and different in the different examples.

Building Design Skills Using Pleasure

1. Create a play experience for yourself and others you know well. Use the design steps of brainstorming, and rank and weigh to create the play experience. Do a written reflection afterwards, addressing the following questions:

   - How was the play experience perceived by adults? By children? If you had both in your group, why the difference?
   - How did the play experience you provided go differently from that planned?
   - What was the most "playful" part?

2. Create a leisure experience for yourself and other adults you know well. Use the design steps of brainstorming, and rank and weigh to create the leisure experience. Do a written reflection afterwards, addressing the following questions:

   - How was the leisure experience perceived by the adults?
   - How did the leisure experience you provided go differently from that planned?
   - What was the most "leisurely" part?

3. Make changes in one of your daily occupations to increase its pleasure level. Remember, the pleasure must come between the beginning and the end of the occupation, not before or after it. Reflect on how difficult or easy this was and where the pleasure came from.

4. Design a highly pleasurable experience for yourself. Use brainstorming, ranking, and a time/task list, and then implement your plan. Pay careful attention to your experience. Reflect on what about it made it pleasurable for you, drawing on the concepts offered in this chapter as needed. Were you more motivated to do an assignment that required you to enjoy yourself than one that did not?

5. Design a highly pleasurable experience for someone you know well. Take the time to go through the process of design: feel ready, investigate the person's perspective on pleasure, generate ideas, choose one, and plan it. Carry out the plan, paying careful attention to how it unfolds. Evaluate your project in three ways: (1) informally interview the person about the pleasure he or she experienced; (2) reflect on what you would have done differently if you had it to do over; and (3) decide what you thought were the greatest benefits to you of doing this design project.

6. Select one of the cases from Appendix A and write two fictitious, brief (one-page limit) reflections by that person about two different occupational therapy sessions: one that used a very pleasurable therapeutic occupation, and one that did not.

7. Record your level of physical activity for 1 week, by noting all your occupations and their lengths, and then ranking them as low, medium, and

POWER BUILDERS

high in physical activity. Look at the pattern. Brainstorm 10 easy ways to increase your physical activity in the next week, and then pick your two best ideas. Do them over 1 week, again recording your occupations. At the end of the second week, write a brief reflection, answering the following questions:

- How successfully were you able to implement your ideas?
- If there were difficulties, what were they?
- Did you feel different after 1 week of higher physical activity?

8. Using one of the cases from Appendix A, create a description of a potential intervention for that person that uses a holiday ritual theme. Brainstorm at least 20 ideas, keeping in mind some potentially important goals for that person.

9. Use a seven-step design process to create and carry out an experience for a group of people that helps them learn about some aspect of pleasure in occupation. This can be done on your own, in a dyad, or in a group.

References

Anderson, R., Crespo, C., & Bartlett, S. (1998). Television-watching is associated with obesity. *Brown University Child and Adolescent Behavior Letter, 14*, 4–5.

Averill, P., Novy, D., Nelson, D., & Berry, L. (1996). Correlates of depression in chronic pain patients: A comprehensive examination. *Pain, 65*, 93–100.

Ayres, A. J. (1972). *Sensory integration and learning disorders.* Los Angeles: Western Psychological Services.

Basmajian, J. (1998). The elixir of laughter in rehabilitation. *Archives of Physical Medicine, 79*, 1597.

Benrud-Larson, L., & Wegener, S. (2000). Chronic pain in neurorehabilitation populations: Prevalence, severity, and impact. *Neurorehabilitation, 14*, 127–137.

Buffum, M., & Brod, M. (1998). Humor and well-being in spouse caregivers of patients with Alzheimer's disease. *Applied Nursing Research, 11*, 12–18.

Changeux, J. (1985). *Neuronal man: The biology of mind.* New York: Oxford University Press.

Clayton, V. (August 27, 1997). Send in the clowns. *Nursing Times, 93.*

Cousins, N. (1979). *Anatomy of an illness as perceived by the patient.* New York: W. W. Norton.

Crepeau, E. (1998). Activity analysis: A way of thinking about occupational performance. In M. Neistadt & E. Crepeau (Eds.), *Willard and Spackman's occupational therapy* (9th ed., pp. 135–147). Philadelphia: Lippincott.

Crespo, C., Smit, E., Troiano, R., Bartlett, S., Macera, C., & Anderson, R. (2001). Television watching in children of the United States. *Archives of Pediatric and Adolescent Medicine, 155*, 360–365.

Cross, G. (1990). *A social history of leisure.* State College, PA: Venture Publishing.

Csikszentmihalyi, M. (1988). *Optimal experience.* New York: Cambridge University Press.

Csikszentmihalyi, M. (1991). *Flow: The psychology of optimal experience.* New York: Harper Collins.

Curry, J., & Gershenson, A. (February 16, 1998). Even at Columbia, gambling and college athletics collide. *New York Times, 147.*

Davison, M., & O'Brien, D. (1997). Humour in midwifery. *Modern Midwife, 7*, 11–14.

Edelman, G. M. (1989). *The remembered present: A biological theory of consciousness.* New York: Basic Books.

Fidler, G., & Velde, B. (1999). *Activities: Reality and symbol.* Thorofare, NJ: Slack.

Fisher, S. (1994). Identifying video game addiction in children and adolescents. *Addictive Behaviors, 19*, 545–553.

Gellner, E. (1988). *Plough, sword, and book: The structure of human history*. Chicago: University of Chicago Press.

Greenfield, D. (1999). *Virtual addiction*. Oakland, CA: New Harbinger Publications.

Guyton, A. C. (1991). *Basic neuroscience*. Philadelphia: W. B. Saunders Company.

Hunfield, J., Perquin, C., Duivenvoorden, H., Hazebroek-Kampschreur, A., Passchier, J., van Suijlekom-Smit, L., et al. (2001). Chronic pain and its impact on quality of life in adolescents and their families. *Journal of Pediatric Psychology, 26*, 145–153.

Martin, J. H. (1996). *Neuroanatomy: Text and atlas*. Stamford, CT: Appleton & Lange.

McCowan, W., & Chamberlain, L. (2000). *Best possible odds*. New York: John Wiley & Sons.

McKeough, D. M. (1995). *The coloring review of neuroscience*. New York: Little, Brown and Company.

McMurray, R., Harrell, J., Deng, S., Bradley, C., Cox, L., & Bangdiwala, S. (2000). The influence of physical activity, socioeconomic status, and ethnicity on the weight status of adolescents. *Obesity Research, 8*, 130–139.

McNeilly, D., & Burke, W. (2000). Late life gambling: The attitudes and behaviors of older adults. *Journal of Gambling Studies, 16*, 393–415.

Morahan, J., & Schumacher, P. (2000). *Computers in Human Behavior, 16*, 13–29.

New York Times (September 9, 1999). Typical drug user is profiled by U.S. Volume 148, issue 51640, p. 25.

Ornstein, R., & Sobel, D. (1989). *Healthy pleasures*. New York: Addison-Wesley.

Phillips, C., Rolls, S., Rouse, A., & Griffiths, M. (1995). Home video game playing in schoolchildren: A study of incidence and patterns of play. *Journal of Adolescence, 18*, 687–691.

Piaget, J. (1962). *Play, dreams, and imitation in childhood*. New York: W. W. Norton.

Pollard, J., Taylor, W., & Smith, D. (2000). Patterns and correlates of physical activity among older adults residing independently in retirement communities. *Activities, Adaptation, and Aging, 24*, 1–17.

Reilly, M. (1974). *Play as exploratory learning: Studies of curiosity behavior*. Beverly Hills, CA: Sage Publications.

Robinson, T., Wilde, M., Navracruz, L., Haydel, K., & Varady, A. (2001). Effects of reducing children's television and video game use on aggressive behavior. *Archives of Pediatric Adolescent Medicine, 155*, 17–23.

Rogawski, M. A., & Barker, J. L. (1985). *Neurotransmitter actions in the vertebrate nervous system*. New York: Plenum Press.

Rose, S. (1976). *The conscious brain*. New York: Vintage Books.

Sandler, H., & Vernikos, J. (1986). *Inactivity: Physiological effects*. New York: Academic Press.

Schultes, L. (1997). Humor with hospice clients: You're putting me on! *Home Health Care Nurse, 15*, 561–566.

Showalter, S., & Skobel, S. (1996). Hospice: Humor, heartache and healing. *American Journal of Hospice and Palliative Care, (7)* 8–9.

Thornton, J., & White, A. (1999). A Heidegerrian investigation into the lived experience of humour by nurses in an intensive care unit. *Intensive and Critical Care Nursing, 15*, 266–278.

Tiggemann, M., & Williamson, S. (2000). The effect of exercise on body satisfaction and self-esteem as a function of gender and age. *Sex Roles, 43*, 119–127.

U.S. Health and Human Services (1999). *National household survey on drug abuse*. (www.health.org/govstudy).

Uren, J. (1998). The canary of health care. *Australian Nursing Journal, 6*, 1–2.

Van Wormer, K., & Boes, M. (1997). Humor in the emergency room: A social work perspective. *Health and Social Work, 22*, 87–93.

Vergeer, G., & MacRae, A. (1993). Therapeutic use of humor in occupational therapy. *American Journal of Occupational Therapy, 47*, 678–683.

Wooten, P. (1996). Humor: An antidote for stress. *Holistic Nurse Practitioner, 10*, 49–56.

CHAPTER 6

Restoration in Occupations

Restorative Activities: The Ancient Beat in the Modern Dance

Restoration from Sleep

Restoration from Eating and Drinking

Restoration from Self-Care Activities

Restoration from Quiet-Focus Activities

Paying Attention to Restoration in the Blend

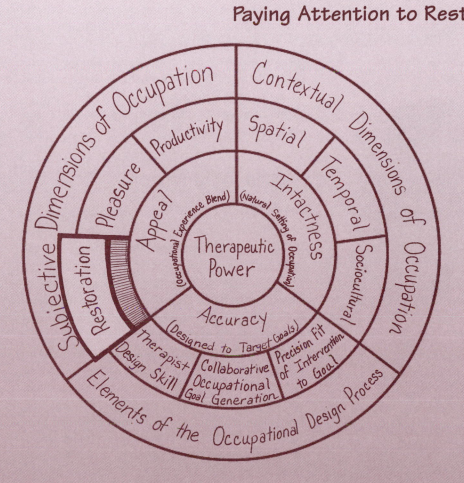

Restorative Activities: The Ancient Beat in the Modern Dance

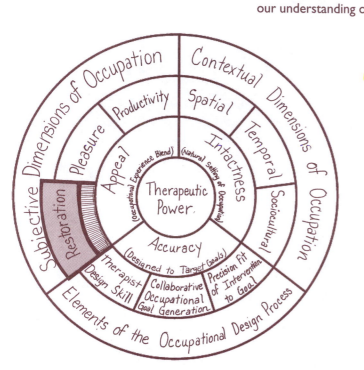

In Western culture, we emphasize the productivity of our occupations, to the neglect of our understanding of their restorative aspects. We judge each other and ourselves by our accomplishments. This is a useful attitude for getting things done. However, it does lead us to ignore the restorative qualities needed in our occupational pattern to maintain our sanity and the energy to work toward our goals. No one can remain task focused all of the time. Have you had times in your life when you had to remain focused on getting some work done and did not have enough time for sleep and relaxation? Remember how you felt after a long period of this lifestyle?

Of the three subjective characteristics of the experience of occupation, restoration is the least recognized in occupational therapy (Howell & Pierce, 2000). In 1922, Adolph Meyer identified rest as one of the primary types of activities with which the new profession of occupational therapy should be concerned. To be true connoisseurs of occupation, in our own lives and in the lives of our patients, we must look at the full 24-hour round of activities in which humans engage. As occupational therapists, we must understand not only where energy is spent, but also how it is created. Highly restorative activities, such as sleep and eating, carry a basic physiologically regulated rhythm within our overall occupational patterns. They are like the bass beat to a song—strong, resonating, and rhythmic. No matter how complex or modern the activities that we passionately pursue in our lives, we all engage regularly in the mundane survival activities that restore our energy. In our clients, the need for improvements in the restorative quality of their occupational patterns can be critical. Without adequate restoration, productivity and pleasure also remain low.

Restoration from Sleep

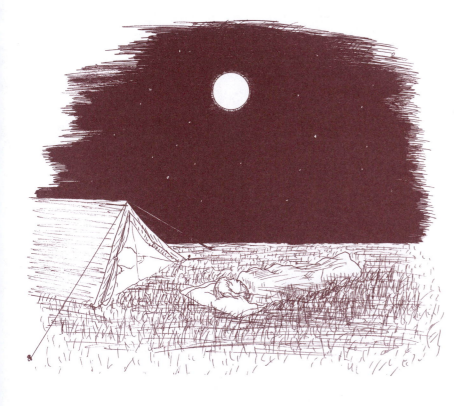

Sleep is the occupation for which the strongest argument for the tie between occupation and health can be made. One of the most obvious patterns in human occupation is recurring sleep. Since the beginning of time, humans have been waking at sunrise and going to sleep at sunset. Our bodies are physiologically entrained to the sun's light. Since the invention of the electric light bulb, however, we have been able to push our waking hours into the time of darkness. We have shift work, late night entertainment, and travel between time zones. Because we value productivity so highly, we limit the time we spend in rest, afraid to "waste time." Since early in the 20th century, humans have had an average of 2 hours less sleep per night than they had been getting in all the eons before (Coren, 1996). What impact does this have on us? Can we really change the pattern of evolution with the flip of a light switch?

A new wave of research on sleep and sleep disorders demonstrates that sleep is not the complete suspension of mental activity, but a unique state of consciousness (Coren, 1996). Without the restful occupation of sleep, humans experience broadly diminishing capacities and loss of the ability to engage in satisfying occupations. In fact, not engaging in the occupation of sleep will soon result in death. The human need for restful occupations is undeniable.

Let's look at how sleep works, what it brings to our lives, and the results of reduced or low-quality sleep. As you learn about sleep, consider your own sleep patterns. If you become a true master of the restorative occupation of sleep, you can enhance your intelligence, creativity, happiness, and health in remarkable ways. In your design of your daily occupational pattern, sleep is the base on which all your efforts are built.

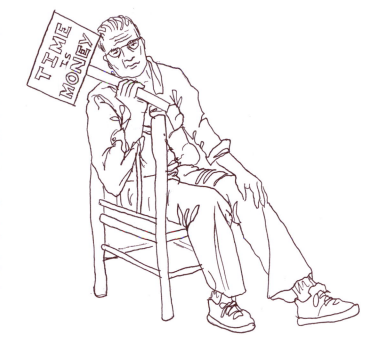

The Architecture of Sleep

Because memory shuts down during sleep, you do not remember much of your sleep experience. There is a pattern in your mental experience of sleep, a structure that sleep researchers call sleep architecture. Sleep is not an even, unchanging experience. It is phased and rhythmic.

Sleep researchers use electroencephalogram (EEG) readings to examine brain activation during sleep. One night's EEG reading is called a sleep histogram. Perhaps the term sleep architecture comes from the way the sleep histogram looks so much like a city skyline, showing the spikes and plateaus of sleep length and depth in the different and repeating phases of sleep.

There are two primary types of sleep—rapid eye movement (REM) sleep and non-rapid eye movement (NREM) sleep. Sleep is usually entered through NREM sleep. REM and NREM alternate over the course of a night's sleep, completing a full cycle through both types in an average of 90 minutes in a healthy adult. As the brain cycles through these phases, we often come to waking consciousness for brief periods, and then sink back into sleep (Hobson, 1989).

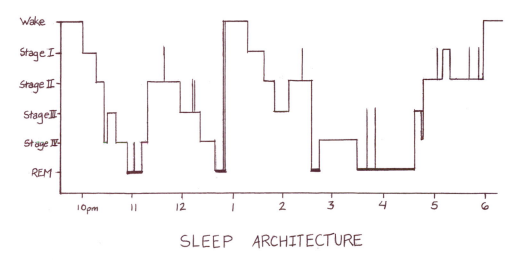

SLEEP   ARCHITECTURE

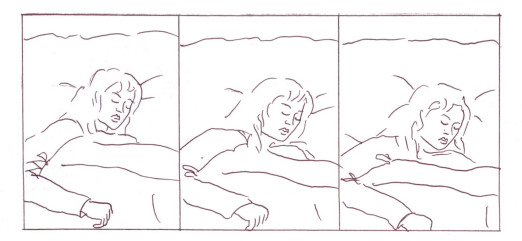

REM Sleep and Dreams

If you could see your own REM sleep on an EEG, you would see strong brain activity, bursts of rapid eye movement, and no muscle tone or body movement. The longest phase of REM sleep would occur around 2 AM, at the nighttime low point of the circadian rhythm. During REM sleep, many neurological processes are inhibited, including body temperature regulation, movement, and memory. It is because of this inhibition that you remember only about the last 5 percent of your dreams. You also don't move around in bed during REM sleep. If you get too hot or too cold, you will change from REM sleep and dreaming to NREM sleep, to restore your body's temperature by moving your covers onto or off yourself during a light sleep state.

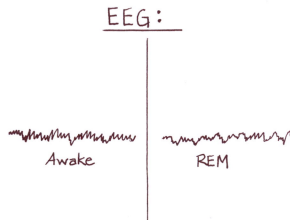

It is during REM sleep that you dream. Sleep researchers believe that REM sleep is essential to waking brain function. Dreams are the brain's way of purging, reconstituting, and reorganizing itself. REM sleep is often called *paradoxical sleep* because its EEG pattern resembles waking more than it resembles NREM sleep. Entry into sleep through a REM phase is not typical for adults, although it does occur occasionally. Have you ever awakened yourself just as you were falling asleep, with a sudden muscle movement, strong visual images, or perhaps a feeling of falling? This is *hypnic myoclonia,* a marker of entering sleep through REM. Frequent sleep onset through REM is usually associated with a large sleep debt or some type of sleep disturbance.

REM sleep makes up about 30 percent of a night's sleep in a healthy adult. That doesn't sound like much, but lack of REM sleep can cause decreased reaction times, depressed mood, disorganized thinking, even hallucinations! Usually, you have about 5 or 6 REM phases in a night's sleep, alternating with longer NREM phases. REM sleep occurs in shorter episodes at the beginning of the night and in longer episodes later in the night.

It is quite possible to sleep a full night and still be REM-sleep deprived. If light, noises, temperature extremes, pets, or a restless bed partner frequently disturbs your sleep, you will pop out of REM sleep and go back to the beginning of your sleep cycle, which begins with NREM sleep. If you are disturbed again before about 1 hour of NREM has passed, you will again restart with NREM, missing REM completely in that second cycle. If your sleep is interrupted regularly, you will become REM-sleep deprived. What is the quality of your sleeping environment? Are you disturbed on a regular basis?

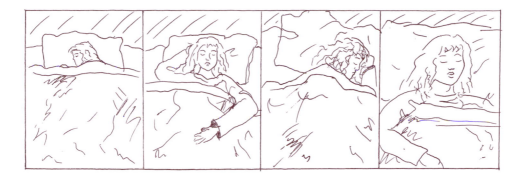

NREM Sleep

If you could see your EEG for NREM sleep, it would look quite different from your REM sleep EEG. You would see slow synchronous waves instead of active spikes. In NREM sleep, the body is active, turning and moving for comfort with a possible change in sleep stage, but without fully waking.

NREM sleep has four stages. Stage 1 sleep is what you might call "dozing off." If someone said your name, you would open your eyes and look around. Stages 2, 3, and 4 are increasingly deeper forms of sleep. It is through the lightest stages, stages 1 and 2, that we usually enter sleep. Stages 3 and 4 of NREM are called *deep,* or *slow-wave,* sleep. If you were awakened from slow-wave sleep, you would display *sleep inertia,* or sleep drunkenness, as you struggled to orient yourself despite your NREM sleep grogginess. During most nights, about 30 percent of sleep is spent in REM, 20 percent in the deep sleep of NREM stages 3 and 4, and 50 percent in the light sleep of NREM stages 1 and 2 (Carskadon & Dement, 1994; Hobson, 1989; Sheldon, Spire, & Levy, 1982).

During NREM sleep, your immune system is much more active than it is when you are awake. It releases waves of interleukins, going about the business of cleansing the body of toxins and invaders. Everyone is familiar with people who seem to be able to postpone getting sick until they have completed that important project at work or passed that exam. They drag themselves around, looking less and less healthy by the day, but still manage to put in long hours to reach their goal. Once it is finished, they fall into bed sick, and we marvel at the perfect timing of their illness. In reality, what is behind this scenario is the effect of a mounting sleep debt. Every day of inadequate sleep degrades immune function and reduces cognitive capacities, making that person more lethargic, depressed, woozy, and slow thinking. Eventually, he or she succumbs to the assault of various bacteria and viruses that a healthy immune system easily fends off on a daily basis. The body then sends the person into sleep and he or she begins to repay the sleep debt that has been accumulated.

Our immune systems use sleep as a weapon against serious illnesses, sending us into twice the amount of sleep as normal. This reduces the demands on our body's metabolism, conserving ener-

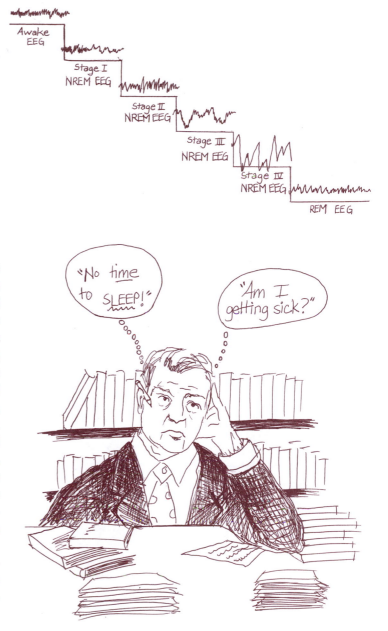

gy. A fever raises body temperature, which destroys many invaders, increasing the rate of immune production during NREM sleep. Doing without sleep leads to illness. Increasing sleep is one of the body's best defenses (Coren, 1996).

Napping

In many cultures, an afternoon nap is nestled in the energy low that normally occurs in all humans at that time of day. In Europe and in Central and South America, the siesta is common. In China, there is the hsiuhsi. Many famous creative geniuses were well known for their habit of napping: Edison, Ford, and Einstein for example. But do you feel guilty if you decide to take a nap in the afternoon? In the United States, afternoon rest and tiredness are not socially acceptable in adults.

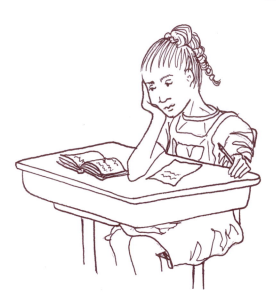

We often attribute our afternoon dip in energy to having just had lunch. Research does not uphold this relationship, however, unless the lunch includes alcohol or the individual is already suffering a significant sleep debt. The dip is just a part of our human circadian rhythms. (Our circadian rhythms are more fully discussed in Chapter 10, The Rhythms of Occupation.) Certainly there is no post-breakfast or post-dinner energy dip. Napping is a healthy and appropriate response to an energy low. It can be extremely restorative to the individual and contributes greatly to cognitive capacities in the remainder of the day. Don't you feel more energetic after a nap?

Infant, Childhood, and Teenage Sleep

Infant sleep is very different from that of adults. Newborns usually enter sleep through REM and sleep about 16 hours a day (Arnoff, 1991). REM is called *active sleep* in infants because facial expressions, slight startles, wriggling, and hand movements often accompany it. Newborns have the largest percentage of REM sleep in humans, approximately 50 percent. One cycle through REM and NREM averages 55 minutes in infancy, as opposed to 90 minutes in adults. Further, infants do not develop con-

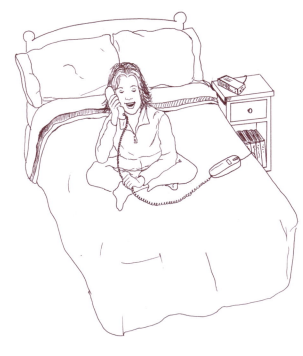

solidated stage 1 and stage 2 NREM EEG patterns until 6 months of age, and even then they are a very small portion of infant sleep. By 8 months, the average total amount of sleep has decreased to approximately 13 hours in a day (Sheldon, Spire, & Levy, 1982).

The sleep of children is different from that of infants and adults, especially in the character of the slow-wave deep sleep, stages 3 and 4 of NREM. In the first deep sleep cycle of the night, typical children are almost impossible to awaken (Carskadon & Dement, 1994). Childhood sleep debt is very common because of overscheduling, stress, or sleeping in noisy environments. Although children need 10 to 12 hours of sleep a night, their schedules often match those of the adults in the household. Sleep debt also looks quite different in children from how it does in adults: a raised level of activity or "hyper-ness," fidgeting when trying to pay attention, difficulty remaining stationary, emotional lability, impulsiveness, and aggression (Coren, 1996). Children with sleep debt have trouble waking in the morning. They remain groggy once they are out of bed. They sleep in on the weekends if possible. If this sounds like a child you know, try an increase of at least 1 hour of sleep per night for 2 weeks. If the symptoms decrease, you can assume that at least some of the problem was sleep debt.

Teenagers are chronically sleep deprived. This is easily demonstrated by noting the difficulties they have in waking, their preference for sleeping during their leisure time, and their tendency to combine late night activities and early morning risings. Many teens sleep as little as 6 hours a night to fit in school, socializing with peers, and a part-time job. This inevitably affects school performance. Teenagers are just learning to take responsibility for self-organization and discipline. It is not surprising that they would struggle, just as adults do, with the difficulty of adhering to a healthy sleep schedule in a culture that values productivity over rest.

Sleep in Older Adults

Healthy older individuals have fairly intact sleep patterns. REM sleep as a percentage of sleep time appears to be maintained well into healthy old age. The efficiency of sleep seems to decrease by about 25 percent, increasing the amount of lighter stage 1 and 2 NREM sleep and decreasing the amount of slow-wave deep sleep (Bliwise, 1994).

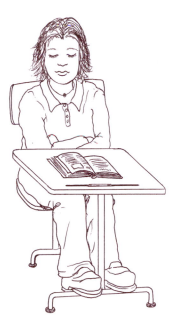

Medical conditions in older people commonly reduce the quality of their sleep. The prevalence of respiratory disorders in older men has strong negative impacts on sleep adequacy (Bliwise, 1994). Approximately half of older people also have periodic leg movements at night, which repeatedly disturb their sleep (Bliwise, 1994; Prinz & Vitiello, 1993). Many medications taken by elders disturb sleep. Other conditions that impact sleep in older adults include gastrointestinal illnesses, asthma, cardiovascular symptoms, nocturia, diabetes, and chronic pain.

Older adults often suffer low-quality sleep as a result of a disruptive sleep environment. Nursing homes are extremely noisy places to attempt sleep, as well as being relatively inflexible in adapting to the differing circadian rhythms of individuals (Schnelle, Alessi, Ouslander, & Simmons, 1993). The commonly occurring respiratory problems of older men disrupt the sleep of their wives. Depression and anxiety secondary to major life changes, such as retirement or loss of a spouse, also result in sleep disruption (Bliwise, 1994).

Older adults face many challenges to obtaining the high-quality sleep necessary to maintain healthy intellectual and immune function. Disrupted sleep and the symptoms of sleep debt are commonly seen in older people. Unfortunately, they are usually dismissed as a typical symptom of aging and go untreated.

Sleep Debt

The typical modern human operates with a consistent sleep debt. Because it is so much easier, in terms of both circadian physiology and cultural constraint, to stay up later than it is to get up later, we push ourselves constantly into sleep debt by extending the length of the day. Our cultural attitude that sleep is just lost productivity helps to make living with a sleep debt seem normal and acceptable.

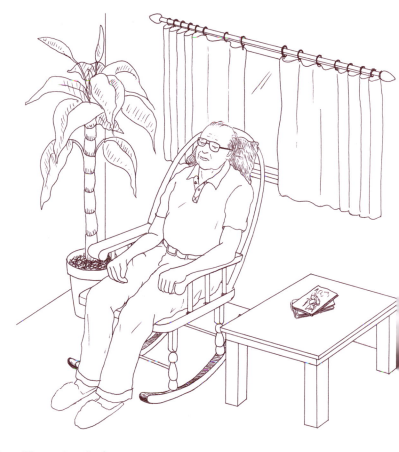

If you are thinking that the loss of an hour's sleep here or there is not a critical issue, consider Coren's (1996) studies of the impact of Daylight Savings Time on highway accident rates. In the spring of the year, much of the United States, Canada, and many European countries set their clocks forward 1 hour on a specified night. This takes 1 hour of sleep from the entire populace. The rationale for this is that it maximizes the available light during the workday. Statistics from Canada

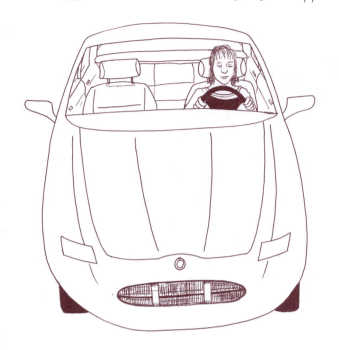

showed a 7 percent increase in highway accident mortalities in the 4 days after the springtime shift. In the fall, when clocks were set back and everyone slept an extra hour, highway accident mortality rates dropped by 7 percent.

People who are suffering a sleep deficit lose vital capacity and endurance, have difficulty maintaining attention, show longer reaction times, and are irritable and moody. Long-standing sleep debt results in depression, loss of motor and visual coordination, paranoia, and hallucinations. Extreme sleep deprivation can result in death through the loss of thermoregulation and the crash of the immune system. In a culture that applauds the ability of high-powered executives to work late into the night, this sounds mildly alarming but only vaguely related to our own lives. However, it does not sound so abstract when you think of the person with sleep debt as your emergency room physician, the night shift worker assembling your car, the exhausted pilot of your red-eye flight, or the tired trucker barreling toward you on the highway! These types of workers typically operate with high sleep debt (Coren, 1996).

Sleep debt can also accrue as a result of environmental disturbances that disrupt the quality of sleep. This is called sleep fragmentation, in which sleep is neither deep nor efficient. One study found that a random selection of parents of 2-year-olds had a significant sleep debt in comparison to childless couples (Coren, 1996). A variety of medical conditions can also contribute to an accumulating sleep debt. Often people who have had poor-quality sleep dismiss it as unimportant because their circadian rhythms provide them with an energy boost in the "no sleep" zones of midmorning and early evening.

The most common test for sleep debt is the Multiple Sleep Latency Test, in which a person is settled in a darkened room and timed to sleep onset several times. The average sleep latency for a healthy adult is about 12 minutes. If it takes you less time than that, consider increasing your sleep time and see whether you feel differently about life!

Sleep Disorders

As a result of a variety of causes, it is possible to have a typical sleep length, yet suffer severe sleep disturbances within certain phases of sleep. Sleep apnea, usually secondary to chronic respiratory obstruction, results in hundreds of brief awakenings during the night. This causes a shift toward the lighter sleep of stage 1 and stage 2 NREM sleep and a loss of REM sleep. With treatment of the airway problem, the sleeper will rebound by sleeping a large percentage of REM sleep for up to a month (Carskadon & Dement, 1994).

Circadian disorders affect sleep. This is especially seen in the tie of peak amounts of REM sleep to the body temperature low in the early morning hours. Disturbance of the circadian pattern, through shift work or jet lag for instance, will disrupt the circadian low and thus decrease the amount of REM sleep (Carskadon & Dement, 1994).

Temperature extremes disturb sleep. Because the brain has limited, if any, ability to thermoregulate during REM sleep, sleeping in too-warm or too-cold conditions will disrupt REM. In these conditions, sleep will shift to NREM to allow the body to either sweat or shiver. Continuation of sleep in such settings will result in a REM sleep debt (Carskadon & Dement, 1994).

Prescribed and nonprescription drugs can alter sleep patterns. Benzodiazepines suppress slow wave sleep. Tricyclic antidepressants and MAO inhibitors suppress REM sleep. Acute withdrawal from these medications can result in a strong rebound of the sleep phase that was suppressed. If REM sleep had been disturbed, hypnagogic hallucinations, or waking dreams, are possible (Carskadon & Dement, 1994).

Sleep disorders also include narcolepsy, or frequent and unpredictable episodes of daytime sleep, and insomnia, in which there is difficulty initiating or maintaining sleep. In recent years, these problems are being successfully treated in sleep disorder units. Sleep medicine is a new frontier, exciting in its capacity to bring us new understanding of the rhythmicity of human occupation and the contribution of rest to daily experience.

Restoration from Eating and Drinking

The Regularity and Quality of Food Experiences

Just as sleep is an ancient human activity pattern without which we could not survive, so are eating and drinking also required to restore our energy for daily activities. Such basic activities as sleep and eating are often overlooked in our study of occupations, as scholars focus disciplinary attention on activities that are of greater complexity or that highlight interesting cultural trends. I would argue, however, that these basic survival activities of eating and sleeping are so critical to survival that they are even more important to our understanding of occupation than are more esoteric explorations of nonobligatory activities in which fewer people participate.

Eating and drinking are so familiar and frequent as to seem commonplace, mundane. Yet meals mark our days with a regular pattern. Sharing meals holds much social mean-

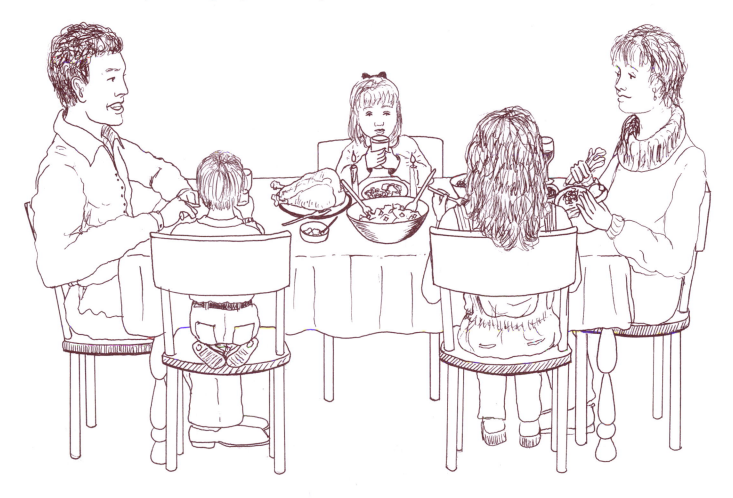

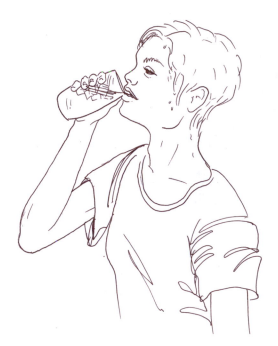

ing. The family is created through shared dining (DeVault, 1991). Our most important religious and national holidays are symbolically marked with special foods and dining traditions. Can you imagine what life would be like if you did not need to eat and drink?

The quality of our meal experiences says much about who we are as occupational beings. Eating alone, eating with the family, eating while driving, eating while watching television, skipping meals, binge eating, eating at your desk, eating out, going on a picnic: all of these say something about what kind of person you are and what kind of occupational pattern you live. Making time to have meal experiences that are fully restorative says that you value restoring your energy and being in a peaceful state. Eating a solitary meal, deeply appreciating a cold glass of water on a hot and physically demanding day, and joining in the celebratory ritual feasts of shared holidays and special occasions are all forms of potentially restorative occupations that include the intake of food energy. Too often, we miss opportunities to be rejuvenated as we feed ourselves. We allow our attention to dwell on things other than our immediate experience, and so miss the benefits of the occupation at hand. Can you think of ways to enhance your restoration by changing your daily experience of food?

Feeding Problems and Eating Disorders

Occupational therapists work with individuals who have problems with eating. Young children with disabilities and developmental problems often have feeding problems. The occupational therapist works with the child and family in different ways, depending on the cause and manifestation of the feeding problem. Feeding problems can also occur in adults as a result of a variety of different traumas or disease processes, such as stroke.

Some individuals in our culture have emotional problems involved with seeking restoration from food. Anorexics experience conflict between the desire for food and the desire for an idealized body image. Anorexia is especially prevalent in young women, who are vulnerable to the strong cultural messages that equate ideals of beauty with

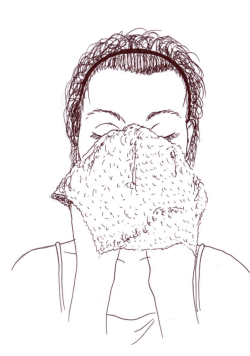

unrealistic thinness. Persons with bulimia go on eating binges and then purge themselves of the food. Others overeat to the point of endangering their health. Although they may receive enjoyment and an energy boost from eating, just as all of us do, perhaps they turn too often to this source of restoration instead of choosing other potentially restorative occupations.

Restoration from Self-Care Activities

As is true of eating, self-care activities can provide us with a little or a lot of restoration, depending on the degree to which we focus attention on the experience. Concentrating on your enjoyment of a refreshing shower, complete with your favorite scents and textures, is a completely different experience from rushing through your morning shower thinking about the problems you will encounter during the day. This is an especially important point for an occupational therapist to understand because it is usually the occupational therapist who assists clients with establishing the most independent possible self-care after a trauma, or despite physical or developmental challenges. Appreciating the restorative, pleasurable, and self-esteem—building aspects of the everyday activities of bathing, toileting, and dressing is essential to the work of an occupational therapist. Acquiring the skills of independent self-care is a marker of the transition from the dependency of childhood to the independence of adulthood.

Imagine that you are an older individual, living in a nursing home. Because the staff does not believe that you are safe standing in the shower on your own, you are given quick sponge baths in bed at mid-morning of each day. This requires you to return to bed during your most energetic time of day, offends your modesty, and makes you more dependent. Now envision an occupational therapist interviewing you about your self-care needs. You say you want to shower on your own. She assesses you by observing you in a mock shower, obtains a shower chair and rails to assist you, and discusses with you the changes you can make in your shower routine to be safer. You obtain your favorite shower supplies. You select early morning for your shower because all your life your morning shower has been the energizing start to your day. The therapist monitors your careful entry into the shower, remains available to your call, and then monitors your exit from the shower. You have a fabulous shower, in spite of being seated instead of standing. You feel stronger, more energized, more in possession of the dignity of a private life, and more independent and confident than you ever did with sponge baths.

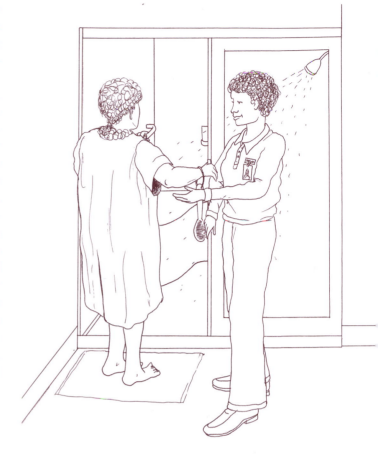

Restoration from Quiet-Focus Activities

We all have favorite quiet pastimes that we turn to when feeling depleted. A quiet-focus activity is one in which you are not very physically active and your attention is highly focused on a limited amount of input. Quiet engagement of our full attention in an undemanding task refreshes us. It is a mini-vacation, in which we turn our minds away from other thoughts and focus simply on the experience at hand. As well as being highly restorative, quiet-focus activities are usually fairly high in pleasure. Which activities are viewed as restorative differs from one person to the next, but doing handwork and hobbies, enjoying nature, reading, television watching, and engaging in spiritual activities are some of the more obvious examples. In each of these, the key to optimizing the restorative quality of the occupation appears to be the mindfulness, or attentiveness, with which it is performed (Langer, 1989). What quiet-focus activities do you turn to for a lift?

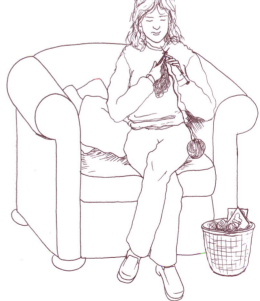

Handwork and Hobbies

Many people relax by losing themselves in handwork and hobbies. People who engage often in such activities report being able to enter flow fairly regularly in this way (Csikszentmihalyi, 1991). Of course, some individuals do not experience handwork and hobbies as relaxing and rejuvenating because they get caught up in emphasizing the productivity of engaging in that particular activity. Handwork and hobbies include the following, as well as many others not mentioned here:

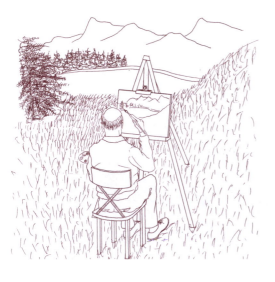

- Sewing, knitting, needlework
- Painting, drawing, coloring
- Stained glass
- Weaving
- Pottery
- Woodworking
- Sculpture
- Model building

Enjoying Nature

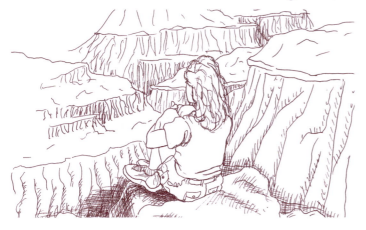

Many people report that nature rejuvenates them. Often they are referring to viewing nature, such as in bird watching, taking a walk, or sitting in a garden. Some people go camping, hiking, canoeing, and boating as ways of being in nature, which may or may not result in a quiet focus activity, depending on how it is done. In my own research (Pierce, 1996) on infant/toddler interactions with their physical environments, there were many instances of either videotaped observations or maternal reports of infants spending time looking at patterns from nature: leaves, shadows, grass, flowers, and sunlight. Mothers reported being able to calm fussy infants or put them to sleep by taking them outdoors. I have often wondered why it is that nature seems rejuvenating to both children and adults. Perhaps something in the simple repetitive visual patterns of nature has a calming effect on the human nervous system. Certainly, being in nature is usually experienced as a reduction of noise and a freedom to pattern our own thoughts away from the tempos, thoughts, and influences of busy environments and other people.

Reading and Television Watching

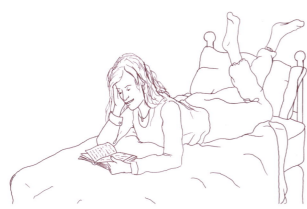

Many people find reading restful. An entire publishing industry thrives on the public's desire for a constant supply of interesting new reading materials. Because reading has been a tradition in Western middle and upper class culture for such a long time, and is associated in our minds with learning, we seem to have no concerns over the amount of reading individuals may do. If they seem withdrawn from the world, spending large amounts of their time reading fiction, we just say they are "bookish" and let it go at that.

But what about television watching? Many have expressed concerns that people are spending too much time watching television. Why do we consider this so much more alarming than reading? The level of physical activity is approximately the same. The plots or primary content of books or television shows are just as predetermined by their writers, although reading may require a bit more imagination to visualize. Perhaps it is the content itself that concerns us because television contains an element of commercialism not found in books. Television also depicts violence and sexuality much more graphically than most reading material. Is there something more hypnotizing, less self-directed, about television watching than there is about reading? Why do we watch so much television? What activities are we doing less now that we did before so many of us had televisions in our homes? How has television watching changed our occupational patterns? Hours of television watching are clearly associated with higher body weight, in both children and adults (Bryant & Bryant, 2001). In our highly work-oriented society, the large number of hours that are spent in television watching is puzzling. We feel guilty spending time in this completely unproductive way, and yet we continue. If it is just for the diversion, why don't we at least do something more active that we enjoy?

One possibility is that television watching is a form of rest very close to light sleep. Consider Coren's (1996) statement that since the invention of the light bulb, humans sleep two hours less per day on average. Is television watching a substitute for the sleep we would be getting if our activities were still ruled by the rising and setting of the sun? A sort of restless sleep, or daydreaming? Watching TV certainly tends to occur at the end of our day, when we are tired. The sun is setting: our ancient cue for sleep. Television watching is passive, like sleep. We sprawl, propped by pillows, on a special piece of furniture called a couch that looks like a cross between a chair and a bed. Often, our attention drifts from the show we are supposedly watching. And certainly, all of us have experienced the surprised realization that we accidentally crossed over into sleep at some point the last show.

Spiritual Activities

What is spirituality? Although different people express spirituality differently, it is a search for the meaning of one's life and a desire for connection to one's self, to others, and to a transcending power or purpose. Some practice their spiritual beliefs within a specific religious tradition that provides guidance for spiritual activities. Others create their own spiritual activities outside of a religious tradition, guided by what seems to work for them. Regardless of whether or not a person's spirituality is guided by a religious tradition, entering a deliberate spiritual experience of inner consciousness is highly restorative. When we meditate or pray, we experience a change in consciousness and physiology. Studies of meditation have documented slowed breathing, reduced oxygen consumption, unique EEG patterns in the brain, and other physiological measures that seem to indicate that, physically, meditation is similar to sleep (Jevning, Wallace, & Beidebach, 1992). The effects of deliberate relaxation, such as in biofeedback, can improve health, suppress pain, and decrease stress. Regardless of the religious or philosophical content to which an individual attends as he or she looks inward, any experience of quiet spiritual attentiveness can be highly restorative. Perhaps the next time you are feeling in need of restoration, you could try a quiet 10-minute meditation to renew your energy.

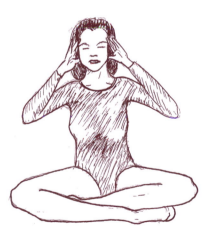

Paying Attention to Restoration in the Blend

Because of our culture's extreme valuing of productivity, most people neglect restoration in designing their occupational pattern. Considering sleep to be nothing more than lost time, they push themselves into sleep debt and lower their life quality. In a rush to get

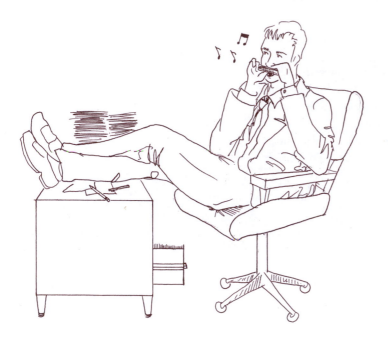

things done, they do not take time to focus on the waking restoration that is available in hobbies, meals, and self-care occupations. We rush from one thing to the next, our thoughts always somewhere else. This leads to lives that can seem unfulfilling, bleak, chaotic, and demanding. A low level of restoration in the occupational pattern is probably much more common than sleep debt, and certainly much less well understood.

It is important to remember that, even in very productive efforts, we can take moments to restore ourselves. McGee-Cooper (1992) calls these joy breaks. It is easy to convince a person who is interested in being productive to take a joy break during his or her work by explaining to the person that this will help him or her to maintain productivity. Taking a break to step outside, make a little music, juggle, or get a drink of water from the cooler will rejuvenate you in your work. Although it is unusual to find an occupation that is high in levels of both productivity and restoration, inserting short restorative occupations into a day of highly productive occupations will help to keep your energy levels up and your emotional experience of the day more positive. Can you think of some short joy breaks that you could design that would quickly restore your own energy when you are trying to complete a high-productivity activity, such as studying?

In your work as an occupational therapist, it will be critical to your treatment design efforts that you understand how the restorative aspect of occupation provides the basis for all we do in our lives. You will see many people who are tired, depleted, and discouraged because of life challenges, health problems, and disrupted occupational patterns. To assist them in rebuilding a satisfying and healthy pattern and to use the restorative qualities of occupation as treatment, you will need to understand this characteristic well. Use the following Power Builders to begin building your capacity to design occupations high in restoration, as well as to enhance the restorative quality of your own occupational pattern.

POWER BUILDERS

Key Concepts for Strengthening Insight into Restoration in Occupations

- REM and NREM sleep
- Napping
- Sleep in infants, children, teens, and elders
- Sleep debt
- Sleep disorders
- Eating and drinking
- Eating disorders
- Self-care activities
- Quiet focus activities

Building Insight into Your Personal Occupational Experience of Restoration

1. Reflect on the following, in discussion with others, as a journal entry, or as a more formal paper or poster presentation:

- What are your favorite memories of sleep as a child?
- What are your favorite memories of eating and drinking?
- What are your favorite quiet focus activities?
- What is the most restorative activity in your present life?
- What is the most restorative occupational experience you have had this week?
- Are you a person who is more restored by nature, handwork and hobbies, reading, television watching, or spiritual activities?
- Are you attempting to get an adequate amount of sleep, or do you tend to be in sleep debt fairly often?
- Are your levels of waking restoration higher or lower than the levels of others? Have there been times in your life during which they have been higher than now? Why? Lower than now? Why?

2. Sit quietly in nature, or sit quietly in a spiritual exercise. Concentrate fully on the sensations for at least 10 minutes. How did you feel afterwards?

3. Figure out a way to find a place and some time for a nap after lunchtime on a weekday. Did it feel strange to try to take a nap, even though you were tired? How did you feel after your nap?

4. Check your sleep debt by keeping track of the following questions for 1 week.

- Did it take you less than 15 minutes to fall asleep at night, once all the lights were out?
- Did you get less than 8 hours of sleep at night?

POWER BUILDERS

- Did you have difficulty waking and getting right out of bed when your alarm went off?

- Did you experience difficulty in maintaining attention because of tiredness?

- On your days off, did you take naps or sleep in later than on workdays?

If you answered yes 10 or more times during 1 week, you are suffering from sleep debt. This is likely to affect your mood, health, and cognitive capacities. Increase your sleep for 1 week and see if you feel more alert, energetic, and happy.

5. Journal your amount of sleep each day and rate your mood, from lowest to highest. Be sure to make your recordings at the same time of day. Perhaps keep your figures beside your bed at night, or where you breakfast, to make it easy to remember to record them. After at least a month, chart your figures and see if there is a pattern of better mood when you are getting more sleep.

Building Insight into Restoration in the Occupational Experiences of Others

1. Do two observations of different people eating in very different settings. (More information on observation skills is in Chapter 17. Be sure you have appropriate permissions to observe, if needed.) Create an observation scheme of at least 10 points, to prompt your full attention to all that is going on before you. Record all you see. Write up or discuss with someone the differences in the degree to which each of the two individuals you observed appeared to be restored by his or her eating experience.

2. Do two observations of different adults engaged in different quiet focus activities. (More information on observation skills is in Chapter 17. Be sure you have appropriate permissions to observe, if needed.) Create an observation scheme of at least 10 points, to prompt your full attention to all that is going on before you. Record all you see. Write up or discuss with someone the differences in the degree to which each of the two individuals you observed appeared to be restored by engaging in his or her quiet-focus activity.

3. Interview someone about the quality of his or her sleep. (More information on interview skills is in Chapter 16.) Create a brief interview schedule before you do the interview, including sleep lengths, disturbances, tiredness, shift work or other night-time scheduling, quality of sleep environment (light in sleep area, noise, temperature, or disturbances). Record responses either in writing or on audiotape. Review the responses after the interview and write a summary (1 to 2 pages) of the main points you discovered about this person's sleep experiences.

4. If you know of someone who has a newborn infant, ask if you can watch active sleep.

5. Interview an occupational therapist concerning the ways in which he or she maintains energy for doing intervention. Remember to ask about the effects of sleep patterns, time of day and energy levels, how breaks are taken, eating and drinking during the workday, and quieter activities of the workday. (See Chapter 16 for more background on interview skills.)

6. Cut out magazine advertisements that show people engaged in highly restorative occupations. What do you assume about their lives and what they are like as individuals by seeing them in this way? Make a collage to share or reflect on, or, with others, tape all the clippings to a wall in groupings and discuss how the experience of restoration might be alike and different in the different examples.

Building Design Skills Using Restoration

1. Assess your sleeping environment in the following areas. Then brainstorm 10 ways to improve it, rank the ideas, implement the top two ideas, and do a written reflection summarizing the expected and unexpected benefits of having done so.

   - Does light come into your sleeping environment? Light disturbs the production of melatonin, on which sleep depends. Can you eliminate or block out the source of the light? Do you have good covers over your windows, so that morning light is prevented from entering the room if you wish to sleep past daylight? Even a small amount of light can alter the depth or type of sleep you are getting.

   - Is noise waking you? If so, is there any way you can decrease the noise level in your sleeping environment? If not, are there ways you can obscure the noise, by using earplugs or another source of soft sounds?

   - Does an individual or a pet interrupt your sleep? Can you do anything to see that their needs are met before you go to sleep, so they don't need you during the night? Can they sleep elsewhere, or could someone else attend to their needs some of the time?

   - If your bed partner snores, he or she may need to see a doctor for chronic obstructive respiratory problems or for allergies. Medical intervention in this area is quite common, and can result in improved sleep quality for both of you.

   - Is the temperature in your sleeping environment comfortable, or do you wake up too hot or too cold? Can this be changed, or bedclothes altered to accommodate the temperature?

   - Is caffeine consumption disturbing your sleep? Are you sleeping restlessly? Add up the amount of caffeine you are presently consuming. Keep a record of your sleep quality for a week. Then cut back a few milligrams and see how it changes. Stopping caffeine intake several hours before sleep will also enhance the quality of your rest.

POWER BUILDERS

- Is your sleep surface comfortable? Is it too hard or too soft? Do you wake with a sore back? Can this be changed?

- Last, can you do anything to enhance your enjoyment of your sleep environment by making it more inviting?

2. Create a shared quiet-focus activity experience for yourself and others you know well. Use the design steps of brainstorming, and then rank and weigh to select the play experience, and then create a simple time/task chart for planning. Carry out the activity you have designed. Do a written reflection afterwards, addressing the following questions:

   - How did adults perceive the experience? How did children? If you had both in your group, why the difference?

   - How did the experience you provided go differently from that planned?

   - What was the most "restful" part?

3. Design and prepare yourself a solitary meal that is highly restorative. You may want to pick a partner who will also be doing this, to compare your experiences. Consider the following in your design process: how to keep the experience more restorative of energy than demanding of energy, what foods and beverages to select, how to prepare them, where to eat, how you want the environment of your meal to be set up, and what day of the week and time of day would be best. Notice how you feel as you begin your meal. Try to remain focused on the moment as you eat. Is this difficult? How many times did your thoughts drift away? Did you feel a restoration of energy from your custom-designed meal? Was it difficult to set aside time for such an experience that was not oriented toward productivity? Describe your experience to your partner, to a friend, or in your journal.

4. Similar to exercise 3, design and complete a highly restorative occupation that is handwork, a hobby, time in nature, a spiritual experience, or a self-care activity. Consider the same questions for this as you would for dining in exercise 3.

5. Brainstorm a list of things you could do in 5 minutes or less to restore your energy when hard at work studying. See who can make the longest list.

6. Create a restorative experience for yourself and other adults you know well. Use a seven-step design process. In your evaluation, address the following questions:

   - How did the adults perceive the restorative experience?

   - How did the restorative experience you provided go differently from that planned?

   - What was the most "restful" part?

7. Make changes in one of your daily activities to increase its restorative level. Remember, the restoration must come between the beginning and the end of the occupation, not before or after it. Reflect on how difficult or easy this was and where the restoration comes from.

114

8. Design a highly restorative experience for yourself. Use brainstorming, then ranking, and then a time/task list; then implement your plan. Pay careful attention to your experience. Reflect on what it was about it that made it restorative for you. Were you more motivated to do an assignment that required you to relax more than one that did not?

9. Design a highly restorative experience for someone you know well. Take the time to go through the process of design: feel ready, investigate the person's perspective on what is restorative for him or her, generate ideas, choose one, and plan it. Carry out the plan, paying careful attention to how it unfolds. Evaluate your project in three ways: (1) informally interview the person about the restoration he or she experienced, (2) reflect on what you would have done differently if you had it to do over, and (3) decide what you thought were the greatest benefits to you of doing this design project.

10. Select one of the cases from Appendix A and write two fictitious brief (one-page limit) reflections by that person about two different occupational therapy sessions: one that used a very restorative therapeutic occupation, and one that did not.

11. Record your quality and quantity of sleep for one week, by noting how much sleep you get and ranking it as low, medium, or high in quality. Look at the pattern. Brainstorm 10 easy ways to increase your sleep quality in the next week, and then pick your two best ideas. Do them over a week, again recording your occupations. At the end of the second week, write a brief reflection, answering the following questions.

    • How successfully were you able to implement your ideas?

    • If there were difficulties, what were they?

    • Did you feel different after a week of higher quality sleep?

12. Using one of the cases from Appendix A, create a description of a potential intervention for that person that uses an eating or quiet-focus activity. Brainstorm at least 20 ideas, keeping in mind some potentially important goals for this person.

13. Use a seven-step design process to create and carry out an experience for a group of people that helps them learn about some aspect of restoration in occupation. This can be done on your own, in a dyad, or in a group.

References

Arnoff, M. S. (1991). *Sleep and its secrets: The river of crystal light.* New York: Plenum Press.

Bliwise, D. L. (1994). Normal aging. In M. H. Kryger, T. Roth, and W. C. Dement (Eds.), *Principles and practice of sleep medicine* (pp. 26–39). Philadelphia: W. B. Saunders Co.

Bryant, J. & Bryant, J. (2001). *Television and the American family.* Mahwah, NJ: Lawrence Erlbaum Associates.

Carskadon, M. A., & Dement, W. C. (1994). Normal human sleep: An overview. In M. H. Kryger, T. Roth, and W. C. Dement (Eds.), *Principles and practice of sleep medicine* (pp. 16–25). Philadelphia: W. B. Saunders Co.

Coren, S. (1996). *Sleep thieves.* New York: Free Press.

Csikszentmihalyi, M. (1991). *Flow: The psychology of optimal experience.* New York: Harper Collins.

DeVault, M. (1991). *Feeding the family.* Chicago: University of Chicago Press.

Hobson, J. A. (1989). *Sleep.* New York: Scientific American Library.

Howell, D., & Pierce, D. (2000). Exploring the forgotten restorative dimension of occupation: Quilting and quilt use. *Journal of Occupational Science, 7,* 68–72.

Jevning, R., Wallace, R., & Beidebach, M. (1992). The physiology of meditation: A review. A wakeful hypometabolic integrated response. *Neuroscience and Biobehavioral Review, 16,* 415–442.

Langer, E. (1989). *Mindfulness.* New York: Addison-Wesley.

McGee-Cooper, A. (1992). *You don't have to go home from work exhausted!* New York: Bantam Books.

Meyer, A. (1922). The philosophy of occupational therapy. *Archives of Occupational Therapy, 1,* 1–10.

Pierce, D. (1996). Infant space, infant time: Development of infant interactions with the physical environment, from 1 to 18 months. *Dissertation Abstracts International.*

Prinz, P. N., & Vitiello, M. V. (1993). Sleep loss in aging. In J. L. Albarede, J. E. Morley, T. Roth, & B. J. Vellas (Eds.), *Facts and research in gerontology, Vol. 7: Sleep disorders in the elderly* (pp. 55–68). New York: Springer Publishing.

Schnelle, J. F., Alessi, C. A., Ouslander, J. G., & Simmons, S. F. (1993). Noise and predictors of sleep in a nursing home environment. In J. L. Albarede, J. E. Morley, T. Roth, & B. J. Vellas (Eds.), *Facts and research in gerontology, Vol. 7: Sleep disorders in the elderly* (pp. 89–99). New York: Springer Publishing.

Sheldon, S., Spire, J., & Levy, H. (1982). *Pediatric sleep medicine.* Philadelphia: W. B. Saunders Company.

CHAPTER 7

Does the Intervention Appeal? Designing with Productivity, Pleasure, and Restoration

Initial Client Picture

Applying Your Estimation of What Will Appeal

Designing with Productivity

Designing with Pleasure

Designing with Restoration

Working on Balance: Is It a Client Goal?

Custom Designing Appealing Therapeutic Occupations

Subjective Dimensions of Occupation
Productivity
Pleasure
Restoration
Appeal
(Occupational Experience Blend)
Therapeutic Power
Contextual Dimensions of Occupation
Spatial
Temporal
Sociocultural
Intactness
(Natural Setting of Occupation)
Accuracy
(Designed to Target Goals)
Therapist Design Skill
Collaborative Occupational Goal Generation
Precision Fit of Intervention to Goal
Elements of the Occupational Design Process

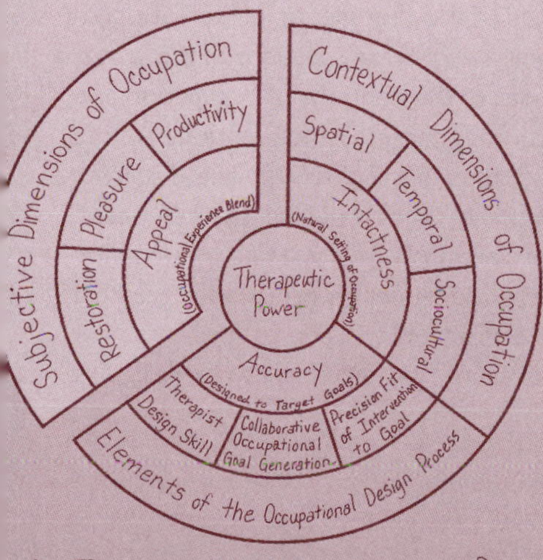

eal + Intactness + Accuracy = Therapeutic Power

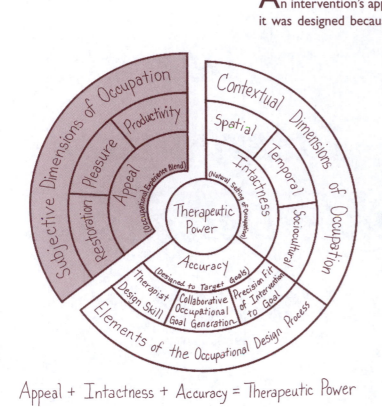

Appeal + Intactness + Accuracy = Therapeutic Power

An intervention's appeal is the degree to which it is attractive to the person for whom it was designed because of its blend of productivity, pleasure, and restoration (Pierce, 1997, 1998, 2001). For example, therapists working with children often use playful therapeutic occupations that are high in the pleasure dimension. Play is engaging for the child, holds his or her interest, makes the child more comfortable and relaxed, and results in a longer involvement before the child grows bored with the activity. To many adults, playful activities can seem frivolous or unlikely to result in important outcomes. For them, more highly productive occupations are appealing and effective. For a client who is emotionally depleted or in recovery from traumatic life events, a quietly restorative experience that moves slowly but surely toward goals may be the most appealing and effect the greatest overall progress.

In this section, you have focused on developing a connoisseur's understanding of the subjective experience of occupation in your own life and in the lives of others. At this point, your grasp of the historical, physical, cultural, and experiential aspects of pleasure, restoration, and productivity is probably far greater than it was before you worked your way through these chapters. It is not that the concepts were really new to you, however, because we all grow up using common sense to create our own occupational patterns. Much of what has been presented thus far should not have felt foreign to you but should have resonated with your own history. But commonsense understanding is not enough. An occupational therapist's understanding of occupation must go deeper if he or she is to apply that knowledge to facilitate changes in the occupational patterns of others. This is not common sense. It takes demanding design work to make real changes in the occupational patterns of an individual. If you can create therapeutic occupations that are highly appealing to your clients, that satisfy the human need to do, and that engage them in a way that touches who they really are, then your clients will really "get" occupational therapy. By studying occupation as you have thus far, you are well on your way to mastery of this disciplinary knowledge of occupation. You have even explored the complicated notion of life balance. Hopefully, you have begun to experiment with your design skills by using the Power Builders, in that way taking some early steps toward the design excellence and reflexivity that will one day be a natural part of your everyday practice.

Appeal is only one of the three primary sources of the therapeutic power of occupation: appeal, intactness, and accuracy. In the following two primary sections of this book, you will have the opportunity to explore the influences of the contexts of occupation and to look more closely at how therapists create accurately targeted interventions. At the end of Section III on the context of occupation, a chapter parallel to this one discusses how therapists can best design interventions within the contexts in which they occur. These are called intact interventions. At the end of Section IV you will find a discussion of how to apply the elements of the therapist's occupational design process for greatest accuracy. For now, however, we will put intactness and accuracy aside to focus on how you can apply your understanding of restoration, pleasure, and productivity by designing highly appealing therapeutic occupations.

Initial Client Picture

Designing for appeal is always custom design. You cannot create an appealing experience without knowing what is attractive to the person for whom you are designing it. So, the first step in designing for appeal—indeed, for almost any effort in occupational therapy—is to get to know your client. Or, in a family-centered approach in which goals are set for the family as much as for the individual, you will need to get to know the whole family. Creating high appeal in therapeutic occupations requires an understanding of the client's activity preferences, current and past occupational patterns, and present energy level and life challenges. This perspective on the individual is then combined with his or her goals to create a custom design of occupational experiences that will be appealing and therapeutic, with just the right blend of productivity, pleasure, and restoration.

The Purposes and Tone of an Initial Client-Therapist Meeting

Initial meetings between the occupational therapist and those he or she serves have several purposes: getting to know each other, exchanging information about what is needed and what the therapist can offer, and completing administrative requirements for intake procedures. This is both similar to and different from the way you get to know others who are not your clients. Conversations with your client should be comfortable and informal, showing respect for the important perspectives on occupational therapy that can be offered by both the client and the therapist. This getting to know each other process should focus mostly on information about the client's needs, current circumstances, and desired changes in occupational pattern. Try to keep the conversation focused largely on the client because this is how you will get the most useful information. Contribute some information about yourself, enough to make your client comfortable by acknowledging commonalities you may have or by making some brief genuine comments on your own approach to therapy. You will probably have to explain briefly what occupational therapy is and can offer in this case.

One of the important topics to explore in an initial meeting is what the goals of intervention should be. You may wish to do a more formal collaborative goal-setting evaluation at this time, or perhaps at your next meeting. (Goal setting is more fully discussed in Chapter 15.) Some clients are very clear on this question of goals; others are not. Do the best you can to get a sense of what the client is hoping to accomplish or change about his or her skills or life. Often, clients will know what is wrong, but not what the answer may be to the problem they are facing. Do not expect the discussion of goals to be a clean, clear-cut process. For the client, "What are your goals for intervention?" is a very big, complicated question.

The Client's Occupational Picture

To gain an understanding of the client, ask open-ended questions about occupational experience, such as these:

- What do you like to do?
- What is your usual routine?
- How has your life changed because of _____ (newly acquired disability, etc.)?
- How do you wish your life to be?
- What do you most miss doing?
- What would you change if you could?
- What is the most important thing for you to be able to do?

- What would you like to accomplish through therapy?
- What are some of the best things you have done in your life?

As you hear the client's story and general goals, you will begin to get a sense of his or her values about occupation. As you listen, ask yourself whether this is a person who is motivated most by things that are productive, pleasurable, or restorative. Add some further questions of your own, in easy nontheoretical language, to test whether your sense of what type of occupation might be most appealing to this person is correct. For some individuals, it is immediately obvious what is going to work well. For others, it may take some exploration.

Applying Your Estimation of What Will Appeal

Once you have gotten a sense of whether the characteristic of pleasure, productivity, or restoration in therapeutic experiences will be most attractive to this individual, you have laid the foundation for designing highly appealing, and thus effective, occupational therapy. You will build on this foundation by using your knowledge of the variety, experience, and meaning of typical human activities to create compelling therapeutic occupations.

Focus on One Characteristic

In your early years of designing appealing interventions, do not worry too much about creating the perfect blend of pleasure, productivity, and restoration. Just focus on the one that you think is most appealing to your client. Try to match your client's preference with an activity that offers high levels of that characteristic. Later, you can try a more subtle approach of blending just the right combination of the three, like a chef adding a combination of seasonings to an entree. Keep in mind that one area in which it is easy to design appealing experiential blends is in the use of games, crafts, and hobbies. The productivity of such activities appeals to cultural values, and the inherent pleasure makes them fun to do. If you can get a good match of skill and challenge, the client is likely to experience flow.

Give Choices

An easy way to strengthen occupational appeal is to identify several activities you think will appeal and then ask your client to choose—or even better, ask the client to provide you with ideas. Be clear that, of the activities you suggest, any choice is equally good, all of them will work, and choice is just a matter of personal preference. Naturally, the person will pick the activity with the most personal appeal.

Refine Appeal

Once you have begun the first therapeutic occupation, observe your client carefully. Was your estimation of what would appeal to him or her correct? There is always room for refinement in this professional judgment as you get to know better the individual's skills, attitudes, and needs. Also, what appeals to an individual can change from day to day, though not usually to a great degree. Making those appeal adjustments is a natural development of your work with each person.

Expertise with Appeal

The more you use occupational appeal in your thinking about intervention design, the easier and more natural it will become, especially if you consistently work with similar groups of clients over a period of years. You will build up a repertoire of activity ideas that offers an appealing blend for these clients. You will constantly be creating new ideas to add to your collection. With experience, the times when you may become most aware of your efforts to design with appeal will be when you encounter clients who do not find your designs engaging, and so are not progressing toward their goals. Such difficult cases happen to all therapists. It's part of the job. Finding therapeutic occupations that really appeal to such individuals will call on all your design skills as you try to find activities that offer just the right blend to individuals who may be in very chaotic life situations. Be patient. Talk with your clients about it. Persevere.

Designing with Productivity

The person who most values highly productive occupational experiences, and thus will work best with therapeutic occupations high in productivity, may indicate such values in several ways. He or she may want to immediately discuss the goals of intervention or will indicate through statements a dedicated willingness to work hard toward goals. A strong Protestant work ethic may also be evident in a client's not wanting to do things that do not produce objects of quality craftsmanship nor to engage in activities that seem frivolous. You may sense a pride in, or a conflict around, work identity.

To design appealing therapeutic occupations for persons who value highly productive activities, you will combine your understanding of productivity with the preferences and interests of the individual client. Each case will be different, but here are a few aspects of productivity that you might consider to spur your design thinking.

Challenge, Arousal, and Flow

For persons who enjoy highly productive occupations, the outcome of the experience is very important. The goal toward which they are striving must be crystal clear. Keep the session challenging. During each intervention, set small, intermediate goals toward which the client can work. Display progress in measurable terms on an easily accessible chart that either you or the client updates regularly. Do not overpraise the individual for his or her hard work, but rather, remark on the successful results of the work he or she is doing.

Consider how you might use flow theory to maximize the appeal of therapeutic occupations. Remember the conditions of flow: clear goals, feedback on relative success, and focused attention within a limited stimulus field. Can you design a therapeutic experience that provides all of these things? Lots of activities can produce flow: games, sports, cooking, paid employment, crafts, art, and even housework, for some people. Remember, what produces flow for one person may not produce flow for another, because flow is a match of perceived skill and perceived challenge.

The biggest problem of productivity-loving clients in occupational therapy is boredom. If the occupational experience is not sufficiently interesting and challenging for a person's skill level, he or she may go through the motions as a kindness to you but will not really be engaged nor progress quickly toward goals. Unfortunately, this happens all the time in therapy. It is difficult to identify and provide activities that match the high skill levels of some persons driven by productivity values. If you keep in mind, however, that the level of stimulation and arousal must be high and that the demand for performance must also be high, you will be able to create designs that are appealing. One way to easily identify challenging therapeutic occupations for an individual is to do therapy that addresses work goals within the environments in which he or she previously worked or wishes to work. Consider also whether your client is living within an environment or a lifestyle that is perpetually boring, such as in a nursing home, unexpected retirement, or schoolwork that is not engaging. What can you do about that boredom to improve the occupational pattern quality for your client?

Working with the Protestant Work Ethic

To use the Protestant work ethic to create appealing therapy, emphasize feelings of doing the right thing, craftsmanship, and pride in a product. The moral goodness of honest, hard work can be remarked on but only in a subtle way that respects the humility of the person. Bragging or praising would be embarrassingly inappropriate. You can convey recognition of hard work without even using words if you think about it: a nod, a raised eyebrow, or a long appreciative look at a product. A comment like "It feels good to work hard, doesn't it?" can go a long way toward supporting a person's feelings of doing what is right by working hard toward his or her goals.

Craftsmanship and pride in product can be easily used in creating a therapeutic occupation that is high in productivity. For craftsmanship, you must look to the quality of the materials and the quality of the production process. If this is an activity with which your client is familiar, it is important to use the craftsmanship rules that he or she holds true. Ask what good craftsmanship is in this case, how the quality of the product is judged, what is "best." Specific praise for the ways in which the product meets these marks of quality as it begins to take shape will emphasize craftsmanship and elicit pride. Such remarks should not be so vague as "Looks great!" Rather, in the example of a woodworking project, you might comment on how nicely the grain shows up as a bowl is taking shape. Pride in a product can also be supported through showing the product in a display case, at an open house or a benefit event, or by making a special effort to get the product out to show to the staff or to the guests, peers, or family members of a client.

Using Work Identity in Appeal

Work identity can be key in the design of appealing therapeutic occupations high in productivity. This is especially true in individuals who have set goals of returning to work or entering a new type of work. The most appealing activities will be those clearly and directly linked with the skills and abilities needed for the work, as long as they are set at an appropriate level of challenge. Goals that are too difficult will be discouraging and can cause a deep questioning of the client's identity as a worker. This is a devastating experience for someone who highly values productivity, although it is sometimes an unavoidable consequence as a person attempts work that is beyond his or her abilities. Goals that are too easy will result in boredom and frustration at not making significant progress toward the desired work skills.

Persons who face unplanned retirement or inability to return to previous work face a more complex question of where they are headed with their work identities. If an individual sets goals to try to resolve this question, the occupational therapist will be a good ally in exploring different options for future productivity. If a new type of employment is sought, intervention is simply a matter of assessing skills, providing opportunities to try out different possible work identities, and then setting goals to acquire the skills necessary for the new work. For unpaid work, such as caring for a family or volunteering, it is important to emphasize the value of the work, and thus the value of that person's identity even though a paycheck is not involved. Once you are sure that your client is valuing the unpaid work to the degree necessary for self-esteem, you can proceed with that person to working on skills and plans for transitioning into or returning to that unpaid work. Be open-minded in your consideration of the many types of unpaid work identity that can be used, including household work, caregiving, volunteering, and study.

Watch for Stress

If you are using high productivity to design appealing occupations for intervention, remember that, taken too far, productivity can result in stress. Be sure the goals you have set with your client are not unrealistically high. Never place a client who enjoys productivity in experiences that are boring, repetitive, or lacking in value. Stress can cause clients to withdraw from intervention or abandon useful goals. Stress can also lower immunity, especially in persons already suffering from illness or life disruptions.

Some clients may have goals specifically targeting stress-management skills. Some characteristics of occupation that may help reduce stress include physical exertion and conditioning, meditation and self-calming, and personal exploration of feelings through journaling. Your client can also work more directly on resolving current life problems that are producing stress, through problem solving and planned action. You may target changes in important daily occupations that will result in reduced stress and increased satisfaction. Altering stressful conditions in home and work environments, such as high noise levels or unsafe work conditions, can also reduce stress.

As you provide intervention to people in future years, many in the midst of very difficult and emotional life changes, monitor your own stress. Protect yourself from burning out as an occupational therapist by setting appropriate limits on your work so that you can continue to provide energetic, authentic, centered, and caring therapy. If you see burnout in therapists around you, perhaps you will have the rare opportunity to design appealing interventions for your fellow workers.

Designing with Pleasure

Occupational therapists have been using the characteristic of pleasure in occupation in a therapeutic way since the start of this field. That is why we are so knowledgeable about crafts and hobbies, the occupations in which people engage just for fun. At some point in the history of our field, occupational therapy attempted to distance itself from its association with play, basket weaving, and other forms of pleasurable activity. We were seeking the easier road of acceptance as a valued profession by fitting into the strong productivity values of the Western culture and strengthening our resemblance to the powerful profession of medicine. Our clients, however, continue to respond best when we use therapeutic occupations that appeal most to them. Indeed, children will hardly engage in therapy unless it is playful. Thus, pleasurable activities have never been left far behind in occupational therapy. The more pleasurable a client finds treatment, the more motivated he or she will be to continue doing it. Clients with a strong Protestant work ethic may feel guilty engaging in highly pleasurable therapeutic occupations, but they may also still progress well in them. Use your understanding of each individual to decide what level of pleasure in therapeutic occupations he or she may find appealing.

Designing with Play and Leisure

Play and leisure are the most obvious places to start in using pleasure to increase the appeal of therapeutic occupations. Begin here by simply asking your client what he or she likes to do for fun.

Much has been written about the types of play and games children enjoy at different developmental stages. For children with disabilities, you may have to experiment a little to find the most appealing occupations because of their possible developmental delays, social isolation from past play experiences with peers, and physical limitations. Pediatric occupational therapists can list many different play activities children enjoy and are always searching for another new game or craft that will support goals frequently set for children with whom they are working. Unfortunately, these therapists are often relatively lacking in a critical perspective on play and can be very susceptible to the media influence of the toy industry in their designs of playful occupations. Nevertheless, pediatric occupational therapy has remained most true to an occupation-based approach to intervention, largely because children are not motivated to engage in therapy in any way other than playful.

In adults, we call fun *leisure*. Leisure includes a rich array of activities from which to choose in designing for high appeal through pleasure: hobbies, crafts, sports, arts, dance, music, entertainment, travel, and others. The possibilities are nearly endless. Once you have a sense of what your client enjoys, you should have no difficulty in coming up with a few good choices. Depending on the goals you are addressing, you may want to involve your client in the preparatory work of finding out what supplies are needed, researching the way the activity is done, identifying or setting up the space where the activity will take place, and directing how the activity happens. Consider whether there are other clients who might also benefit from the same activity. Perhaps an ongoing group focused on this particular leisure activity would be successful. A good example of an ongoing activity group that supports healthy aging is a mall-walking group.

Appealing Sensations

Occupational therapists are fairly knowledgeable about sensory systems because of their study of anatomy and neurology as well as their understanding of sensory testing and use of sensory integration theory to facilitate changes in function in children with disabilities. Although these theories are useful, they do not specifically focus on pleasurable sensation. Sensory pleasure can be included in an occupation through limbic arousal and relaxation, taste and smell, touch, movement, vision, and hearing.

Regardless of what type of sensory input you use to enhance the appeal of an intervention, it is important that the sensory input be provided at the appropriate level. Do not confuse overstimulation with a pleasurable experience. Observe clients carefully when using sensory approaches. Watch for signs of nervous system overload: flushing, paling, nausea, dizziness, hyperactivity, emotional over-reactivity, and withdrawal or refusal to participate in an activity. You want to use enough sensation to give pleasure but not enough to be overwhelming to the person. Populations that may be in need of special consideration regarding sensory input are those with brain injuries, sensory deficits, and sensory processing problems, and individuals in medical isolation.

Limbic arousal and relaxation are most strongly seen in thrill seeking, entertainment suspense, competitive games, and activities that require strong physical exertion. Within this list of possibilities, there are options for those who are young and old, or physically fit and physically disabled. Consider how much a client is maintaining a minimum of physical activity and, thus, a minimum amount of arousal and stimulation to the muscles and joints of his or her body.

The most obvious activities you can use to enhance pleasure and appeal through taste and smell are cooking and eating. Unlike many leisure activities, cooking and eating are familiar activities in which nearly everyone has some basic skills for his or her age. This is why so many occupational therapy departments have kitchens. The possibilities for individual and group activities that include cooking and eating are nearly endless, and such activities are almost always popular with both clients and staff. Cooking has the added advantage of combining well with productivity values. Other ways to include smell in therapeutic occupations are by incorporating various aromas in the space or materials used—for example, mint-scented play goop, aromatic candles, working under pine trees, and sharing memories triggered by smells.

Touch and texture can be pleasurable enhancements of appeal. Again, much has been written in sensory integration regarding the use of touch, pressure, proprioceptive and tactile input, and therapeutic aims. Remember, use these sensory inputs with caution, taking care not to overstimulate. Tactile input can be especially stimulating in some individuals. Tactile sensation can be provided through textures of foods, activity materials, objects with which the client comes into direct skin contact during activities, or therapist-provided brushing or massage. Proprioceptive input, which is neurological information about joint position and traction, can be provided through jumping, hanging by the arms, pulling or carrying things, being overlaid with weighted covers, doing heavy work, and other activities that exert significant forces on the more proximal joints and surrounding muscles of the neck, shoulders, arms, and legs. Most people find proprioception very pleasurable and calming. Few find it overstimulating.

Human touch is an important feature of therapy but must be used with subtlety. Variation among cultural attitudes and in individual responsiveness to professionals touching clients is great. Use this with care and only when your client welcomes it. You will be able to tell by asking or by observing reactions to a slight touch on the hand or shoulder. Being careful about the appropriate use of touch is critical to respecting your clients, whether they are children or adults. Touching an individual who does not wish to be touched is an invasion of body space, although there are occasions when it may be required. If it is necessary to touch a client, even though this may make him or her uncomfortable, ask permission first and warn the client just prior to doing so. If you do use touch in your interventions, be sure it is increasing, not decreasing, the appeal of the intervention. Be sure you restrict your touch to socially acceptable areas of the client's body, such as a hand or shoulder, unless the client indicates otherwise.

Simple movement can feel good, especially to a person who does not get to do this enough. Movement can be easily incorporated into many different types of activities. Consider whether your client is getting enough physical activity on a regular basis. If not, and he or she is able, include physical activity in the therapeutic occupations that you offer. Activities that use physical movement include dancing, sports, walking, and games, to mention only a few.

Vision and hearing can be used to enhance pleasure in many ways through such visual games such as puzzles, video games, and crosswords. Arts and crafts activities often have a largely visual component, as does much of entertainment. Watching nature is generally pleasurable for people. Travel is very visual. Reading is visual, but in a way that produces the pleasure more through the cognitive processes regarding what is read, rather than through the visual imagery it provides. Hearing, through listening to or creating music, rhythms, and stories, can enhance pleasure and appeal.

Humor

The best way to include humor in intervention is to be humorous yourself. This may take some practice because you can feel you are swimming against the tide of opinion that professionals must act very serious and distant. Actually, this serious and distant approach is probably more about professional power than it is about what is good for patients. I have never seen a humorous occupational therapist who was not completely appreciated and beloved by staff and clients alike for his or her efforts to bring fun into therapy. Although people may laugh and shake their heads at your approach, they never seem to object to it. A moment of shared laughter can go a long way toward easing tension, making clients and staff more comfortable, and reducing stress during difficult situations. You can bring laughter into therapy through jokes, silly costuming, and laughing at yourself. Be careful not to laugh at others or to make jokes that use other people or groups as the butt of the jokes. Try to develop your sense of timing so that your humor is regarded as helpful, rather than disruptive or disrespectful. Laughter is also especially useful for alleviating stress and burnout in yourself and other staff with whom you work.

Using humor is perhaps easiest with children. They love to laugh, dress up in costumes, and pretend. For kids, humor can be silliness, comical reactions to things they do, and acting playfully yourself. Humorous activities with children include pretending to be or move like a person or an animal, surprising someone, making up and performing simple or planned-out puppet shows and plays, and doing simple pratfalls and slapstick. These activities will work with some adults also. With both adults and children, humor is easily available through comedy movies and stand-up comedians. There are also several adult games, such as charades or silly relay races, that can provoke a lot of hilarity. Use your imagination, watch for laughter around you, and take a humorous attitude yourself, and you will increase your skills in using humor to enhance the appeal of your interventions.

Using Meaningful Ritual in Intervention

Therapeutic occupations offer many opportunities to use meaningful rituals, drawing pleasure into the experience through the deep resonance the ritual holds for the individual. The most obvious type of ritual used in therapy is engaging in different types of seasonal, cultural celebrations, such as creating and displaying holiday decorations, fixing or eating special holiday foods, or making holiday gifts. Every cultural holiday has unique activity traditions. In your own culture, you probably already know what these are. Take care, however, not to assume that the meanings they have for you are the same as those they hold for your clients. They could, in fact, have negative associations and cause distress for some individuals. Also, clients come from different cultural traditions, with which you may or may not be familiar. The best course is to include your client in selecting holiday-centered activities that truly increase the degree of pleasure your client experiences in the occupation.

Some clients may be responsible for participating in or creating specific rituals important to them in their lives: a daughter's wedding, a Jewish family's Sabbath meal, a student's graduation ceremony. These occasions are more likely to appear as goals of intervention than as modes of treatment. Yet, it is important that the therapist recognize the motivation and identify importance of such rituals to the person he or she is treating. This is especially true of those special rituals, called *rites of passage,* which mark important milestones in a person's life.

Personal rituals might be called rituals with a small *r*. They are not cultural or seasonal celebrations with meanings widely understood by others, but smaller routines that individuals develop to transition from one mood to another, or from one part of their day to another. Examples are sitting down and going through the mail at the beginning of the work day, taking a long bubble bath to relax after a stressful week, and taking a break from work to step outside and look around. Many small personal rituals center around self-care, rest, or the more routine and quiet aspects of work life. These rituals can be used in treatment in various ways—by collaboratively creating them with clients as ways to strengthen or change the pleasure in a problematic occupational pattern, as stress reducers, or as ways to enhance the pleasure of a self-care activity. Brief personal rituals can also be created as moments to visualize a client's successful performance of a skill to support his or her success.

Replacing Chemical and Activity Addictions with Other Pleasures

In the case of chemical and activity addictions, such as substance abuse, obesity and bulimia, pathological gambling, and technology addictions, pleasure is primarily applied in attempting to develop occupational experiences that produce enough enjoyment for the client that he or she can replace the dangerous behaviors by fulfilling that addictive need for enjoyment. This is a challenging form of occupational therapy. It requires strong communication with, and commitment from, the client to develop occupational preferences that are sufficiently rewarding to challenge the place of the addictive behavior in the occupational pattern. These approaches are best developed by therapists with a strong grasp of occupation-based practice in a setting that provides long-term engagement with the client and within a social group that supports the efforts of the client to make changes in his or her lifestyle.

Designing with Restoration

The idea of using restoration in therapeutic occupation, as a way to increase the appeal of interventions, is probably the greatest theoretical stretch when considering the use of productivity, pleasure, and restoration. The values of productivity in Western culture are so strong as to render concerns about restorative experiences nearly invisible. Despite the fact that sleep, eating and drinking, self-care, and quiet-focus activities are central to our survival and mental health, they have not been researched or theoretically developed to any great depth in occupational therapy. Let us explore here briefly what use might be made of such activities in creating therapeutic occupations that are appealing and effective.

Attending to Sleep as the Base of the Occupational Pattern

The take-home message about sleep is that it is the base of the entire occupational pattern. Without a certain adequacy of sleep, other aspects of the occupational pattern decline—capacity for completing desired tasks and goals, health, and cognitive ability. So, to do occupational therapy well, it is important to understand the full 24-hour cycle of your client's occupational pattern. Ask every client about sleep quality, environment, and schedule. If problems are evident, explain your understanding of the importance of sleep as a base for other occupations. Discuss with your client whether he or she would like your help in working on sleep quality. If the answer is yes, begin with a self-report sleep environment assessment and a review of sleep schedule. Patients who are especially at risk for sleep problems are those with respiratory or psychiatric disorders; those who are overweight; teenagers; children on busy family schedules or showing behavior problems; children taking methylphenidate (Ritalin) or with attention deficit or hyperactivity disorders; parents of young children; caregivers; patients in intensive care units; and shift workers.

It is probably not possible to blend a little sleep into other therapeutic occupations to increase their appeal. Sleep is one of those very basic activities that you cannot easily combine with any other. For this reason, it is difficult to argue that sleep can increase the appeal of a therapeutic occupation. Sleep comes into intervention more as a direct goal, as a place to address the overall quality and balance of the occupational pattern. Improving sleep quality may be the first necessary step in assisting a client to reach a level of cognition and energy that allows other areas of occupation to be addressed. Occupational therapists can also greatly assist clients by engaging in general programmatic attention to the environmental sleep conditions in healthcare settings such as neonatal intensive care units, pediatric and adult intensive care units, psychiatric hospitals, and nursing homes.

Eating and Drinking as Interventions

As just discussed under the pleasurable contributions of taste and smell to appeal, eating and drinking are familiar and important activities for nearly everyone. Because they are so central and generally valued, they are powerful avenues for intervention. Eating and drinking can serve as intervention goals, as the primary activities within which eating and drinking abilities are addressed, as activities within which many other goals can be addressed, or as additions to another activity to enhance its enjoyment. All occupational therapists should be familiar with these easily understood and widely accepted activities as a mode of intervention. These activities are done by everyone every day, are flexible in complexity and degree of preparation and equipment required and are fairly inexpensive, can be engaged in alone or with others, hold great meaning, and are usually regarded as restorative to body and mind. No matter what the population or setting may be, eating and drinking are usually appealing modes of intervention—something that can be said of very few activities.

Making Self-Care a Restorative Experience

Basic self-care activities of bathing, grooming, toileting, and dressing are a mainstay of occupational therapy. Often they are a primary reason for referral to occupational therapy. Like eating and drinking, they are done daily by nearly everyone. Yet they are not always viewed as restorative to energy. Some individuals see self-care merely as necessary maintenance. But those who are prevented from engaging in these activities will quickly feel uncomfortable, drained of energy, and unready to engage in other activities.

For those individuals who find some self-care experiences restorative, they can be used as activities within which to work on other goals. For example, for an elderly woman who just does not feel ready for the day until dressed in the gown she has picked herself from her closet, reducing left-side neglect and improving dressing skills can be worked on during her morning dressing routine. For a busy executive working on stress-management skills, taking the time to step into his executive washroom and splash water on his face between meetings could be an excellent way to quickly unwind and refresh himself.

Another way to use understanding of self-care to enhance restoration is to insure that, when you are working on self-care activities with clients, you inquire how they usually do such an activity, what supplies and methods they prefer, and what is most restorative about that experience for them. In this way, you can know how to make this intervention more restorative and avoid the dehumanizing effects of requiring your client to adhere to self-care procedures that are dictated by the institution.

Using Quiet-Focus Handwork and Hobbies

Quiet-focus handwork and hobbies, such as knitting and stamp collecting, offer many possibilities for intervention. Given the right match of skill and challenge, clients tend to experience flow, which provides an enjoyable escape from daily worries and the pressures of dealing with a disability. Many of these quiet activities are easily portable and can be used by clients in a hospital room or clinic setting, at home, or in the community. Quiet-focus activities are especially useful as interventions for clients, such as those who are quite elderly or severely depressed, who are low in energy, or who do not have the ability to engage in highly demanding forms of intervention. Using a quiet-focus activity allows them to engage in therapeutic occupations at a slow but steady pace, rather than withdrawing from intervention completely.

Bringing Nature into Therapy

Because many people find nature restorative, think about how you might use nature in interventions to enhance their appeal. This approach should be especially effective for clients who have indicated their enjoyment of nature. Nature can be used in intervention in two different ways.

Nature-oriented activities can be used as the primary mode of intervention. Gardening, for example, is the most popular adult leisure activity in the United States, and works well as an intervention. In fact, it works so well that occupational therapy's neglect of this activity as an intervention has resulted in the birth of a whole new field: horticulture therapy.

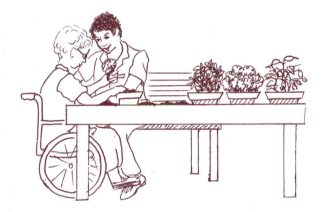

Nature can also be used as a setting, or to add appeal to a treatment setting. That is, you can move your interventions into nature, or you can bring some nature into where you are doing interventions. For example, studies of the relaxation that people experience from watching tropical fish has led many doctors to add fish tanks to their offices.

Can Reading and Watching Television Be Interventions?

Although reading and watching television are certainly restorative, I am not sure that there are many ways in which these activities can be made use of as therapeutic modalities. Certainly, educational content pertinent to a client could be provided through watching television. Perhaps a reading group would be useful as the basis for discussion of particular emotional and life issues, such as dealing with grief. Including such highly restorative activities in an overly demanding occupational pattern could certainly be a goal of intervention.

Spirituality Activities in Occupational Therapy

Spirituality is a source of energy that comes from inner beliefs about life's meaning. For some individuals, spirituality is a set of activities existing within the framework of a religious community. Often, these activities include gathering regularly with others to worship, study, or discuss religious beliefs; observing religious holidays; praying; or adhering to certain proscriptions about lifestyle. For other people, spirituality is more loose—it is meditation or prayer or ritual without belonging to a larger group, or just regularly doing things that are personally renewing. Still others do not engage in any activities they would identify as specifically spiritual.

Spiritual activities are important in occupational therapy in several ways. Clients may set goals of engaging in specific spiritual activities that, because of disability or resources, they are not currently able to do. Understanding a client's spiritual beliefs can be as important in grasping that person's occupational pattern as is understanding his or her cultural background. Many areas of intervention, especially 12-step substance-abuse programs, use a specific set of religious practices and beliefs to support the client as he or she tries to adhere to a changed lifestyle. Finally, if agreeable to the client, spiritual activities can be used as an avenue for working on intervention goals, such as using seated prayer for working on sitting tolerance.

Staying in touch with your own spiritual health and beliefs can make you a better therapist. At times, working with individuals who are going through tumultuous, and sometimes sad, times in their lives requires great strength and calm on the part of the therapist. Clients often look to the therapist for encouragement and a bright smile when things seem very hard for them. You must have energy reserves you can call on if needed, and know how to use your own spiritual practices to calm and renew yourself when life at work gets tough. Therapists are privileged to share life experiences with many people who are working to triumph over negative life events. They share with them the ups and downs of determined life development and reconstructions of self. It is a growth-promoting, but emotionally demanding, type of work.

Intervention Breaks and Wrap-ups

During highly demanding intervention sessions, consider what you might do to create a truly refreshing intervention break. In treatment, both the therapist and the client tend to be focused on working toward the goals, and the client can become completely exhausted or stressed by pushing so hard toward the desired outcomes. Rather than just stopping briefly and then resuming, consider what might really give this particular client back enough energy to get the most out of the remainder of the session. Would it be sharing a joke, a cookie, a trip to the drinking fountain, a step outdoors, a little music? As occupational therapists, we may think too much about where the client's energy is headed, rather than whence it comes. Try giving some real thought to the intervention break, and you are likely to increase the overall results of your sessions, despite the time lost for that quick restorative break.

As with the intervention break, give some consideration also to how you end your intervention sessions. Allow a little wind-down time. Exchange some observations with the client about how the session went and what might be good to do next time. As you wrap up the session, how could you make this ending a bit more restorative? Sit down, perhaps, if the session has been upright and active. Or laugh if it has been serious. Have a cup of tea. There are many brief activities that could be used during the session wrap-up to leave the client feeling somewhat restored, instead of being quickly transitioned out the door with little opportunity to catch his or her breath or experience closure to the work of the session and readiness to move on to his or her day.

Working on Balance: Is It a Client Goal?

One of the things that may become evident in discussing possible outcomes of therapy is that the client has problems in life balance. As he or she, or a family member, describes current and previous occupational patterns, your own knowledge of human occupation will provide you with a comparative frame within which to view the picture they are providing. You may immediately sense, for example, that this person overemphasized productivity to such a stressful extent as to result in the present injury. Or you may see a person without life goals, constantly seeking momentary pleasures but finding it difficult to survive without solid employment skills. You may suspect that this person is chronically tired and sleep deprived. There are many instances in which persons with congenital, chronic, or newly acquired disabilities and their families deal with the demands of their situation by leading a life that is out of balance. Sometimes, they will openly acknowledge this problem. Sometimes, they seem relatively unaware of it. Often, they feel it just comes with the territory.

If you suspect a life-balance problem, use open-ended questions to inquire carefully whether or not your client and significant others also see this problem. Remember, there is no right way to live a life, no correct balance between pleasure, productivity, and restoration. There is only the question of whether the client and family are finding the balance that suits their values. Life-balance problems will be resolved in working with an occupational therapist in two simple ways: either the client wants to set goals that address life balance or he or she does not. If the problem is something your client wants to address, then you can develop a goal together that describes the desired occupational pattern and progress toward it. For example, a recovering alcoholic may set a goal of engaging in pleasurable activities that do not involve alcohol on a daily basis for 1 hour. As another example, a very productivity-loving person who has entered an early retirement because of disability may set a goal of exploring, selecting, and developing a satisfying role as a valued community volunteer. If the client does not wish to change occupational balance, however, you will not address it unless the life-balance problem is so extreme that his or her immediate safety is at risk.

Custom Designing Appealing Therapeutic Occupations

Remember, if you can custom design therapeutic occupations that hold strong appeal for individual clients, you will achieve greatness as a therapist. Think about pleasure, productivity, restoration, and balance as you get to know and design for your clients. Observe carefully how they work. Refine your designs, using a single characteristic with strong appeal or a more sophisticated, blended approach. You will make it look easy, although it is not, because of how quickly and willingly those you serve take up and engage in the activities you provide. If you are really good, your clients will progress rapidly toward their goals, thinking that all the credit is due to their own ideas and work. Do not locate your measures of success in how well other team members understand and appreciate what you do. A true understanding of the successful application of occupation is far beyond common sense. Those in other professions cannot be expected to possess this perspective. The successes of your clients are your successes. Celebrate them. Revel in them. Reflect on them. Grow as a designer through them.

POWER BUILDERS

Key Concepts for Strengthening Insight into Designing for Appeal

- The client's occupational picture
- Designing with one characteristic: restoration, productivity, or pleasure
- Challenge, arousal, and flow
- Protestant work ethic
- Work identity
- Stress
- Play and leisure
- Sensations
- Humor
- Ritual
- Sleep
- Eating and drinking
- Self-care
- Quiet-focus handwork and hobbies
- Nature
- Spirituality activities
- Intervention breaks and wrap-ups
- Balance

Designing Appealing Occupations for Yourself

1. Reflect on the following, in discussion with others, as a journal entry, or as a more formal paper or poster presentation:

- What is the perfect challenge in your life right now?
- What goals do you have in your life right now?
- Which of the three primary characteristics presently motivate you to pursue your goals?
- Could you use a better blend of characteristics to make working toward your goals more appealing?
- How does your work identity as a student support or not support your progress toward your goals at different times?
- Is your life balanced? If not, what is out of balance about it? What could you do to change it?

2. Design for yourself the perfectly balanced week. Use the time/task method to list everything that must be included. Sketch it out on a piece of paper in a time-log format.

3. How could you make studying more pleasurable? Brainstorm 50 ideas, select one using a ranking exercise, plan and implement it, and write a reflective evaluation of how well it worked.

Building Insight into Appeal in the Occupational Experiences of Others

1. Create a demonstration of one humor technique that might be useful in occupational therapy, using literature search, boiling down a definition, listing five ways to do the demonstration, or picking one through a simple ranking. Make a plan for giving the demonstration using a time/task table and a Gantt chart. Give the demonstration. Have the person rate your effectiveness on a paper feedback form that uses criteria from your definition.

2. Activity Interview. Pick an activity that you enjoy and that people will feel comfortable discussing. Find someone to interview who also engages in this activity but is as different from you as possible in his or her experience of it. Areas in which you might look for difference with an interviewee include gender, ethnicity, age, lifestyle, level of experience in the activity, paid versus leisure engagement in the activity, and usual degree of enjoyment. Try to select someone who is fairly articulate. This exercise will also give you a chance to practice your interviewing skills that are so essential to your success as a therapist.

   - Once you have decided on the type of activity and selected your interviewee, prepare for your interview. An audiorecorder is easiest because it leaves you free to attend to the person you are interviewing. Take extra batteries and tapes. You can also take notes on the answers to your questions, but this will be more difficult to do well, and the information will not be as rich.

   - Interview the person you have selected on the pleasurable, productive, and restorative characteristics of his or her experience of the activity. Be ready with a list of probes in each of these areas: prompts to help explore aspects of each characteristic. Probes are easy to generate by skimming through the chapters you have just read and picking out the main concepts. Remember to talk as little as possible during the interview. It is not a conversation. The less you speak, the more you will hear. Use your body language to show that you are listening, with a nod, a smile, or leaning forward.

   - With 24 hours, record your personal reflections and observations about the person you interviewed, generally what was said, and what insights you gained. It always seems that you will remember and can wait longer than this, but it is not true. The details fade very quickly. Transcribe the taped interview in full, or in primary phrases. If you recorded your interview in written phrases, you will need to transcribe it more fully within 24 hours.

   - Write summaries of the person's perspective on the pleasure, productivity, and restoration of his or her experience of the focus activity. Comment on how your experience of that activity differs. Describe how your thinking about the occupation has been changed or expanded. Other ways to do this, instead of writing it, are to explain it to someone and to make a poster display of what you discovered.

POWER BUILDERS

Building Design Skills That Insure High Appeal

1. Select a case from Appendix A. Create potential treatment goals if they are not provided in the case. Design a therapeutic occupation for that individual that you believe offers maximum appeal, through use of the productivity, pleasure, and restoration characteristics. Refer to Chapter 2 for reference on working through the design phases, if necessary. Of course, you can actually perform the phases only from acceptance to idea selection, and then you can make plans only for implementation and evaluation. You may wish to write an analysis of your design process, a description of the treatment you designed, a fictive scenario of how the treatment session went, or a fictional reflection by the therapist on how satisfied he or she was with the session.

2. To sharpen your skills further, do the previous exercise with a very different case. Notice how much therapeutic occupations with high appeal differ from one individual to the next. Write, or describe to someone, why the designs came out differently.

3. Here is a fun variation on using the presenting cases to practice designing for maximum appeal. It is somewhat like a game of telephone and is done in a group. Select a case and read through it. Write down an idea for a therapeutic occupation that would seem to fit that individual's needs and interests. Pass your idea (or several ideas at once) around the group, each person trying to improve on the appeal of the design. Once the idea has gone through at least four sets of revision, share it with the group and discuss why you thought of the changes that you felt would increase the appeal of the occupation.

References

Pierce, D. E. (1997). Sources of power in therapeutic applications of object play with young children at risk for developmental delays. In L. D. Parham & L. Fazio (Eds.), *Play in occupational therapy practice*. St. Louis, MO: Mosby.

Pierce, D. E. (1998). The issue is: The treatment power of occupation. *American Journal of Occupational Therapy, 52*, 490–491.

Pierce, D. (2001). Occupation by design: Dimensions, creativity, and therapeutic power. *American Journal of Occupational Therapy, 55*, 249–259.

Designing for Intactness:
Spatial, Temporal, and Sociocultural Dimensions

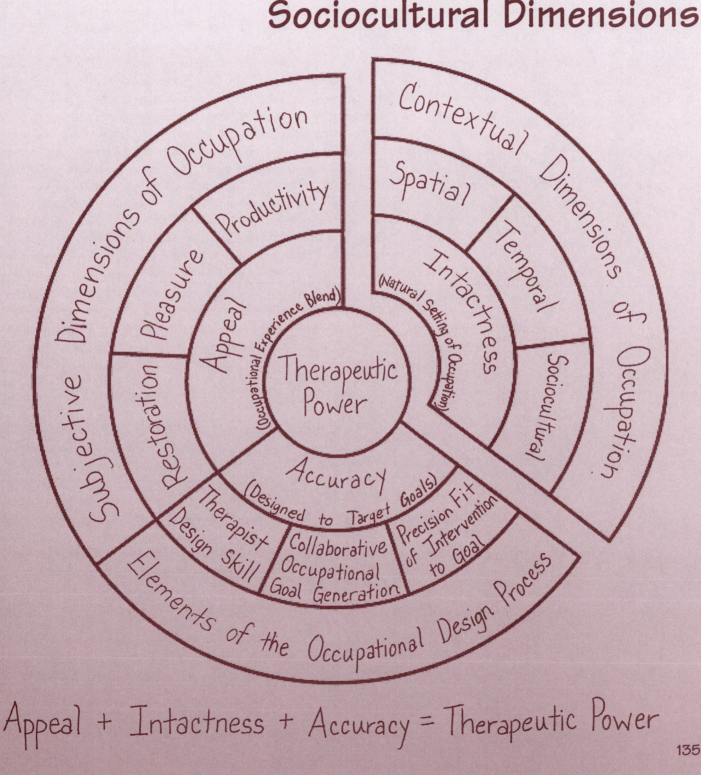

Appeal + Intactness + Accuracy = Therapeutic Power

In the previous section, Section II, you focused on developing your understanding of how occupations are experienced by yourself and others, as well as looking briefly at how the characteristics of that experience can be used to design a more appealing intervention. Now, in Section III, you will look even deeper into occupation by examining the contexts in which it occurs. Whereas the concepts of Section II may have seemed fairly straightforward and familiar, the concepts of Section III will be interestingly novel. Although we are usually aware of how pleasurable or productive we may find an occupation, we are often relatively oblivious to how the time, place, and social setting in which we do occupations shapes our experience. And certainly, we think only infrequently of the degree to which the evolution of the human brain and body and of human culture shape our everyday lives. Yet it is the essence of being human to experience our lives in this uniquely human way, and not in the way that other animals might. Parallel to the chapter on appeal in Section II, this section ends with a chapter on the design of powerful therapeutic occupations through intactness, or the use of natural contexts for intervention. This section is my favorite because I am so intrigued by how evolution, time, space, and sociocultural conditions influence us. I hope you enjoy using it as much as I have writing it. So, to begin with the broadest stroke, the most basic foundation of our daily lives, let us enter a brief exploration of human evolution, provided here for us by Dr. Ruth Zemke, a renowned occupational scientist.

CHAPTER 8

The Evolution of Today's Occupational Patterns

Ruth Zemke, Ph.D., OTR, FAOTA

Adaptation and Evolution

Human Evolutionary Adaptation

Tools, Technology, and Occupation

The Evolutionary Template of Today's Occupational Patterns

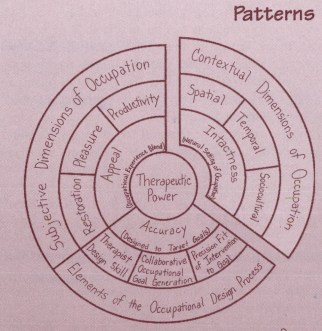

Appeal + Intactness + Accuracy = Therapeutic Power

Adaptation and Evolution

The concept of adaptation was introduced by Charles Darwin as a key to the process of evolution. Evolution generally affects species over extensive periods of time. Adaptation in evolution is a change in a species, but the concept is also used to consider change in individuals. Whether measured in eons or in days, adaptation is based on the potential of living things to grow and develop and, through that development, to change. Evolutionary adaptation focuses on the outcome of a better "match" between the species and environment. Developmental adaptation focuses on the changing structure and function of the individual interacting with the environment. Human occupational adaptation focuses on individuals as agents of changing competence in interaction with the environment.

Evolutionary adaptation results from the process of natural selection. Any adaptive process (evolutionary, developmental, or occupational) is based on selection and requires three things: (Edelman, 1992)

- Variation—a variety of elements from which selection can occur

- Interaction of the varying elements with the environment, producing differing outcomes

- Differential reproduction of successful outcomes

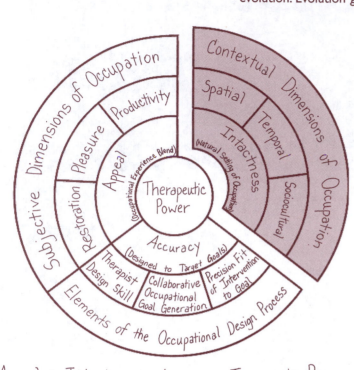

Appeal + Intactness + Accuracy = Therapeutic Power

In evolutionary adaptation, natural selection acts on a variety of structures (genetic and morphologic) and functions that have different effects on the environment. The successful outcome of staying alive and reproducing results in increased numbers of offspring with qualities that are better matched to the environment. On the other hand, those organisms that don't fit so well with the environment decrease in numbers through death or less successful reproduction. The frequent result of evolutionary adaptation is an organism's precise fit into a particular ecological niche.

Actually, humankind's best evolutionary adaptation may be its adaptability! Primates, in general, and humans, in particular, are known for their nonspecialized bodies and flexible behaviors. A great amount of adaptation occurs through changing the physical environment with tools, shelters, crops and herds, and clothing. This means that primates and humans can more readily adapt to environmental change than organisms that are uniquely matched to a specific environmental niche. Thus, selection processes have used our great human diversity and our nature as occupational beings (interacting with the environment) as prime elements in our successful adaptation to a constantly changing world.

Human Evolutionary Adaptation

The evolution of the occupational human was shaped by relationships between walking upright, hand structure, brain structure, hand-eye coordination, and conscious use of objects as tools for occupation. The order of development and reasons behind these adaptations are unknown, although many hypotheses exist.

Primates are predominantly tropical tree-dwelling creatures. They have four limbs with five digits on the extremities and more mobile thumbs and big toes. Instead of claws, they have flattened nails and more sensitive pads on the digits. They have less of a snout (resulting in less skilled sense of smell) than other creatures; placement of the eyes toward the front allows binocular vision. The brain size is such that infants must be born relatively undeveloped. That is, they are more dependent at birth than most other creatures, and they have a very long period of development before maturity. This developmental period allows potential for a lot of learning, or adaptation, by individuals as they mature (Zemke & Horger, 1995).

We humans have four limbs, but how is our forelimb (our hand) unique? Limbs are frequently used for locomotion, and primates are predominantly *quadripedal,* using all four limbs for locomotion. However, many primates are mobile in trees. Because tree dwellers are farther away from their enemies and their prey, they need highly developed vision more so than a well-developed sense of smell. Their descendants may have used these visual abilities in combination with increased manipulation skills. The long arms and mobile shoulder joints of the tree-dwelling primates give them ground mobility, in which the majority of the body weight is supported by the hind limb. That is, they are more bipedal and upright: the knuckle walking of the great apes (such as chimpanzees) reflects this. Only the human is habitually *bipedal,* walking upright on two hind limbs, freeing the hands. The mobile upper extremities of primates assist in *arboreal locomotion* (swinging through the trees) by padded fingers and a *semi-opposable* thumb (one that can almost touch the ends of the fingers) that provide a firm grasp of various-sized branches. These same sensitive fingertips are not just aids in exploring and learning about objects. The hand, in combination with the eye, can be a primary way of knowing objects in the world around us and of interacting with them in occupation.

Evolution of the Hand

The skillful hands of humans have several important differences from those of other primates (Lewis, 1989). Changes in bones at the wrist increase forearm rotation (*supination*), allowing objects to be turned as they are brought close to the eyes for examination. This freedom of rotation is less stable for quadripedalism, but *brachiation* (swinging from branches) and bipedalism do not require such stability. Bipedalism frees the hands for carrying things. Primates living in trees have the beginning of opposition, which is improved even more in monkeys and apes. Longer thumb bones and additional thumb muscles improve the strength of our power grip and stability of the extended thumb against which the fingers can act. A saddle-shaped joint allows the rotation of the thumb for *opposition* (ability to touch the thumb and fingertips). Straight finger (*phalangeal*) bones, rather than the curved ones of brachiating primates, with broad flat ends, allow a precision pinch or grip. This enables us to manipulate objects skillfully while they are held between the thumb and fingertips. These differences enable us to use our hands for more than hooking over branches in a simple power grip, pinching objects between the thumb and the side of our index finger in a lateral pinch grip, or cupping them in one or two hands. They enable not only a precise thumb-to-fingertip pinch that allows skillful manipulation of a sewing needle, but also the complex manipulation as we "hand"le a small object such as a key in *haptic* sensory exploration, a combination of touch and manipulation.

Early human ancestors (*hominids*), such as those represented by the 3-million-year-old fossilized remains known as *Lucy,* had strong hands for using simple tools in pound-

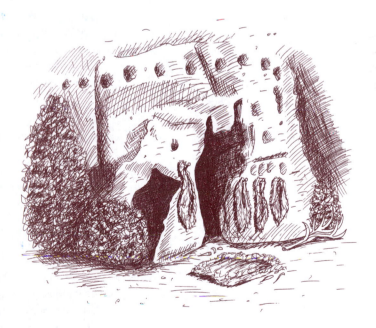

ing or digging, but not for precision handling. Fossils found in South Africa, which date back about 2-1/2 million years, also have the hand structure of a potential tool user and tool-maker. The long thumb had the saddle-shaped joint for opposition, and the straight bones of the fingers were broad at the tips. Two-million-year-old bones found at Olduvai Gorge in Tanzania, East Africa, had simple pebble tools nearby. Louis and Mary Leakey, who discovered them, named these fossil remains *Homo habilis*, or "handyman." It is not at all surprising that hominids were identified through occupation even millions of years ago because it was the adaptive interaction through occupation of the existing structures of hand, eye, and brain that shaped them.

Hand: Tool of the Mind

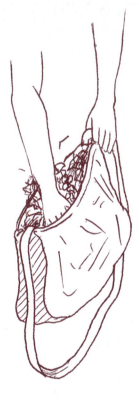

Structure alone cannot explain the skillful adaptive ability of the human hand engaged in occupation. Most of the elements of the hand structure are available to other primates. However, along with the minimally necessary hand structural elements described above was the human nervous system that controlled them. The nervous system is plastic. That is, it changes with experience. Its plasticity is a major source of human adaptability. From conception, individual cellular structures differ with our differing DNA, and the unique history of each developing embryo forms in time and with experience. Even our brains, with similar structures and familiar form, are shaped individually through an adaptive selectionist process in which our interactions with the intrauterine and later the extrauterine environment determine which cells will function and which will remain unused and die away. Thus, for the hand-eye-brain connection, determining which changes came first and which later is like trying to sequence the chicken and the egg.

Important changes in the brain occurred as the hand was freed from quadripedal locomotion and became an interface between the hominid and the environment (Paillard, 1993). In the human brain, the cortex or surface of the brain includes areas of cells that control movement. This motor cortex uses almost one-third of its area for direct control of voluntary movements of the hand and fingers. Through this greatly enlarged control system and a similarly large sensory area for the touch information from the hand, the fine motor skills for the extensive dexterity of the human hand make possible occupations requiring delicate control and skill. As in our arboreal ancestors, an important portion of the neocerebellum of the brain controls the placement of the hand in space for reach, grasp, and transport of objects. It is also involved in the links that initiate skilled sequences of movement (such as playing the piano or typing) and support eye-hand coordination.

Closely related to the development of hand function through changes within the brain were changes in vision. Binocular vision (with better depth perception for distance) has been proposed as a vital element in the ability to imagine the three-dimensional nature of objects and, thus, to encourage their exploration through manipulation of all sides of the object. In primates, different parts of the brain are responsible for vision relating to the space of the environment, the position of body parts within that space, and in particular, the position of the hand in nearby space. In fact, some neurons fire only when the hand is grasping an object and others only when it is actually manipulating something. Although human skill learning depends heavily on visual information, the information for skilled control is usually from touch or the actual sensations of the skilled movement itself (*kinesthesia*). Thus the brain has developed extensive areas in which a variety of sensations (visual, tactile, and so forth) are related to movement sensations, in what are called *association areas*. This multimedia association in humans is much greater than that available to other primates. Through this association, the sensation of skilled action in occupation is incorporated into the control system for that action. Similarly, the multimedia perception of our actions is reflected in the premotor part of the brain's structure for initiating action. That is, there is a functional organization for relatively specific actions such as a particular form of grasp or bringing the hand to the mouth in eating. In other words, our brains are organized for functional occupation, not for muscle contraction or biomechanical aspects of movement. In just this way, our ability to use tools as an extension of our bodies and minds became possible.

In most animals, the brain functions in reaction to environmental stimulation. However, the human brain has developed extensive ability to perceive time and to link the past, present, and future to our actions. Such an awareness of the effect of action on the environment in the individual's past history becomes an important part of our planning for future goals and affects our actions in the present. Thus it is not so much the structures of the hand and eye or their neurological connections within the brain as it is the occupational goals and meanings of our skilled actions that are the real evolutionary success of the adaptive human. The long-term goal of the concert pianist to produce wonderful music is what makes possible the extensive learning and practice over time that develops the skills needed to reach the goal. Although it is possible, structurally and functionally, for many human hands to perform similarly, it is the occupational meaning to the individual that causes a few to acquire the hand coordination of the pianist.

As the hand changed over evolutionary time, it freed the mouth from its role in environmental interaction. Just as the sense of smell became less important with increased vision, the ability to taste and feel objects with the mouth is of slight importance in comparison to the information obtained from manipulation. In individual development, we see the infant move from early mouthing exploration of objects to later, skilled in-hand manipulation. The functional asymmetry of the brain, with the right hemisphere organizing object position in and movement through space, allows the left hemisphere to organize the elements of and movement through language. Elements and sequences of movement, especially for manual dexterity, are controlled by the right hemisphere, allowing the left to control the elements (vocabulary) and sequence (syntax) of language. Both are vital to the human's ability to make tools and use them functionally.

Dr. A. Jean Ayres, an occupational therapist, defined *praxis as the ideation, planing, and execution of movement* (1985). Similarly, we may think of speech as ideation, planning, and execution of language. Praxis is the language of action, just as speech is the language of words. Just as praxis supported the human's simple hand and development of tool use, language may have assisted us in taking tools from the hand and developing technologies such as machines and computers.

Tools, Technology, and Occupation

Objects can become tools—extensions of ourselves that increase our effective interactions with the environment. Our prehensile skills in gathering and manipulating objects meant that human tool use went far beyond that of the other animal tool users. Our mind meant that we could become toolmakers, and our technology stretches from the first use of sticks and rocks as the simplest technological toolkit for improving the success of our daily occupations of food gathering or hunting, to the complexity of our using the atom. Tool technology has increased the power available to humans in their interactions with the environment, from the addition of a rock for pounding to harnessing of the atom for production of nuclear power (Bunch & Hellemans, 1993). Human use of technology as a physical tool for interaction with

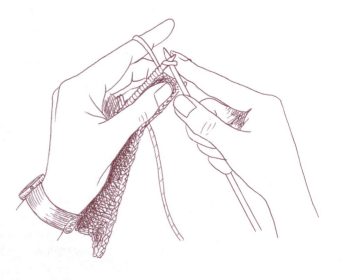

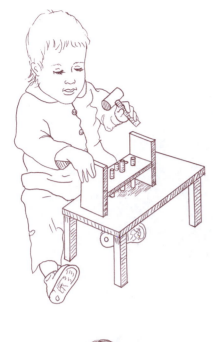

the environment can be seen as an adaptive selectionist process. New technology offers a culture an additional variation on its traditional ways of interacting with the environment and one that appears to be more successful than what has been previously available. Cultural adaptation occurs by training the young, through play and education, to use the technology. This selects and reproduces the successful adaptive technology in future generations.

Tool Use and Toolmaking

Many animals use found objects for tools. Along the central California coast, a favorite tourist attraction is watching the sea otters, floating on their backs, using flat rocks balanced on their chests as anvils on which to hit abalone shells and crack them open for luxurious dining. Many birds use similar techniques, holding a snail in their beaks and pounding it on a rock to break its shell into pieces, or conversely, picking up a rock in their beaks and dropping it on the shell. Such tool use is an example of using the materials that exist.

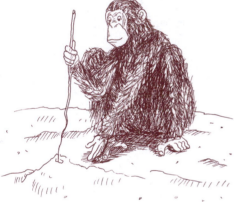

Dr. Jane Goodall, the famous anthropologist and occupational therapy faculty member at the University of Southern California, has described tool use in the chimpanzee community she observed for over 30 years at Gombe Reserve in Tanzania (1986). Chimpanzees "fish" in the termite mounds by selecting twigs of the appropriate length and thickness, stripping off excess leaves, and then poking the twig into the mound. When it is pulled out, some termites can be found clinging to the twig, and they become snacks for the chimps. Such tool use is the more complex modification of existing materials.

These forms of tool use and tool modification (Napier, 1993) are not uniquely human occupations, although human hand-eye coordination may make the task easier. However, toolmaking is an activity in which a naturally occurring object is changed to use in a way that is not a part of its natural form (Napier, 1993). It is a process in which the goal tool is not a *percept* (a representation of a concrete external thing), but a *concept* (a representation of an abstraction of a thing). The resultant tool is a memory or idea in the mind of the toolmaker and is not evident on looking at the original object.

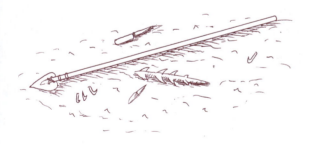

That is, a *made* tool exists first in the mind of the maker and only later in the hand. Technology further differentiates between primary and secondary tools, and that classification also depends on the mind of the user. A *primary* tool is one that is applied directly to the task, such as a knife used for killing an animal for food. A *secondary* tool may look the same (another knife), but it becomes secondary when it is used to shape a simple spear for killing animals for food. In other words, classifications of tools are not based on the objects themselves but on the purpose that the mind of the maker has for it. As such, our hands can be seen as simple or complex tools of our mind, as primary or secondary ones, depending on the particular occupation and the meaning and purpose we have in mind for them.

Ancient Technologies

Stone Age Technologies

Making simple tools was guided by the meaning and purpose of daily occupational needs of early humans and handcrafted in a variety of ways. Because of their slow perishability, rocks provide some of the earliest records of human tool use and modification, and of toolmaking. The Stone Ages of hominid evolution are identified by these tools. Simple peb-

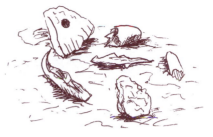

ble tools—stone choppers formed by striking off a chunk or flake to form a relatively flat edge for pounding or a sharp edge for cutting—were found with remains of *Homo habilis* from about 2-1/2 million years ago. Tools called hand axes were found with fossilized remains of *Homo erectus,* from about 1 million years later. This general-purpose tool had two surfaces flaked away, providing a better cutting edge, with the natural shape of the stone providing a smooth rounded surface for a handheld power grip. About 500,000 years ago, *Homo erectus* had tool kits consisting of a variety of flakes from such stone working. These more specialized tools might have been used to scrape hides for use as coverings, to slice or cut hides or food into pieces, and even to use as spokeshaves, the tools that shape a branch into a spear.

Old Stone Age *Homo habilis,* according to fossil records, were gatherers of roots, vegetables, and fruits. They may have hunted small animals but were probably scavengers of larger animals. Activities of daily living were primarily about obtaining sufficient food. Gathering, scavenging, and some hunting by all available individuals were needed. During daylight, focused work was necessary to maintain life. However, increased climate variation produced several thousands of years of *glaciation* (so-called "ice ages"), followed by longer periods of more temperate interglacial periods. Although interglacial periods had more lush vegetation and better animal food supplies in the temperate zones of earth, they produced desert-like conditions in more equatorial areas where hominids had flourished. As competition for food and water increased, migration into the temperate zones of Europe and Asia occurred. However, this migration introduced needs for adaptation to new vegetation, animals, and seasonal changes. Such needs may have been better met by skilled tool users, including the later species of our genus *Homo.*

In addition to *Homo erectus*'s skilled use of flake tools, there is evidence that *Homo erectus* were the first creatures on earth to control fire, one of the defining characteristics of humanity. However, there is no indication that they were able to start fires as needed. Members of this species built shelters that allowed them to live in the colder climates of the temperate zone, an important adaptation.

The knowledge and skills required for stone chipping are evidenced at several levels. There appear to have been master crafters who produced the best results and another level of tool makers who produced more varied results but the highest production. A low level of skill, probably of learners, is also evidenced. The basic conditions for reproducing the skill of the stone knappers or any other occupations are the availability of a skilled model, the ability to observe and learn, and manual skill. Language is not necessary, although gestures for communication would be helpful. All of these conditions appear to have been widely present in our ancestors, even in the Stone Ages.

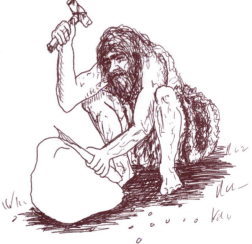

The Neanderthals, although not ancestral to modern humans, are what we commonly picture as cavemen. They were a European race of hunters who lived about 75,000 years ago, and used a variety of general tools such as hand axes and flake tools for spearheads and knives. They also flaked more specialized tools for dismembering and cutting up the carcasses and skins of successfully hunted animals. They used the hides for clothes, blankets, and shelters constructed from wood or mammoth tusks and covered with skins, with hearths for warmth. They stored food, cared for each other (one fossil is an individual with severe arthritis), and buried their dead with ritual. Their lives were very hard, but social grouping and the development of a shared culture show that it was meaningful to them.

About 35,000 years ago, another race of *Homo sapiens,* Cro-Magnon, appeared and supplanted the Neanderthals, possibly because their more adaptive brain developed the use of speech. A vast technological leap forward also occurred as their large brains and dexterous hands refined stone technology through the development of blade tools. These fine stone tools were useful for arrowheads, harpoons, and points on spears. As they developed agriculture and farming, the use of domesticated plants and animals as a means of survival began, and the stone tools became farm tools such as sickles.

Biodegradable Tools and Materials for Occupation

There is no reason to believe that the first tools had to be stone ones. Tools used even today by tribal peoples include biodegradable materials such as digging sticks of wood, containers of woven grasses, thongs from the stems of plants, and other tools of bark, bone, antler, horn, teeth, and leather. Surely those materials were used by Stone Age hominids as well, even if no evidence has survived the passage of time. Probably wood, plant parts, animal parts, and clay were first used in their original forms. Early spears and harpoons had the stone points fastened onto them. The materials for handles and bindings were biodegradable so that only by studying the stone blades can we surmise that they were formed to fit between split wood shafts or provided a groove to accommodate lashing. With increased planning skills (that is, the ability to use the past to attempt to control the future, a temporal adaptation), modification of the forms probably occurred, followed by actual toolmaking. The ancient woodworker was probably much more knowledgeable of raw materials, choosing a tree that required the least shaping and joining. In contrast, today's woodworker tends to work from a selection of standardized wood stock, using an extensive array of tools to "put it together" again.

Other forms of occupation that have been lost to time include basketry. Most peoples of the world were engaged in basketry when the European cultures met them. It seems probable that these skills extend back into prehistory. Basketry has primarily been a craft of women, perhaps because it can be set aside and picked up later with little disruption, as has been true of many women's occupations. It probably used materials that were associated with women's food-gathering activities, rather than men's hunting tasks for which the stone points of male craftsmen might have been used. Baskets were tools that extended the use of the hands for carrying, collecting, and storing loose items such as foodstuffs and seeds (and babies who might wander off). Most ancient basket remains give evidence of decoration via patterns of weaving or use of dyed materials. The combined meaning of such an occupation as basket weaving was already overlapping any possible role definitions—it was productive, pleasurable, and perhaps restorative as experienced by the weaver, and it provided a useful object with a variety of symbolic levels for interpretation by the observer. Weaving of fabric from wool and flax was a late Stone Age technology, and we have every reason to believe that variations in yarn were used for decorative and symbolic purposes as well.

Leatherwork was probably produced by people since the first hunters killed animals for food. Hides might have been used for shelter, bedding, and body covering. Awls for piercing leather and needles that could have been used for joining pieces are among Paleolithic finds. The tanning of leather is a complex process that, in many cultures, developed as a necessary but low-caste occupation, partly because of the nature of the materials (skins of animals) and their accompanying smells.

Ceramics were probably one of the first synthetic materials developed by human technology. The step from sun-dried adobe clay bricks to ceramics is not so great as is the control of fire, which made ceramics possible. Once the clay is heated and the water is driven off, the process becomes irreversible. About 50,000 years ago, ovens that might have been kilns existed. The non-nomadic life of agriculture was suited to this development more than was that of hunting. Hand shaping of clay for pottery was the technique available until the technology of the potter's wheel developed about 5000 years ago. Ceramic body ornaments were also common, and the decoration of pottery for daily use seems to arise naturally out of the plastic nature of the clay and the symbolic thought processes of humans.

The Metal Ages

The so-called metal ages (Bronze Age, Copper Age, and Iron Age), about 6000 or 7000 years ago, incorporated the agricultural revolution and the beginnings of what we call civilizations. For the average person, pottery and ceramics were still dominant and much more important to daily life than metals, which were used mainly by soldiers and technicians such as builders. Politically, civilizations arise when numerous villages are gathered under the control of a regional ruler. These rulers can have direct effects on technology and its use. They can order large numbers of people to work together on projects such as the pyramids. They support the development of labor specialization. With specialization, the gradual development of towns and cities, with their different needs from agricultural communities, occurs. Rulers may engage in warfare, which has been suggested as a major source of technological change throughout the ages, including in our contemporary society. The metal ages were the beginning of known history when written language was developed as a form of communication. With the rise of towns and cities and specialization of labor within them, the storage of food and materials and trade of resources for products and vice versa required more extensive record keeping than simple tally marks.

The Industrial Revolution

The use of tools has always been considered an extension of or increase in human abilities: the stone axe with handle offered more power and a harder and sharper surface than the human hand, leather and cloth provided more warmth than a cover of skin alone, and the forces of nature, water, and wind also were controlled as tools for human occupation. The waterwheel provided more power for grinding grain and powered saws for cutting building materials. Great ships using the wind in their sails explored the globe.

In the history of technology (Bunch & Hellemans, 1993), we see the changes as exponential. That is, across millions of years, we see evidence of slow adaptive changes. This is followed by a period of just thousands of years in which metals began to be used. Then, as we consider the Industrial Revolution, we speak of technological change and changes in occupations (through tools and materials) within about 150 years.

The Industrial Revolution may be defined in several ways. If it is the beginning of using power sources other than human and animal, then it is early in the evolution of the hominid, with the use of tools themselves. If it is viewed as the use of machines, then even the simple wheel defines its beginning. If it is defined by a major change in materials, then the metal-age production of iron would qualify. If the definition of industrialization is linked to the place and standardization of human occupation, however, we see the mid-18th century as a starting point. Textile workers, or weavers, started using a new shuttle that allowed them to weave so fast that they ran out of yarn. Invention of the spinning jenny solved the problems of increasing production of one type of yarn that was needed, but the second type of yarn production was increased by the use of another machine, the water frame. The water frame was too large and too expensive to put in the cottage of the weaver, so factories were built where textile weaving took place within a standardized workday, synchronized to the needs of the materials and machines, not the people.

With the use of the gaslight in the early 19th century, workers' schedules were not limited by shorter winter daylight, and round-the-clock production made better use of the factories, if not of the second- and third-shift workers. Jobs opened up, and cities grew. Industrial society moved from a closeness with nature, which had been the occupational rhythm of the hunter-gatherer and agricultural societies, to one with sharp divisions between work, rest, and play. The concept of balance of work, rest, and play that is mentioned in early occupational therapy literature reflects the labor movement's pressure to limit work to an 8-hour day, with 8 hours for sleep and the other 8 for self-care and play. A major byproduct and exemplar of the industrial age is the automobile, stamping the assembly-line method of industrial production as the primary one.

The Electronic and Information Age

The 20th century can, for the most part, be technologically considered the electric and electronic age. The Industrial Revolution began regional pollution of waterways and land, and the use of coal for generating electricity began to pollute the air. Anyone living in Los Angeles today and struggling with the smog problem may need to be reminded that early 20th century London had hundreds of smog deaths each year from the coal burned for heating and generating electricity. Our awareness of the byproducts of our technological advances (such as smog) and their effects on our occupations (reduce auto trips, don't play outside) has improved significantly as have many of our efforts to maintain our environmental health.

The communications improvements with the telephone, radio, and television, and technological gains from the vacuum tube through the transistor and printed circuit board formed the basis for the later third of the century's becoming known as the information age. The computer is a major tool of this information age and the World Wide Web, the sign of its exponential growth. Linked globally by fiber-optic satellites, our communications are truly beginning to connect the world.

The Evolutionary Template of Today's Occupational Patterns

Although we usually do not recognize it, human evolution has placed a broad template on our daily experiences that cannot be avoided. The facts that we walk upright, are tool users, have slow-maturing young, and use lots of material objects for our survival seem so familiar that we do not even recognize how unique and different from other animals on this planet we are. But, so what? What difference does it really make to us as people or as therapists? The answer to that, of course, is that it only makes a difference if we are looking for ways to be truly great therapists. When you see a person who, through an acquired disability, is deprived of abilities so central to our human evolution as are eye-hand coordination and upright walking, then you will see how this strikes at the very humanness of that person. When, through economic hardship, a person is without shelter and homeless on the streets, you will see the pain of falling outside the template of human evolutionary adaptation. A sense of this basic evolutionary stage on which our lives are acted gives us as therapists a sense of the importance to humanness of regaining these key capacities.

Key Concepts for Strengthening Insight into the Evolution of Human Occupations

- Adaptation
- Natural selection
- Bipedal stance
- The human hand
- Eye-hand coordination
- Tools and technologies
- Shelter, clothing, fire
- Stone tools
- Basketry, woodwork, leatherwork, and pottery
- Metal and the wheel
- Industries
- Electronic and computer work

Building Insight into the Evolutionary Template Shaping Your Own Occupations

1. Reflect on the following, in discussion with others, as a journal entry, or as a more formal paper or poster presentation:

- Are you a computer user? How does using a computer affect your writing style?
- Have you noticed a change in awareness of time when working on the computer?
- Do you think communication options such as the Internet are positive or negative influences of today's technology?
- Close your eyes and use your hands to explore something in your environment. Pay close attention to the sensory experience of exploring with touch. What have you learned that you could not know from vision?
- What are some occupations you enjoy in which the use of your hands is as important as the use of your eyes?
- Write about an experience you have had adapting to a new environment, such as moving to a new residence or visiting another country. What are some of the adaptations you made to this environment?
- What are some of the things you do frequently that use the power grip of your hands? What things require precision grip? What occupations require skilled control of fingers and hand for movement or manipulation?
- Scout leaders suggest that hikers should carry a bag with 10 basic survival items for back-country hikes. These are small survival tools.

POWER BUILDERS

What are some of your "survival tools" for your daily life? What are some of your favorite tools? What daily occupations are they used for?

- What do you think the daily round of occupations entailed for Stone Age hominids? How were their occupational patterns different from our own? How were they the same?

- Think about the effect of the industrial age on daily occupations. Have you ever worked other than a dayshift or known about the life of someone who did? How does it affect one's habits or produce a need for creative designing of occupational routines?

- Have you ever worked on an assembly line or known someone who did? What ways do people use to adapt to the controlled sequence of the assembly-line activity?

- Have you spent time as an automobile commuter, or do you know someone who has? What forms of occupation are nested within the commute?

2. Make something of wood, leather, or basketry materials, using no more than two modern tools. What would it be like to do this with only flint tools?

3. Go into a usual workspace for yourself, such as your kitchen or study. Sit down on the floor, giving up your bipedal posture. How well does the space fit you now that you are a quadripedal being? What would have to be changed to make it functional for you again? Are there some activities you would no longer be able to do?

4. Study or draw your hand for 15 minutes minimum.

5. Sit and watch a fire for 15 minutes minimum.

Building Insight into How the Evolutionary Template Shapes the Occupations of Others

1. Spend 15 minutes watching an infant use his or her hands. Write an accurate description (no more than 1 page single-spaced) of how this infant uses his or her hands, including types of grasps, objects with which the infant interacts, how the rest of the body supported or did not support the hand use, and other points you notice.

2. Interview someone who has recently moved concerning what adaptations of occupational pattern had to be made to fit the new space, how objects (such as furniture, utensils, television) had to be placed differently and the effects this had, and other observations of how the relocation has changed daily life.

3. In a group, construct a shelter from tarps, blankets, cardboard boxes, and other large pieces of flat material that you can find (bringing tents is cheating). Spend the night in your constructed shelter. In the morning, share your thoughts about what it would have been like to live nomadically in Neolithic times, and what it would be like to live homeless today. Which does the group think would be a better life?

4. Do an observation of a craftsperson who works in basketry, wood, leather, or clay for a minimum of 1 hour. Use an observation guide that cues you to observe hand use, stance, eye-hand coordination, tools and materials, and products. Write up your observation.

5. Go on an expedition, either on your own or with a group, to an industrial worksite of some kind. (Get permission if necessary.) Observe for a minimum of 1 hour. Use an observation guide that cues you to observe hand use, stance, eye-hand coordination, tools and materials, and products. Write up your observation.

6. Do an observation of an occupational therapist. Use an observation guide that cues you to observe hand use, stance, eye-hand coordination, tools and materials, and products. Write up your observation.

7. Assemble a group of clippings from magazines and newspapers illustrating hand use in all its varieties. This can be done as a group, posting the clippings on a wall or bulletin board for discussion, or on your own and used to create a collage.

8. Take away your vision, either through taped-over glasses or a blindfold. Try to do something that is very routine for you and does not seem to depend entirely on vision, such as brushing your teeth. This is how it feels to fall outside the evolutionary template for smoothly performing everyday occupations.

9. Spend 1 day keeping track on a small pad of all the machine-manufactured items with which you come into direct contact. At the end of the day, count them. Compare results with someone else's.

10. Select a case from Appendix A. Write an essay describing how this person with the same disability in prehistoric times would have lived.

11. Put socks over your hands for 3 hours and do not use them. Discuss this experience with others.

12. Select a case, a disability narrative, or an occupational narrative from Appendix A. Select one of the following aspects of the human evolutionary template, and write an essay analyzing its importance in the life of the individual described in your selection (no more than 2 pages double-spaced): eye-hand-brain coordination, tools and materials, adaptation to change.

Building Design Skills Using the Evolutionary Template

1. Use a seven-step design process as you create a wood, leather, basketry, or clay product that you have never tried before. This can be done on your own, with a group going through all the phases together, or a group sharing their experiences as each does the phases independently.

2. On your own or in a group, use a seven-step design process to create and provide a learning experience about some aspect of the human evolutionary template to a person or group.

POWER BUILDERS

3. For this Power Builder, you will need some type of nonbipedal movement device (scooter boards or wheelchairs, for example). On your own or in a group, create and carry out the following definition: "Provide an obstacle-course experience for nonbipedal humans." Use the following design strategies: brainstorming, simple ranking with three criteria, time/task, and reflective discussion on the design process itself.

4. Select a case from Appendix A and plan treatment for that individual that focuses on either eye-hand coordination, tool use, or adaptation to change. Use the following steps: write a goal, brainstorm at least 20 ideas for intervention, rank and weigh with 3 criteria, and end with a brief description of the materials and tasks required to carry out the intervention.

5. Make one improvement in one of your usual occupational spaces, such as your kitchen, bathroom, or study area, using all the following strategies: brainstorm, rank with two criteria, use a time/task chart, and write reflectively on how well it worked based on your criteria.

6. Perform an ergonomic assessment and write-up of an individual's work area, using a seven-step design process and producing a written recommendation for changes in the workspace.

References

Ayres, A. J. (1985). *Developmental dyspraxia and adult onset apraxia.* Torrance, CA: Sensory Integration International.

Bunch, B., & Hellemans, A. (1993). *The timetables of technology. A chronology of the most important people and events in the history of technology.* New York: Touchstone Press.

Edelman, G. M. (1992). *Bright air, brilliant fire. On the matter of the mind.* New York: Basic Books.

Goodall, J. (1986). *The chimpanzees of Gombe.* Cambridge, MA: Harvard University Press.

Lewis, O. J. (1989). *Functional morphology of the evolving hand and foot.* Oxford: Clarendon Press.

Napier, J. R. (1993). *Hands* (rev. ed.). Princeton, NJ: Princeton University Press.

Paillard, J. (1993). The hand and the tool: The functional architecture of human technical skills. In A. Berthelet & J. Chavaillon (Eds.), *The use of tools by human and non-human primates* (pp. 36-46). Oxford: Clarendon Press.

Zemke, R., & Horger, M. (1995). Hands: Tools for crafting human adaptation. Lesson 1 in C. Royeen (Ed.), *Hands on: Practical interventions for the hand.* AOTA Self-paced clinical course. Bethesda, MD: American Occupational Therapy Association.

CHAPTER 9

The Spatial Dimension of Occupations

The Body as the House of the Occupational Self
The Occupational Environment
Material Culture as Human Adaptation
Social Meanings of Occupational Spaces
Treatment Space

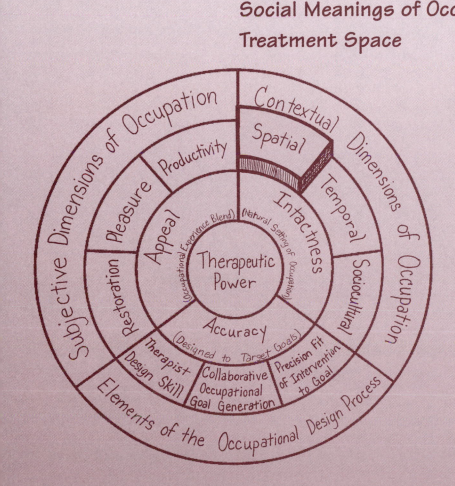

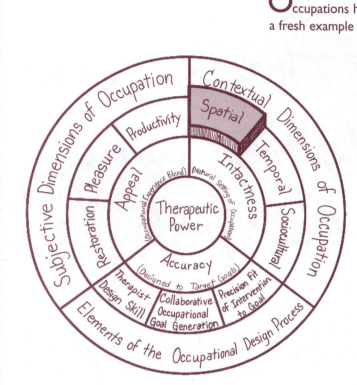

Occupations have a spatial dimension, or shape. It is easiest to see this shape by using a fresh example from your own experience. Think of something you did today—anything at all. Now, first consider the body from which you are acting, your own body. Were you energetic, tired, focused, brain weary, standing up, lying down, moving around, feeling a variety of sensations? Were you disabled or restricted from your usual abilities in any way? If you mapped out your movements from the beginning to the end of the occupation, what would be the shape of that movement? Is the movement a single point for no motion while you sat and read, or a zigzagging and overlapping line for all the movements around and about your kitchen as you cooked up a big pot of spaghetti? All of our occupations are experienced from the base, or house, of our own bodies and their conditions at that time. This is a part of what makes each occupation unique. Now, think of the conditions of the environment in which the occupation occurred and how they affected your experience: light, sound, smells. Consider all the human-made and natural objects involved in the occupation: tools, your clothing, the building, maybe a vehicle. Were you sharing space with others? How close did you stand, how often did your gazes meet, what was the social meaning of the space? In the one occupational experience that you picked to think about, all of these aspects of its spatial dimension make important contributions to its shape.

To be a masterful practitioner of occupation-based intervention requires a sophisticated understanding of the spatial dimension of occupation. The shape of occupations often goes unseen and unused in intervention. The

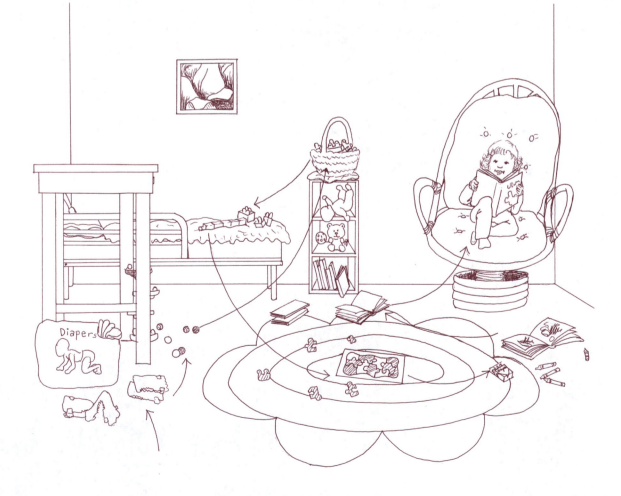

spatial dimension of occupation is so familiar that we cannot recognize and apply it without good theoretical training. If you can begin to see the shape of your own occupations and from that build insight into the shape of others' occupations, you are well on your way to expert and effective therapeutic interventions that use the spatial dimension to meet the needs and goals of your clients.

The Body as the House of the Occupational Self

Each of us is housed within a physical body. We see our bodies as the location of our selves. Gazing out from the vantage point of the physical body, we perceive the world around us in relation to our physical capacities to perceive, move through, and make use of the spaces and objects surrounding us. Physical evolution has provided us with a perspective on the world that is uniquely human. We do not hear or smell as well as dogs, yet we do have quite sophisticated senses of vision and touch. The most basic aspect of the spatial dimension of our occupations is our experience of those occupations from the standpoint of a physical body.

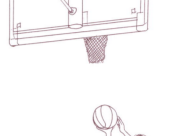

Vision: The Spatial Sense

Vision is the primary sense of spatial perception. Gaze leads our interactions with the physical world. Walking upright, we can see long distances from the vantage point of height. We can see things from different angles as we travel through, across, under, over, and around them. James Gibson (1986), at the peak of a distinguished career of research into visual perception, proposed a revolutionary ecological approach to visual perception. His theorized that it is not simply the processing of visual stimuli that results in our understanding of the environment and its objects. Rather, Gibson proposed that we actively discover the properties and uses of the physical environment through our interactions with it as we engage in everyday activities. In contrast with more traditional neurophysiological explanations of perception, Gibson's active and ecological view of perception is highly congruent with an understanding of the engaged and spatially contexted experience of occupations.

We Meet the World with a Hand

If vision is our primary sense of spatial perception, then the hand is our primary physical interface with the spaces and objects around us. Our opposable thumb provides such dexterity for interacting with the physical world that humans have evolved a complex culture of object making and using. The density of sensory receptors in our fingertips supplies a rich flow of information about the texture, temperature, and shape of the objects and surfaces with which we interact. Our eye-hand coordination is highly sophisticated, allowing us to bring objects up to the eyes and turn them for inspection and to complete intricate manipulations of objects. The human hand is a miracle of functionality. It allows a variety of types of grasps for different situations: fingertip pinch, power grasp, palmar grasp, key pinch, and tripod grip. The complexity of human culture depends heavily on the

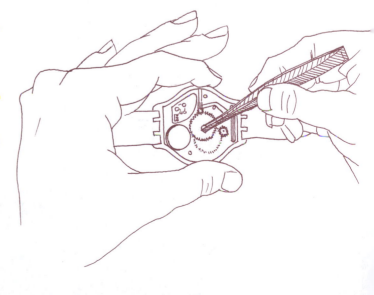

abilities of the human hand to serve as a sophisticated physical interface of the human body with the material world (Pierce, 1996).

Embodiedness

Our physical bodies interact with the spaces and objects around them without a need for us to conceptualize those actions. It is through the hand that humans contact and make use of the physical world. Over development, through years of experience with physical action, we acquire an "embodied intelligence" (Benner & Wrubel, 1989, p. 42) that knows how to perceive, move through, and interact with the world. Expert therapists display this sort of phenomenological knowing in their abilities to accomplish complex therapeutic tasks in seemingly effortless ways (Mattingly & Fleming, 1994). When asked to explain what they are doing, it is difficult for them to put it into words because it is a physical knowing, rather than an abstract reasoning process. This ability of the body to intelligently act within the physical environment is taken for granted until it is disrupted.

Of course, each person has his or her own distinct makeup of physical skills and limitations. The physical bodies of individuals differ greatly because of gender, growth and aging, illness, and disability. In Western culture, we tend to think of the adult male as the standard for a "typical" physical body and all other physical makeups as variations or somewhat deviant from the norm. Thus, infants are viewed as still too small and unskilled, women as weak and hormonal, elders as less fit than they should be, and a person with a disability as less deserving of inclusion in the social world. Yet, the unique embodiedness of each of us offers a one-of-a-kind perspectives on the world.

The type of work done by an individual can have physical effects on his or her body. For example, in a study of police and clerical workers, significant differences were found in levels of stress and arousal on work and nonwork days (McLaren, 1997). In research on assembly-line workers, physical positions and spatial arrangement of workspaces had a significant effect on back pain and health (Duquette, Lortie, & Rossignol, 1997). Many groups of workers have clearly identified risks of physical injury related to the type of activity in which they are engaged on the job.

In occupational therapy, we often work with individuals who are stigmatized for the ways in which their bodies differ from the norm. They often have less power over their lives than others do because of prejudice brought on by their illnesses or disabilities. It is critical that occupational therapists work through and beyond these common attitudes of their own cultures, to truly understand what it is like to live from within the house of a client's particular body and know how to assist in overcoming any barriers that are preventing that client from engaging in occupations important to him or her. In helping a person with a newly acquired physical limitation, it is critical for therapists to comprehend, empathize with, have patience with, and assist wherever possible in the emotional and functional demands brought on by these limitations. Despite our differences, we all share

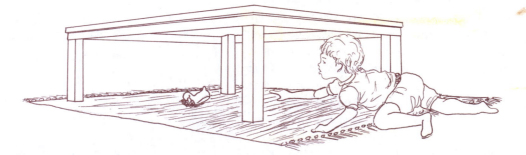

the same basic necessity to sense, move through, and interact with the spaces and objects around us to engage in occupations (Murphy, 1987; Sacks, 1993; Zola, 1982).

Working on Physical Function

Occupational therapy intervention often uses valued occupations to produce therapeutic changes in the physical body, especially following a suddenly acquired disability, such as from a stroke or traumatic brain injury. This type of practice is often labeled as using a *traditional, physical disabilities,* or *biomechanical* approach to treatment because these approaches emphasize physical change. Thinking of an individual's intervention needs primarily in terms of the physical capacities of his or her body is highly congruent with a medical model of thinking about clients. Changes in physical function tend to be more highly valued within the medical world of hospital-based practice than are changes in the ability to engage in occupations specifically valued by the individual. Physical disabilities practice is often highly appealing to new therapists because our culture so highly values the medical perspective on illness and healing, giving status to those who can produce such physical changes in people. Also, biomechanical goals, such as improving the range of motion in a joint, are appealing in their clarity, concreteness, and measurability. However, as therapists gain experience and are ready for more complex challenges in their practices, they tend to take a more holistic and functional view of changes in physical ability and also to evolve a more occupation-based approach to goal setting with clients.

Activities of Daily Living

A group of activities that are primarily concerned with immediate physiological space are self-care activities. These include bathing, toileting, grooming, dressing, and other seemingly simple things we do each day to care for our bodies. Activities of daily living (ADLs) are an area of expertise for which occupational therapists are well known. Although such routine self-care occupations can seem mundane and commonsense, the loss of abilities to engage in such basics of everyday life can severely impair an individual's function, self-esteem, and independence. Because their abilities to do self-care activities are so critically important to our clients, occupational therapists cultivate a specialized understanding of ADLs and the adaptations that can make them possible.

The Occupational Environment

The spatial dimensions of occupation are far more complex than the simple measures of height, width, and length with which we would describe the spatial dimensions of, for example, a room. Occupational therapists must understand human bodies and spaces to such a degree of sophistication that their designs of the spatial context of interventions will increase their positive effects. That is, decisions about where to treat, the conditions of that environment, the objects that need to be available or that present barriers, and the social meaning of that space to the individual play a critical role in the success of the intervention. Developing a sophisticated view of environmental space requires an understanding of the multisensory nature of spatial experience, the way spaces fit or do not fit the physiological dimensions of different individuals, the way in which human skills for negotiating spaces develops, the unique human activities that emphasize the exploration and enjoyment of the spatial environment, and some of the more common ways in which occupational therapists intervene by adapting the spaces of occupations.

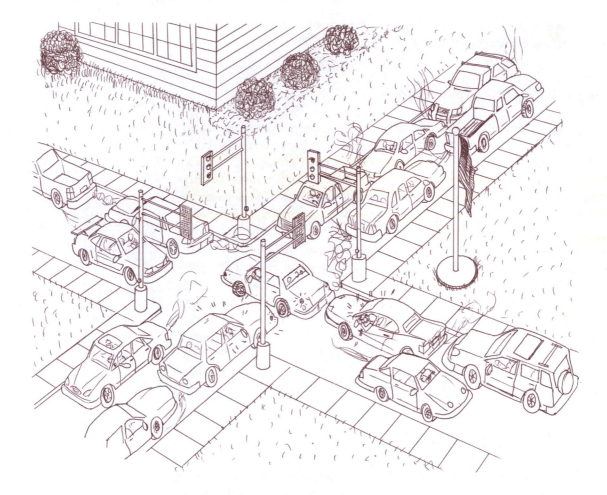

The Effects of Environmental Qualities

In the field of environmental psychology, much research has been done into the qualities of spatial environments and how they affect experience (Gallagher, 1993; Hiss, 1990; Holohan, 1986; Oborne & Gruneburg, 1983). The focus of this research has been on how workers are affected by types and levels of sound, various toxins or pollutants, light conditions, and safety and risk involved with equipment and manufacturing processes. These studies demonstrate the multisensory nature of the spatial dimension of occupation. As an individual engages in an occupation, the experience that he or she has is not simply affected by the size of the space, but also can be influenced by how the space is lit, its air quality, noise levels and distractions, and the stress of hazards. A study of noise levels in emergency rooms, for example, found that the noise levels approximated those determined to cause consistent feelings of annoyance and stress in the workers in those settings (Buelow, 2001). To experience the degree to which the environment affects your mood, simply pay attention to how you feel when in different settings over the course of a day in which you are doing some traveling. Try an open park, an industrial area, an urban center with tall buildings, a suburb, and a roadside along a field.

Environmental Affordances

Another aspect of the spatial dimension of experience is the opportunities, or "affordances" (Gibson, 1986) that the environment provides to a particular individual. Gibson described the meaningful environment in terms of mediums, surfaces, and affordances.

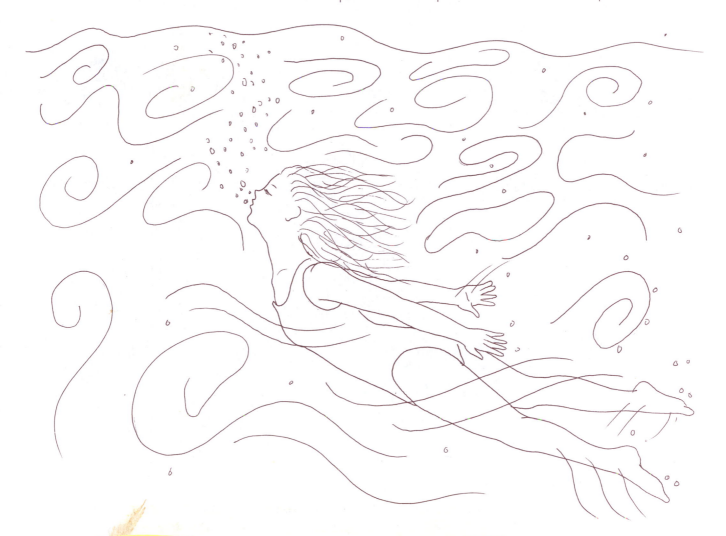

Mediums include liquids, solids, and gases. Each medium offers special characteristics in terms of breathing, locomotion, transmission of light and sound, chemical diffusion, and gravity. For example, water affords humans movement and buoyancy, but does not afford humans air for breathing. Where two mediums meet, such as where earth and air meet, there is a surface. *Surfaces* are the areas of the environment at which most perception and action occur. You could say that all the action is happening at the surfaces. *Affordances* are the specific opportunities that a surface provides to an animal or a human. For instance, a large and level piece of ground affords humans support. It can be stood on, walked or run on, and danced on. It cannot, however, be dipped into, poured, or waded through, as could an air-water surface.

An occupational therapist must also understand that affordances differ for different individuals. The affordance depends on the embodiment, perception, and developmental history of the individual. The same grassy hillside in a park may constitute for an infant a green blur of no particular meaning, for a 10-year-old an exciting surface to roll down, for a young couple a place to lie on a blanket together, and for a person in a wheelchair an impossible barrier.

Mapping and Negotiating Space

Skills for negotiating the environment complexify with development. The child's perspective on surrounding space changes from an *egocentric* reference system, relating object

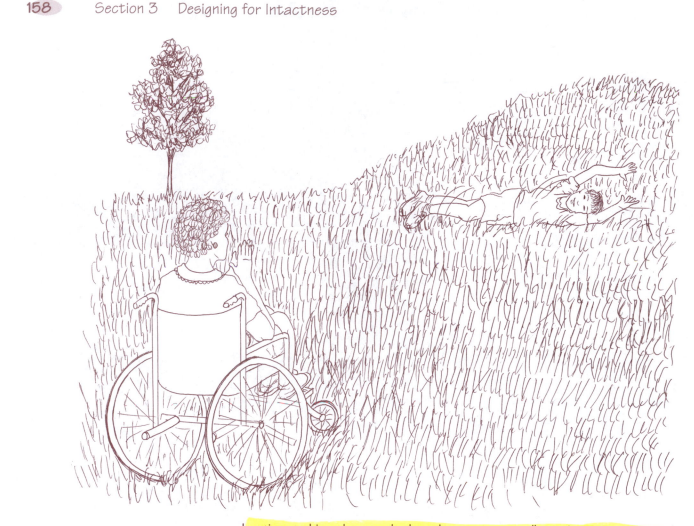

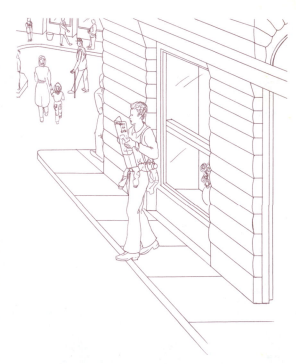

locations to his or her own body as the center, to an *allocentric* system, representing space in terms of a layout of the environment unrelated to the individual. Adults hold a fully coordinated reference system, in which they visualize the locations of themselves and others within large, abstract cognitive maps (Heft & Wohlwill, 1987; Piaget, 1952, 1962). Research on the development of spatial perception in infants, children, and adults demonstrates that they actually understand the world, not abstractly, but occupationally. That is, they recognize spaces as sites at which a certain activity takes place, know the paths between activity sites, and know that the maps are larger representations of how to move from one activity site to another (Hart, 1979; Moore, 1983; Pierce, 1996).

Two interesting sets of human activities seem to focus on spatial experience: those that emphasize viewing and visual sensation, and those that emphasize spatial negotiation or way-finding. Viewing occupations can be observed in the fascination of an infant with a crib mobile, children watching television, or adults viewing art in a museum. Humans seem to delight in seeking patterns in visual experience. Way-finding activities, such as hiking, driving, sailing, and mountain climbing, also emphasize visual input but include some spatial negotiation as well.

Ergonomics and Accessibility

The expertise of occupational therapists in the spatial dimension of occupational experience is especially useful in prevention of workplace injuries and architectural adaptations to home and work environments to improve accessibility for individuals with disabilities. *Ergonomics,* or the *kinesiology* of human occupation, is an area of specialization in occupational therapy. Therapists specialized in ergonomics often try to prevent repetitive motion injuries in workplaces by altering the ways in which equipment, computer workstations, and assembly-line workspaces are laid out. The advent of the Americans with Disabilities Act (ADA), which requires public places to be accessible to individuals with disability, has increased the numbers of occupational therapists doing accessibility work. Some occupational therapists are collaborating with architects, assisting them with the requirements of the ADA, special accommodations for elders, and other architectural accessibility and safety issues. The concept of universal design, creating spaces that fit and are accessible to all people, resonates equally for architects and occupational therapists (Mace, 2001). Occupational therapists also commonly do safety and accessibility assessments for individuals returning to home and/or work with newly acquired disabilities, such as spinal cord injuries. Such assessments often result in recommendations for changes in architecture, the addition of ramps, the reduction of safety hazards, and the addition of adaptive equipment to enable daily function in occupations important to the individual. Adaptations to the spaces of institutional settings, such as assisted living centers for elderly persons, can also improve the fit of the environment to the needs of individuals.

Material Culture as Human Adaptation

The space of human occupations is not empty. It is filled with meaningful objects. Humans have evolved a complex material culture as a way of adapting to the challenges of the environment (Chapple & Coon, 1942; Hodder, 1989). No less important than our bipedal stance and sophisticated neocortex is the evolution of a mode of living unique in the degree to which it depends on the creation and use of objects. No other animal depends on "stuff" for its survival as much as humans do. This material culture, its symbolic meanings, and its processes for manufacture are passed down and improved from one generation to the next. Thus we commonly interact with a wide variety of things in everyday human life: clothing, shelters, vehicles, tools, toys, crops, foods, medicines, domesticated animals, written documents, aesthetic and symbolic objects, and many others.

Tool Use and Dedicated Activity Spaces

Humans are tool users. Tools extend the capacities of the human body to act on the world. The variety of human tools today is enormous, from the tools of a mechanic, to those of a surgeon, to those of a computer graphic artist, to those of a mother. For a particular activity, a space will often be organized that includes the tools, large furnishings, and spatial qualities that support that work. For the mechanic, this may be a set of tools, a tool chest, a car lift, a garage, and the heat, lighting, and electricity required. For a mother of an infant in Western suburban culture, the tools will probably include toys; infant feeding and diapering supplies; various infant positioning devices such as a bouncer, high chair, and swing; infant furniture such as a bed and changing table; probably a stroller and a car seat for outings; and a home space that is conducive to infant health, sleep, and safety. People's dedicated workspaces and the tools they contain are typical examples of the way in which activities frequently engaged in occur in a spatial context that has grown up and developed around them. Just as the

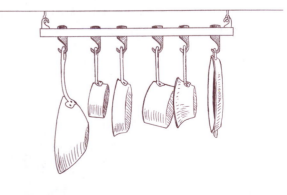

skills of the individual develop into the ability to engage in a certain type of activity, so too do customized activity spaces naturally develop where occupations occur. For this reason, attempting to engage a person in an occupation outside of the space in which it naturally or usually happens will be difficult, inauthentic, and interrupted by efforts to adapt to an impoverished setting.

Toys

The objects and spaces of childhood play are especially intriguing in the way they support and advance development. Bruner (1972) has argued that play is an evolutionary mechanism to bring the human infant to species-typical functioning, after being born necessarily immature to fit the infant brain case through the narrow upright pelvis. The abilities to use tools and solve problems develop best in the nonthreatening, novelty-seeking, fun activities of childhood play. Occupational therapists who work with children depend heavily on the objects and spaces of childhood play to assist them in working toward developmental goals. A pediatric occupational therapist is rarely without a bag of toys. Knowing which toys advance which skills and changing play activities to keep the child interested and engaged are the art of intervention with such young clients. Unlike adults, children are not likely to engage in a therapeutic occupation just because the therapist believes it will help them reach therapeutic goals. If it is not play, they are likely to refuse. This tendency of children to be more self-directed has exerted an irresistible pull on pediatric occupational therapists toward the use of whole occupations that are meaningful to their clients.

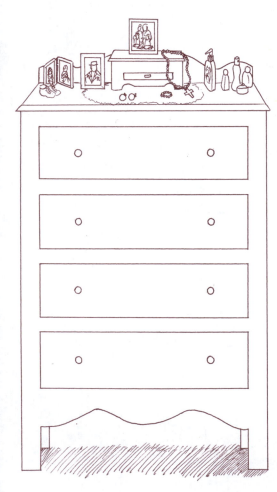

Symbolic Objects

Many of the objects in people's lives have great symbolic value and meaning for them (Csikszentmihalyi & Rochberg-Halton, 1981). When you enter someone's home, you will usually see these symbolic objects on display: family heirlooms, art, collections, and photographs. If you were to ask, you would hear the story that goes with each object. The variety and types of objects you see give you a feeling about who people are, their histories, and what they hold dear. Usually we think of these symbolic objects as being in the living room, on the mantel, or on the walls of the dining room or the kitchen. A similar perspective can be used to gain an understanding of individuals through objects in other, less public spaces. What a teenager picks to put on his or her bedroom walls, the items displayed in a basement workshop, or the furnishings of an office or break room say a lot about the people and valued occupations of that space. Occupational therapists learn to be acute observers of spatial features of the environment. Even when you are in a nursing home, where there may be room for only a couple of treasured items, asking about those objects or photos is an excellent start on building rapport with a client and beginning to understand him or her as an occupational being.

Mapping Routines onto Spaces

An interesting aspect of the spatial dimension of occupational experience is the way in which we map our routines onto familiar spaces in our homes and workplaces. Not only do these frequently repeated activities have a general sequence that is little changed from one time to the next, but also the locations of the objects that support routines within our usual spaces are highly predictable. In fact, this is what makes routines effective. Once we map our routines onto a space, object locations become predictable. We do not have to search for our toothbrushes or decide where to store them after we brush our teeth. Once established, a routine for where things are found and kept is easily followed, freeing our minds to think of other things during routine activities. This is why moving, natural disasters that destroy homes, or having to leave one's home to go to a skilled nursing facility can be so disruptive. Not only does the new space require mapping by the individual to way-find in the environment, but new routines must also be constructed and mapped onto the new space.

Most human occupational experiences include the use, creation, or maintenance of objects. Some activities that are particularly focused on interactions with objects include arts or crafts, different types of manufacturing and construction, cooking and housework, yard and building maintenance, and repair work. Reflecting a strong materialistic value set, Western culture is typified by individuals spending extensive amounts of time involved with the objects they own. What those objects are, and the occupations in which they are used, can tell the observant occupational therapist a significant amount about any individual.

Social Meanings of Occupational Spaces

Just as objects are imbued with history and value by the persons who use and display them, the spaces in which we live, work, and play also come to hold great personal significance for us. The space becomes a place filled with memories and associations (Rowles, 1991; Rubinstein & Parmalee, 1992). We shape the space to reflect who we are. Often our identities are strongly tied to the places in which we have grown up or worked for a long time, or where we engaged in particularly significant occupations in our lives. People who are displaced from places in which they have spent a long time can feel great loss. The destruction of a church, factory, farm, or home is more than the loss of the physical structure. That can be replaced. The true loss is of the ability to relive in that place all the routines and memories and experiences that occurred there. The places in our lives are a part of how we exist in the world, how we typically engage in and experience occupations. That is one reason why it is difficult to understand an individual's occupations when they are seen outside of those places, such as when a therapist assesses a client in a clinic. Without understanding the places in which the person is most accustomed to doing things, the therapist's understanding of how those things are done is necessarily limited.

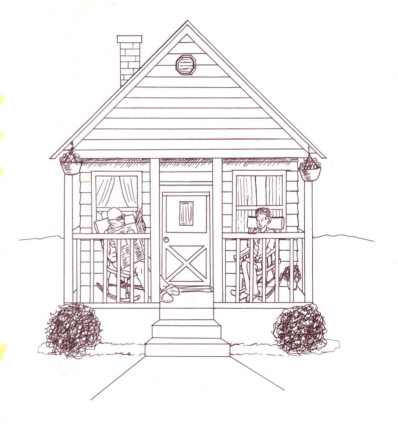

Public and Private, Sacred and Profane Space

Cultures share a recognition of which spaces are public and which are private (Hall, 1982). Think of the spaces in which you have spent time today, from waking up until now reading this page. There are probably very few people whom you would have felt completely comfortable having in your bedroom this morning as you slept. You may have been in a store, library, or restaurant today, however, where it would have made little difference to you if strangers came and went while you were there. Certain spaces are also considered sacred, in which only certain occupations can be appropriately engaged. For instance, it is not generally considered acceptable to play poker on a church altar or to set up a picnic in the middle of a baseball game. Sensitivity to the public/private and sacred/profane natures of occupational spaces is critical in practice. Although occupational therapists must sometimes work with occupations that are quite intimate, such as dressing and bathing, an awareness of the degree to which the therapist is being invited into an individual's private space can suggest ways of putting that individual at ease, such as by approaching the private space gradually and including a close family member for support.

Social Density of Space

Another especially social feature of the spatial dimension of occupational experience is the degree to which the occupational space is shared with others. The social density of a space can range from complete solitude to stressful overcrowding (Calhoun, 1962; Sarton, 1973). Depending on the individual and what he or she is doing, different social conditions of the space are desirable. For instance, concentrating on writing a book seems best done in solitude without the distractions of interacting with, or hearing the conversations of, others (Woolf, 1929/1981). Watching a baseball game, however, can be even more fun in the middle of a crowd of fans. In between, some things are best done with just a few people, or even with one other individual. If the person doing the activity feels that the social density of the space is about right, then it is. If he or she feels that the space is underpopulated or overpopulated, however, that mismatch will interfere with the occupational experience. A good example of this is the overcrowding of classrooms. Occupational therapists working with children with attention, learning, and behavioral problems in the schools know all too well how differently a child behaves and functions in a quiet room with the therapist, in a small quiet group of children, and in an overcrowded and noisy classroom.

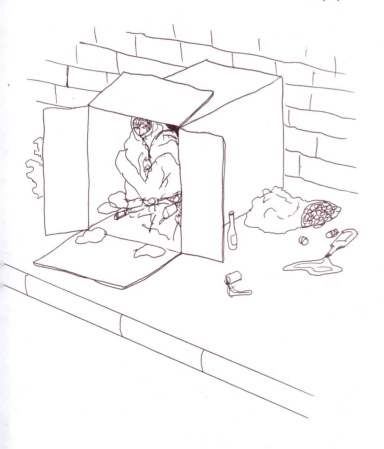

Space as Social Status

The amount and quality of the spaces we are given are also clear indicators of social status in Western culture. The big corner office with windows, the house on the ocean, the reserved table in front of the dinner speaker: all of these placements of individuals show they are considered important by those around them. In contrast, think of how unvalued you feel when crowded in a plane or subway, in a small cubicle without real walls, or in a small apartment with no open views. Space is accorded to those with power, money, and influence. Consider how a high-status executive who is accustomed to plenty of premium space must feel when he or she ends up in a shared hospital room. Imagine the feelings of the newly homeless.

Proxemics

An understanding of *proxemics,* the study of body language and proximity, offers many insights into the spatial dimension of an individual's occupational experience (Hall, 1982). Over years of practice, occupational therapists become highly skilled observers of proxemics. Body language can express mood, receptivity, engagement, level of comfort, and many other feelings important to the success of an intervention session. Eye contact and physical distance are primary indicators of comfort and attentiveness between individuals. Of course, these vary between cultures, so one must be informed as to the appropriate proxemic behavior in the culture of individual clients in order to judge the meaning of their proxemic responses. Eye contact and physical touch are especially variable between cultures. *Mirroring,* or taking on the same posture of another individual, is a particularly potent indicator of engagement and interest in another person. Occupational therapists, either intuitively or deliberately, use proxemics both as a way of communicating their own moods and feelings regarding the client's intervention and a way of interpreting the occupational experience that the client is having during the intervention.

Treatment Space

Just as you can tell a lot about a client by paying attention to his or her living space, so too can you tell a lot about an occupational therapist by his or her treatment space. Is the treatment space out in the community, within the natural settings of clients? Or is it a clinical space, designed more for the convenience and economies of the institution than for the effectiveness of intervention and comfort of patients? What kind of equipment and materials are used, and what kinds of activities do these imply as the primary modes of intervention? If you were to ask the therapist to describe his or her treatment space, to what degree would the client's perspective on that space play a part?

Occupational therapy and occupational science are only beginning to explore the spatial dimension of occupation. For this reason, the ideas presented here are not yet being applied to the fullest degree on behalf of those to whom we provide service. Each occupational experience has many spatial features. It has a rich shape. Comprehending this shape and how it may be enhancing or detracting from the quality of therapeutic occupations can be a powerful expertise. A silent observation by a master therapist of a therapeutic occupation as it occurs could expertly and immediately take in the impacts of physical embodiedness, environmental qualities, material culture, and the social meanings of space. This broad understanding of the spatial aspects of occupation can then be used to adapt the spatial dimension to better assist the client in engaging or re-engaging in valued occupations.

Treatment space must become, in our minds, not occupational therapy departments in healthcare facilities but the client's perception of physical, environmental, material, and social spaces during intervention. Treatment space must become the way in which we use space to effectively treat. The spatial dimension of occupation offers us rich and varied sources for comprehending our own occupational natures as well as greater intervention power as therapists to assist our clients.

POWER BUILDERS

Key Concepts for Strengthening Insight into the Spatial Dimension of Occupation

- Vision as spatial sense
- The hand as the human interface with the physical world
- ADLs
- Embodiedness
- Qualities of environmental space
- Affordances
- Mapping and negotiating space
- Ergonomics
- Accessibility
- Material culture
- Tools
- Symbolic meaning of objects
- Spatiality of routines
- Public/private, sacred/profane space
- Social density of space
- Space as indicator of social status
- Proxemics

Building Insight into the Spatial Dimension of Your Own Occupations

1. Reflect on the following, in discussion with others, as a journal entry, or as a more formal paper or poster presentation:

- In what type of space do you study or read best?
- What works well, or does not work well, in how your kitchen space is set up?
- What is the most threatening space you have been in during the last month, where you felt most at risk and ill at ease?
- What viewing and way-finding occupations have you experienced in the last month?
- Analyze how the space you are in now affects experience, shapes behavior, and communicates meaning.
- Describe an important place in your life, either now or previously.
- Observe a space you call your own. What are the most meaningful objects in that space, and why?
- If you were stranded on an island, what 10 objects would you wish to have with you?
- What are the most crowded and the most solitary spaces you have been in this month?

- Select an object that is important to you and describe its meaning.
- What is your favorite tool, and why?
- Describe the most private and the most sacred spaces in your present life.

2. Take a walk in a natural or urban setting. Attend carefully to the spatial qualities and objects around you. How do they affect you in sensory, emotional, and behavioral ways?

3. Take a walk, as in exercise 2, at two different times, once in daylight and once in the dark. How are the spaces and the experiences different?

4. Spend 1 hour without using your hands.

5. Brush your teeth in the kitchen instead of the bathroom. How is it harder to do in a place that is only slightly different? How is your tooth brushing routine not well mapped onto the kitchen space?

6. Using large cardboard boxes, a selection of markers, and some tools, work in a group to construct a space that has a particular use and social meaning.

7. Try an activity you have never done before. What are the spatial aspects of this new activity that are important for you to understand and master to do the activity?

8. Draw your perfect space. What would it look, sound, and feel like?

9. List all the spaces you use in 1 day from beginning to end. Rate them on a scale, according to how public (5) or private (1) they were. What patterns do you see? (This activity can also be done for 1 week to highlight patterns more strongly.)

10. Draw a map, using one long uninterrupted line delineating your path through all the spaces you used today. What patterns do you see? (This activity can also be done for 1 week to highlight patterns more strongly.)

Building Insight into the Spatial Dimension in the Occupations of Others

1. Take a walk, as in exercise 1 in the preceding group of Power Builders. At some point, impose a hearing or visual impairment on yourself through the use of earplugs or taped-over glasses. How was the experience of walking in that space different because of your changed embodiedness?

2. Make a peanut butter sandwich while wearing a blindfold.

3. Negotiate a space you often use, but in a wheelchair.

4. Use smell, sound, lighting, texture, spatial arrangement, and other features to alter a space to which you or others are accustomed. Observe the differences in behavior caused by your changes to the space.

5. For 1 hour, in a place where lots of people are milling around, stand 2 inches closer to people than you usually would. Observe their reactions and your feelings.

POWER BUILDERS

6. Discuss how, in an occupation or disability narrative from Appendix A, the embodiedness, qualities of the environment, material objects, and/or social meaning of spaces is shaping the occupational experiences of the person described.

7. Using your best observation techniques, and focusing on the spatial dimensions, record observation notes on an individual or group of individuals engaging in an activity of interest to you for a minimum of 1 hour. If the occupation is usually brief, do repeated observations over 1 hour. What patterns did you observe?

8. Develop an essay on the spatial aspects of an activity in which you are particularly interested. This can be done from reference materials, observations of yourself or others, and/or interviews.

9. How might the identity of an occupational therapist be indicated and reflected in the spatial aspects of his or her occupations during work hours? Consider embodiedness, environmental qualities, material culture, and social meanings of space.

Building Design Skills Using the Spatial Dimension

1. Observe an occupational therapist during an intervention. How is he or she using objects and spaces in the session to reach goals? How might the objects and spaces be impeding the intervention's goals?

2. In a group, put all the key concepts provided at the beginning of this chapter's Power Builders on slips of paper, and then have everyone draw one. Create a Power Builder that will help someone else gain insight into this aspect of the spatial dimension of occupations.

3. Do as for exercise 2; then brainstorm (as a group or on your own) as many different Power Builder ideas as you can to provide an experience on a single key point.

4. Your supervisor has just told you that you have been selected to design the space for a new intervention program. Do a benefits analysis to identify some motivational energy to help you accomplish this project in a satisfying way.

5. Use a seven-step design process (the implementation phase may have to be fictional) to create a new treatment space for a population of interest to you. Keep uppermost in your mind the spatial experience of your clients in this design process.

6. Do a balloon analysis of the spatial aspects of an imaginary vacation you would like to take.

7. Using the priorities exercise, write a definition of your perfect home.

8. In a classroom, use the ideation and idea selection phases to identify a change in the space that would make it a better learning environment.

9. Do a time/task chart and implement the idea from exercise 8.

10. Using the following definition, evaluate your usual cooking area on these spatial qualities. "A great cooking area will be the right height

and size to fit me, allow me to see everything I need easily, provide effective tools and tasty ingredients in a convenient way, be safe, and have enough room for cooking and serving a group of people comfortably."

11. Use a seven-step design process to create and use a space for a real event, such as a meeting, an outing, or a celebration.

12. As a group, or individually, use a seven-step design process to create an experience that teaches another person, or a group of persons, about some aspect(s) of the spatial dimension of occupation.

13. Select a written case from Appendix A and speculate on which spatial factors may be important in understanding and addressing goals with this individual.

References

Benner, P., & Wrubel, J. (1989). *The work of care.* New York: Addison-Wesley.

Bruner, J. S. (1972). Nature and uses of immaturity. *American Psychologist, 44,* 1–11.

Buelow, M. (2001). Noise level in four Phoenix emergency departments. *Journal of Emergency Nursing, 27,* 23–26.

Calhoun, J. B. (1962). Population density and social pathology. *Scientific American, 206,* 139–148.

Chapple, E. D., & Coon, C. S. (1942). *Principles of anthropology.* New York: Henry Holt.

Csikszentmihalyi, M., & Rochberg-Halton, E. (1981). *The meaning of things: Domestic symbols and the self.* Cambridge: Cambridge University Press.

Duquette, J., Lortie, M., & Rossignol, M. (1997). Perception of difficulties for the back related to assembly work: General findings and impact of back health. *Applied Ergonomics, 28,* 389-396.

Gallagher, W. (1993). *The power of place: How our surroundings shape our thoughts, emotions, and actions.* New York: HarperPerennial.

Gibson, J. J. (1986). *The ecological approach to visual perception.* Hillsdale, NJ: Lawrence Erlbaum Associates.

Hall, E. T. (1982). *The hidden dimension.* New York: Anchor Books.

Hart, R. A. (1979). *Children's experience of place.* New York: Irvington.

Heft, H., & Wohlwill, J.F. (1987). Environmental cognition in children. In D. Stokols & I. Altman (Eds.), *Handbook of environmental psychology* (pp 281–328).

Hiss, T. (1990). *The experience of place.* New York: Vintage Books.

Holohan, C. (1986). Environmental psychology. *American Psychological Review, 37,* 381–407.

Hodder, I. (1989). *The meaning of things: Material culture and symbolic expression.* Boston: Unwin-Hyman.

Gibson, J. J. (1986). *The ecological approach to visual perception.* Hillsdale, NJ: Lawrence Erlbaum Associates.

Mace, R. (2001). *Definitions: Accessible, adaptable, and universal design.* www.design.ncsu.edu:8120/cud/pubs/center/fact_sheets/housdef.htm.

Mattingly, C., & Fleming, M. (1994). *Clinical reasoning: Forms of inquiry in a therapeutic practice.* Philadelphia: F. A. Davis.

McLaren, S. (1997). Heart rate and blood pressure in male police officers and clerical workers on workdays and non-workdays. *Work and Stress, 11,* 160–174.

Moore, G. (1983). Knowing about environmental knowing. In J. Pipkin, M. La Glory, & J. Blau (Eds.), *Remaking the city: Social science perspectives on urban design.* Albany, NY: State University of New York Press.

Murphy, R. (1987). *The body silent.* New York: Henry Holt and Company.

Oborne, D., & Gruneburg, M. (1983). *The physical environment at work.* New York: John Wiley & Sons.

Piaget, J. (1952). *The origins of intelligence in children.* New York: International Universities Press.

Piaget, J. (1962). *Play, dreams, and imitation in childhood.* New York: W. W. Norton.

Pierce, D. (1996). Infant space, infant time: Development of infant interactions with the physical environment, from 1 to 18 months. *Dissertation Abstracts International.*

Rowles, G. D. (1991). Beyond performance: Being in place as a component of occupational therapy. *American Journal of Occupational Therapy, 45,* 265–271.

Rubinstein, R. L., & Parmalee, P. A. (1992). Attachment to place and the representation of the life course by the elderly. In I. Altman & S. Low (Eds.), *Place attachment* (pp. 139–163). New York: Plenum Press.

Sacks, O. (1995). *An anthropologist on Mars.* New York: Vintage Books.

Sarton, M. (1973). *Journal of a solitude.* New York: W. W. Norton.

Woolf, V. (1929/1981). *A room of one's own.* New York: Harcourt, Brace, Jovanovich.

Zola, I. K. (1982). *Missing pieces: A chronicle of living with a disability.* Philadelphia: Temple University Press.

CHAPTER 10

The Temporal Dimension of Occupations

Biotemporality
Sociotemporality
Subjective Time
Orchestrating Occupations within the Flow of Time
Broad Temporal Patterns of Occupations
Using Time

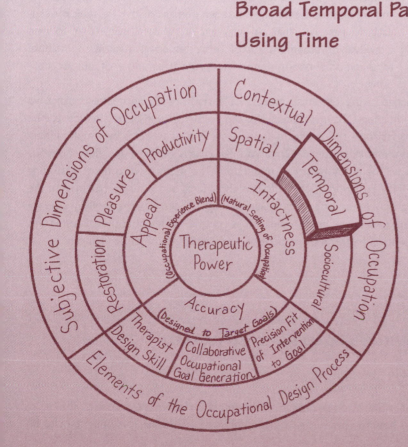

> *The culminating feature of evolution is man's capacity of imagination and the use of time with foresight, based on a corresponding appreciation of the past and of the present. . . . The whole of human organization has its shape in a kind of rhythm. It is not enough that our hearts should beat in a useful rhythm, always kept up to a standard at which it can meet rest as well as wholesome strain without upset. There are many other rhythms which we must be attuned to: the larger rhythms of night and day, of sleep and waking hours, of hunger and its gratification, and finally the big four—work and play and rest and sleep, which our organism must be able to balance even under difficulty (Adolph Meyer, 1922/1977, pp. 639–640).*

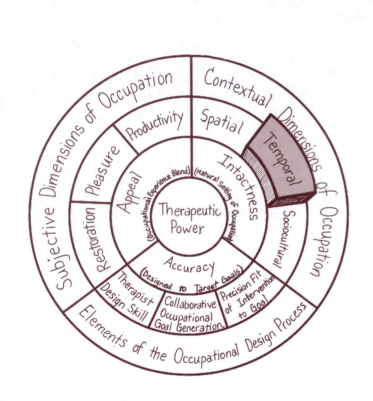

Just as each of our occupational experiences has a certain shape, each human experience of doing has a unique temporal rhythm. Each day's occupations accumulate like beads on a string. As each day's string of experience is laid alongside the previous day's, patterns emerge. Those temporal patterns show who we are in our day-to-day lives and are unique to each of us. In a sense, they create us. Our bodies respond to strong biotemporal cues, yielding occupational patterns that follow the sleep-wake cycle and change with the seasons. Our social world synchronizes much of our occupational experience to mesh with the patterns of others, through the use of clocks, calendars, and cultural expectations for the time at which certain things are done. Each occupational experience has its own subjective temporal characteristics, such as a beginning and an end, the speed at which it seems to be happening, and the length it lasts. We orchestrate our occupational experiences into a pattern across time by anticipating, planning ahead, using familiar routines, and keeping our general goals in mind. Just as chimpanzees have typical patterns determined by daily life in the chimpanzee community and by developmental age, modern humans also have typical occupational patterns that fit into a cultural synchrony that follows individual development. All of these temporal qualities contribute to the moment-to-moment and year-to-year flow of our occupations.

Facilitating change in the temporal aspects of an individual's occupations can have powerful therapeutic effects. To understand the temporal rhythms of occupation to the degree required to facilitate those effects, however, it is best to start by simply understanding your own temporal patterns. Once you can clearly observe and describe your own patterns, you will be ready to try to understand the patterns of others. Analyzing the patterns of an individual who does not follow the typical occupational patterns of the culture, such as a shift worker or a person whose life has been disorganized by a newly acquired disability, requires even greater skill. Most complex of all, of course, is using this insight into the temporal patterns of occupation to facilitate therapeutic changes.

Biotemporality

Brain Dynamics Underlying Circadian Rhythmicity

Occupations occur within strongly repeating biotemporal rhythms regulated by the brain. Before delving into how the brain regulates our biological rhythms, it is important to be familiar with some basic language used in the study of biotemporality. Although the primary human biotemporal rhythm is the circadian (meaning "around the day"), other important rhythms are shorter or longer than the circadian rhythm (Moore-Ede, Sulzman, & Fuller, 1982; Pierce, 1997) (see Table 10.1).

Table 10.1	**Biotemporal Rhythms of Differing Lengths**	
Rhythm	**Length**	**Examples**
Ultradian	less than 1 day	Heart rate, breathing
Circadian	24 hour	Sleep/wake
Circaseptum	7 day	Weekday/weekend
Menstrual	28.5 day	Menstruation, ovulation
Circannual	1 year	Body temperature regulation, sesonal variation in activity levels/types

In addition to language describing rhythms of different lengths, language is also used to describe the characteristics within a rhythm (see Table 10.2).

Table 10.2	**Descriptive Characteristics of Biotemporal Rhythms**	
Term	**Meaning**	**Example**
Period	Length	24-hr period of the circadian rhythm.
Frequency	How often recurring	The circaseptum rhythm occurs 52 times per year.
Oscillation	Pattern within 1 period	In the circadian, typically, from deepest sleep, around 2:00 AM, to highest energy late morning, and back to deepest sleep at 2:00 AM.
Phase	A part of a rhythm	In the circadian, the after-lunch energy dip is a phase.
Amplitude	Distance between highest and lowest points	In the circannual rhythm, in people new to Alaska, low energy and high sleep need in winter change to high energy and low sleep need in summer.
Zeitgeber	German for "timegiver"	In the circadian, light and dark regulate the rhythm environmental cue.

All biotemporal rhythms have all these characteristics. They show interesting patterns in their typical, as well as their disrupted, states. Here, however, let us focus on the strongest biological regulator of human occupational rhythms, the circadian rhythm. As is discussed more fully in Chapter 6, the relatively new field of sleep medicine has contributed greatly to our understanding and valuing of the circadian rhythm in recent years.

The human temporal sense operates through the interactions of the pineal gland, the eyes, and the suprachiasmatic nuclei (SCN). The SCN are found within the hypothalamus above the optic chiasm. They receive information from the retina and transmit it by an indirect route to the pineal gland. Descartes once called the pineal gland the third eye and seat of the soul. It exhibits many structural similarities to the eyes. The pineal gland and the eyes, to a much lesser degree, secrete melatonin, which influences the SCN. Melatonin regulates circadian rhythmicity and annual rhythms in reproductive activity (Armstrong & Redman, 1993). Abnormal melatonin production has been found in sleep disorders, seasonal affective disorder (SAD), depression, and bipolar disorders (Thalen, Kjellman, & Wetterberg, 1993). Melatonin levels are highest during darkness. Light exposure suppresses melatonin production. The structure of this anatomical pathway highlights the degree to which circadian rhythms are entrained to daylight (Moore-Ede, Sulzman, & Fuller, 1982; Swaab, Fliers, & Partiman, 1985).

Moore-Ede, Sulzman, and Fuller (1982) model the physiological dynamics of the human circadian system by describing two primary pacemakers, called *X* and *Y*. The dynamic tension in the interactions of the two pacemakers results in a circadian rhythm that can flexibly accommodate the demands of daily life yet pulls strongly back toward the natural 24-hour rhythm. Some of the differences in how X and Y operate are shown in Table 10.3.

Table 10.3	**Characteristics of the Two Pacemakers, X and Y**	
	X	**Y**
Location	A group of metabolic rhythms	Suprachiasmatic nuclei (SCN)
Physiological	REM sleep, body temperature	Sleep-wake timing, skin temperature
Indicators	Hunger/thirst	Activity patterns
Natural period	Strictly 24 hrs	Naturally lengthens from 24 to 40 hrs
Zeitgeber response	Little response, unless exactly 24 hr zeitgeber	Very responsive to light/dark and activity rhythm

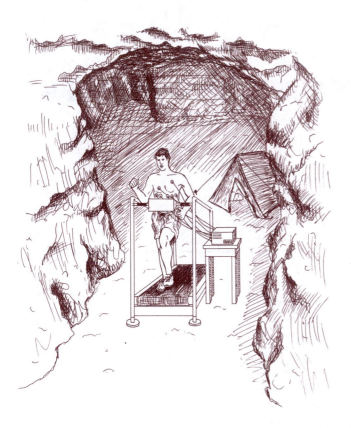

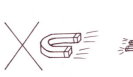 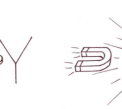

Much valuable research regarding the interactive operations of the two pacemakers X and Y has been done by studying human subjects who willingly placed themselves in cueless environments, such as caves, for extended stays. X and Y have different locations, indicators, natural periods, and responses to zeitgebers. The natural period of X's cycle is 24 hours, whereas Y, if allowed to run free in a cueless environment, will lose synchrony with X within a few days and gradually lengthen its period, reaching up to 40 hours in length (Aschoff, 1989; Moore-Ede, Sulzman, & Fuller, 1982). The difference in the degree to which the two pacemakers are affected by the environment is also striking. Y is easily entrained by zeitgebers of light and social activity. X is fairly impervious to zeitgebers, unless they are provided at exactly X's 24-hour period. For example, a weak zeitgeber of the natural 24-hour period of X will entrain body temperature (an X indicator), but not rest/activity (a Y indicator). However, a strong zeitgeber of 28 to 32 hours will entrain rest/activity (Y), but not body temperature (X). For X, the period of the zeitgeber is critical, and there is a resistance to zeitgebers of other lengths. For Y, the intensity of the zeitgeber is more important (Moore-Ede, Sulzman, & Fuller, 1982).

The difference in the two internal pacemakers sets up an adaptive tension between X, Y, and the environment. X and Y are affected not only by the environment but also by each other. This is called *internal coupling.* X's pull on Y is four times greater than Y's effect on X. Because Y is more susceptible to environmental cues, X's strong pull on Y counterbalances environmental influences, preventing Y's oscillations from being too easily disturbed by zeitgeber changes and thereby altering the rhythms of the entire circadian system. Y's susceptibility to zeitgebers pulls X to adapt to changes in the environment (Moore-Ede, Sulzman, & Fuller, 1982).

It is possible for the two pacemakers to become desynchronized from each other. Persons whose circadian rhythms have become desynchronized will experience sleep difficulties, health problems such as ulcers and insomnia, tiring, dangerous decreases in performance, and difficulty matching prevailing social schedules (Moore-Ede, Sulzman, & Fuller, 1982).

Circadian Influences on Occupational Patterns and Vice Versa

Based on this understanding of how the brain creates the circadian rhythm, consider how circadian rhythms create a template for our occupational experiences every day. This pattern is so familiar to us as to be almost invisible. It typically looks like this: wakening awareness, high cognitive capacity until late morning, slight decline in energy in a post-lunch dip, a moderate recovery of activity level and capacity in the afternoon and evening, gradual decline until sleep, and then the alternations of rapid-eye movement (REM) and non-REM sleep until waking again. This circadian rhythm is reflected in variations in perception, attention, problem solving, optimism or pessimism in viewing problems, day-dreaming, physical response to drugs, activity levels, and many other variables (Fraser, 1987; Giambra, Rosenberg, Kasper, & Yee, 1988; Raviv & Low, 1990; Teterina, Volkov, & Moldova, 1989; Thayer, 1987).

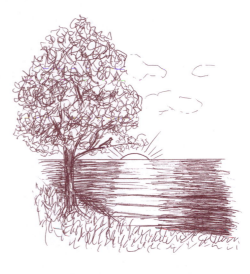

Some individuals exhibit lifelong, synchronous, healthy sleep-wake schedules that appear advanced or delayed in comparison to a typical schedule. "Larks" awake early and go to sleep early, and "owls" awake later and go to bed later. Because these rhythms are so biological, both groups have great difficulty understanding the odd patterns of the other and tend to view each other suspiciously. Requiring a lark and an owl to share sleeping space can be disastrous! Even though extreme lark or owl patterns can seem odd to us, as long as regular circadian rhythms, health, or personal happiness is not disturbed, they should not be a concern (Buela, Caballo, & Garcia, 1990; Mecacci, Zani, Rocchetti, & Lucioli, 1986; Moore-Ede, Sulzman, & Fuller, 1982; Wilson, 1990).

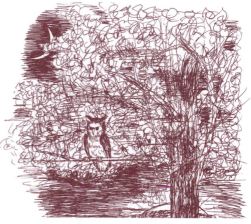

Infant Biotemporality

In the human infant, circadian regularity is thought to precede the capability to entrain to environmental zeitgebers. In utero, the infant is subject to the circadian rhythms of the mother through cross-placental transmission. The infant's sleep-wake pattern is rhythmic and repetitive at birth. However, the newborn does not immediately entrain to the cues of the environment. As new parents know, infants initially have a short sleep-wake cycle, alternating between wakefulness and napping around the clock. The periods of sleeping and waking lengthen over the first few months. This free-running rhythm may appear in the early months to reach synchrony with the rest of the family, with the baby sleeping at night. In actuality, this early matching rhythm is merely a congruent free-running oscillation that matches for a few nights to that of the rest of the household's sleep-wake cycle. Then, inevitably, the oscillations continue into completely incongruent patterns, to the despair of the baby's sleep-deprived parents. By about the 20th week of life, however, the human infant begins to achieve true synchrony through entrainment to light and social cues (Moore-Ede, Sulzman, & Fuller, 1982).

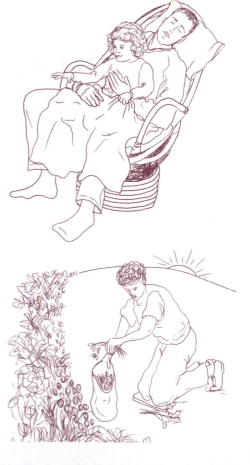

Biotemporal Rhythms in Elderly People

Research shows that the circadian rhythms of well elderly people are generally healthy. Studies have also found similar activity levels but earlier waking and sleeping times in elderly people compared to young adults. This is often considered a phase advance (discussed in the next section) in relation to the norm, but may result from generational differences in lifestyle (Katzman & Terry, 1983; Mason, 1989; Mecacci, Zani, Rocchetti, & Lucioli, 1986; Minors, Rabbitt, Worthington, & Waterhouse, 1989).

Quite different findings exist for institutionalized and ill elderly persons. The phenomenon of *sundowning* (increased confusion and restlessness at dusk) is often observed in older persons with dementia or other organic impairments (Evans, 1987). One study found a decrease in the volume and cell number of the SCN in elderly individuals, especially those with Alzheimer's disease (Swaab, Fliers, & Partiman, 1985). Another study found a significant level of disruption in the rest-activity cycle of Alzheimer patients on sedatives (Witting, Kwa, Eikelenboon, & Mirmiran, 1990). Katzman and Terry (1983) consider some of the biotemporal disturbances experienced by elderly individuals to be due to normal neurological changes of aging, depression, lack of control over environmental zeitgebers, or loss of important social zeitgebers because of isolation. These circadian disorders often go unaddressed in elderly people.

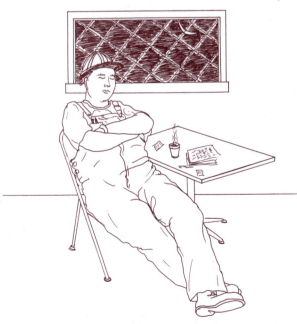

Disorders of Circadian Rhythmicity

Disruptions of the circadian system can also result from alterations in occupational patterns and contexts. Jet lag forces the human system to reset to new environmental cues. It is physiologically easier to adapt to flying to an earlier time zone, responding to a later-occurring set of zeitgebers (light and social cues). This is called phase delaying and is easy to do because of the natural tendency of Y to free-run into longer periods. Phase advancing, which occurs when one flies eastward across the United States, is more difficult and requires a greater number of days in which to adjust. The treatment recommended for jet lag, if one wishes to entrain body time to local time, is to seek the strongest available zeitgebers. That is, synchronize your occupational pattern with the period (dawn and dusk timing) of daylight and join in the activity patterns of others. This provides the strong cues to entrain Y and the exact 24-hour period to entrain X (Moore-Ede, Sulzman, & Fuller, 1982; Redfern, 1989).

Shift-work research shows the negative health effects of attempting to maintain a work schedule contrary to zeitgebers: stomach problems, sleep disorders, and work errors. People who are engaging in high activity during the time of day that is usually biological "down time" may also experience social stress because of isolation. In the case of serious health concerns, the recommendation is to leave shift work. If shift work is not discontinued, then the worker should try to maintain a regular sleep-wake schedule to maintain a synchronized set of biological rhythms. The most difficult schedule to adjust to is the weekly shift rotation, which should be avoided if possible (Adams, Folkard, & Young, 1986; Colquhoun, 1985; Moore-Ede, Sulzman, & Fuller, 1982).

Three types of circadian disorders have been identified: phase, period, and amplitude disorders. These disorders are treated in sleep-disorder units and offer an interesting new area of practice to occupational therapists who are interested in working in broad interventions to support the temporal regularity of occupational patterns.

Phase disorders, caused by extreme advance or delay of circadian rhythms in relation to the norm, are most often seen in psychiatric illness. It is suspected that circadian phase disorders are not simply a result of psychiatric illnesses but may also be a contributing factor in the disease process. For a person who is severely phase-delayed, such as someone coming off an extended period of night-shift work, the treatment is to phase delay the individual's activity pattern a small amount each day, gradually pushing bedtime around the clock until the rhythm reaches synchrony with the environment. By lengthening each day by about 20 minutes, the natural tendency of Y to free run can be used to support this adjustment (Moore-Ede, Sulzman, & Fuller, 1982).

Period disorders are disturbances in the length of the circadian oscillation. They are most often seen in individuals who are blind or are on free-running circadian rhythms. It is not surprising that persons with blindness would have difficulty regulating circadian rhythms in the absence of the strong zeitgeber of light. It is also possible that the damage that produced the blindness could extend to the pacemakers, especially Y, located in the SCN. Consistent free-running rhythms can also be caused by isolation from social cues in a reclusive lifestyle (Moore-Ede, Sulzman, & Fuller, 1982).

Seasonal affective disorder (SAD) is a winter depression tied to circadian rhythms, hypothesized to result from inadequate light cues in the environment. Unlike other depressions, it is strictly seasonal and will dissipate on its own in early spring, as the light increases and days lengthen. Along with depression, SAD symptoms include increased appetite for carbohydrates, snacking and weight gain, daytime fatigue, anxiety, and increased sleep duration. Persons with SAD are now being successfully treated with light therapy (Terman, 1994).

Sleep-disorder clinics offer an area ripe for development of innovative occupational therapy practice. More importantly, many of the clients served by occupational therapists exhibit clear symptoms of undiagnosed sleep disturbances and disorders. Sleep disturbances are especially prevalent in children with neurological and learning disabilities, in adults with respiratory dysfunctions, and in elders in institutional environments. As the premier professionals knowledgeable about patterns of activity, it is our responsibility to help clients understand that interventions are available by referral and that some of the other problems they are experiencing are probably being exacerbated by disrupted sleep. If families or individuals are interested in working with their current occupational therapists on an additional goal of improving sleep quality, it is appropriate for the therapist to offer environmental and temporal recommendations, sleep-quality tracking systems for periodic review of this goal, and any other interventions that may support progress toward enhanced sleep quality.

Sociotemporality

Just as biotemporal rhythms exert a strong shaping force on our occupational patterns, sociotemporal rhythms mold our patterns so that they fit smoothly with the patterns of others in our culture and surrounding life world. Biotemporal and sociotemporal rhythms work in synchrony. Just as you are beginning to feel hungry in the evening, the family will begin to converge around routine dinner preparations, and the meal will occur with minimal decision making about whether it is the right time for a shared meal. The culture in which each of us lives provides many supports for these social rhythms in the forms of calendars, clocks, socially accepted schedules, and a shared history of activities regularly occurring at expected times.

Calendars

The annual calendar is such an accustomed regulator of our life patterns that we are fairly oblivious to how much it influences us. We forget that patterns such as resting and socializing on the weekend, working Monday through Friday, and sharing traditional holiday events are not facts of nature, but social conventions. We depend completely on the calendar to coordinate our activities with others and organize our daily lives.

The origins of the modern Western calendar reach back to the schedule, or *horarium,* used in Benedictine monasteries. The horarium orchestrated the lives of the Benedictines, so that all were engaged simultaneously in shared daily and seasonal rhythms of activity, such as a time of day to wake, read, and attend mass, a time of the week to wash out the beer jugs, and a time of the year to celebrate Easter and Christmas (Zerubavel, 1981). The Benedictines showed unusually strong temporal symmetry: doing the same activities at the same time.

The modern Gregorian calendar is also very much rooted in strong Jewish and Protestant traditions regarding the importance of the Sabbath, a day devoted to religious observance and spiritual renewal. Rituals mark the beginning and ending of the Sabbath as sacred time, different from the profane time of the rest of the week. In both traditions, there were activities you did not do on the Sabbath and activities you did only on the Sabbath. The Sabbath was not only a day of the week but also a particular pattern of activities over the week. For people who are not strict in their observance of a Sabbath, there is still this sense of sacred and profane time, during which you do and do not do certain activities (Rybczynski, 1991; Zerubavel, 1981). For you, what activities are sacred to a certain time, and are rarely displaced by the profane, everyday activities of other times of the week?

Weekday and Weekend

The rhythm of the 7-day week seems very natural: days of work and days of rest. It has an even stronger impact on modern everyday life than seasonal changes. In the 18th century, the seasons shaped activity patterns more forcefully than they now do. At different times of the year, one wore different clothes, ate different foods, lived in different parts of the house, did different agricultural work, engaged in different types of recreation, and got up and went to bed at different times. Since those days, the Sabbath day of rest has grown into a full weekend. For a time, people had a half day of work on Saturday, often a market day. Now, most people consider Saturday a day of leisure, a day off from work, although they may use it to do marketing and errands and household chores. Today, the beat that we feel in the rhythm of our lives is not the seasons, but the alternation back and forth between weekend and weekday. We look forward to weekends as a time of freedom and leisure. If you asked what day is the beginning of the week, most people today would answer "Monday," although the calendar still clearly shows Sunday as the beginning of the week. We work hard all week for the reward of the weekend. The values behind such an expectation of when work and leisure occur strongly reflect the values of the Reformation and Protestantism, as discussed in Chapter 4 on productivity.

Other calendars were not structured as a 7-day week. Most well-known of these is the French Revolutionary calendar, which was used from 1793 to 1806. This calendar was formulated on several principles: alignment with rhythms of nature, rational numbering, and an emphasis on revolutionary time instead of religious time. Each day was made up of 10 hours, of 100 minutes each. Each day of the week was named for its place in the 10-day cycle: *Primidi, Duodi, Tridi, Quartidi, Quintidi, Sextidi, Septidi, Octidi, Nonidi,* and *Decadi.* The 10 days made up 1 week, or decade. Decadi, the 10th day of the week, was a rest day. This cycle completely disrupted the 7-day rhythm of attending church. The Sunday Sabbath and many saint's days of the Catholic Church were thus eliminated. However, the fact that the new week required 9 days of work before a day of rest occurred did not increase its popularity with the people. In the revolutionary system, 3 weeks made up a 30-day month, of which there were 12. (The extra 5 days were grouped together at the end of the year.)

MAY

Sunday	Monday	Tuesday	Wednesday	Thursday	Friday	Saturday
		1	2	3	4	5
6	7	8	9	10	11	12
13	14	15	16	17	18	19
20	21	22	23	24	25	26
27	28	29	30	31		

The calendar year started on the autumnal equinox, called New Year's Day, on what the Gregorian calendar called September 22. The 12 months were named for the seasons: *Vedemaire* (vintage), *Brumaire* (mist), *Frimaire* (frost), *Nivose* (snow), *Pluviose* (rain), *Ventose* (wind), *Germinal* (seeds), *Floreal* (flowers), *Prairial* (meadows), *Messidor* (harvest), *Thermidor* (heat), and *Fructidor* (fruits) (Rybczynski, 1991, p. 92). Although the French attempt to revolutionize, rationalize, secularize, and naturalize the annual calendar was not long lasting, it certainly pointed out to many the arbitrary and culturally created nature of the Gregorian calendar.

FLOREAL

Primidi	Duodi	Tridi	Quartidi	Quintidi	Sextidi	Septidi	Octidi	Nonidi	Decadi
1	2	3	4	5	6	7	8	9	10
11	12	13	14	15	16	17	18	19	20
21	22	23	24	25	26	27	28	29	30

Culturally Accepted Schedules

Today's calendars do not require such symmetry in our everyday patterns as the Benedictines experienced, or the orderly naturalness attempted by the French. Certain settings, however, do require a highly synchronized and symmetrical, hour-by-hour schedule of activities; for example, the military, schools, and factories. When occupational therapy began as a profession in the early 1900s, concern was raised about the dehumanizing effects of industrialization's increasing regulation of daily occupations. That concern with how humans use the time of their lives remains at the core of occupational therapy's philosophy. Sharing such rhythmic, regulated patterns of action does tend, however, to create a feeling of social solidarity in the participants. In some ways, calendars and socially accepted schedules also provide us with great freedom to act in ways highly differentiated from each other. By relying on these social mechanisms to hold the times at which we will share activities such as meals or holidays with other people, we are freed to do highly individualized activities in the intervening times. Without the calendar and a culturally accepted schedule, we would have to stay in each other's vicinity constantly, waiting for the time that seemed right for everyone to begin shared activities.

Clocks

The effects of clocks and watches on our occupational patterns are analogous to the effects of the calendar. For thousands of years, people had only sundials to measure the passing hours. Later, water clocks extended timekeeping through the night, tracking the passage of 1 hour at a time by the movement of water through an aperture. Then the hourglass was used to measure 1 hour at a time. Around the 14th century, monastery clocks, working by the use of weights, marked 1 hour and were used to ring the bells to mark the hour of the day. Both within and outside the monastery, and later the cathedrals, the ringing hours regulated the activities of all those within hearing. The word *clock* is derived from the Dutch word *clok,* which means bell (Levine, 1997). A Dutch mathematician named Christiaan Huygens perfected the first pendulum clock around 1700. New words such as *speed* and *punctuality* then began entering the English language. Soon after this, the forces of the Protestant work ethic and growing industrialization, combined with such inventions as wristwatches and time clocks, introduced the minute-by-minute measuring of time that we live by today.

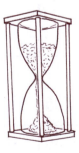
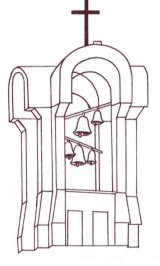
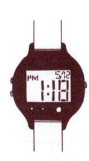

Clocks, calendars, and the weekend-workday rhythm combine to give us a sense of when it is time to work and when is time for leisure. Another interesting extension of this pattern is a sense of public time and private time. Public time is out in the world. Private time is when one is home for sleep and the intimacy of a shared lifestyle with loved ones. We understand when is public time, when a phone call or visit is appropriate, and when is private time, when such socializing is not acceptable. If a next-door neighbor began mowing the lawn at 2:00 AM, you would consider it a rude intrusion into your private time. If a friend unexpectedly knocked at your door at 5:00 AM on a Sunday morning, you would wonder if it were an emergency.

Cultural Differences in Time Use

Of course, it is important to recognize that attitudes toward time are very cultural. The present discussion largely reflects typical values of Western cultures. Levine (1997) describes how many cultures are not so oriented to clock time, but live instead on "event time" (p. 81). That is, daily life is organized not by the date on the calendar or the time on a clock but more in terms of the activities that need to be done or the expected events of the day. The day moves through the sequence of those events, rather than around the circle of the clock.

Another way to view cultural differences in the experience of time is what Hall (1983) terms *M-time* and *P-time*. The Western system is monochronic (M-time), emphasizing efficiency of time use, doing one thing at a time, and being strictly observant of time commitments. Polychronic time (P-time), on the other hand, encourages doing multiple things at once, values being with people and involved in events important to them, and is experienced as more fluid and adjustable. P-time is most frequently seen in more agricultural societies, where the length of the day and the tasks to be done far outweigh the time on a watch or the date on a calendar. Even in Western culture, M-time seems to dominate in business settings and solitary work, whereas P-time works better at home in the midst of the multiple activities of family members. Children, certainly, are naturally on P-time, and think of time in terms of the length of experience of typical activities. Thus, when a child asks how long until dinner, her mother may answer, "about as long as it takes you to get your bath."

Economic View of Time

In Western culture, "time is money." We have a very economic view of time as a precious commodity that should be invested wisely. Some of this attitude is rooted in the Protestant work ethic's moral valuing of productivity. *Taylorism,* the efficiency theory behind factory organization in the early 1900s, has also permeated our societal perspective, pressing us to use time in ways that produce the greatest results possible within the time expended (Taylor, 1911/1967). One of the problems with an economic view of time is the pressured feeling it can produce in people. This results in cultural phenomena such as hurry sickness and workaholism. Of course, some people are "faster" and some "slower," but try the assessment in Table 10.4 to see whether you are living dangerously fast.

According to Levine's time urgency assessment, are you a dangerously hurried person (1997, p. 21)? Another side effect of this hurry and pressure to be productive with our time is that, because we consider our time so valuable, it is difficult for us to enjoy our leisure time or get adequate rest (Levine, 1997; Rifkin, 1987; Schor, 1992). Unfortunately, many people try to redress their low-quality leisure experiences by spend-

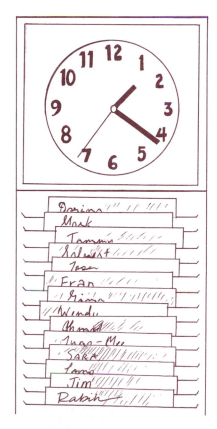

Table 10.4   Assessment of Time Urgency and Personal Pace

Concern with clock time: Compared with most people, are you particularly aware of the time on the clock? Do you, for example, frequently glance at your watch? Or, on the other hand, are you someone who frequently forgets the time or even what day of the week it is?

Speech patterns: How rushed is your speech? Do you tend to speak faster than other people? When someone takes too long to get to the point while speaking, do you often feel like hurrying him or her along? Are you a person who accepts interruptions?

Eating habits: How rushed is your eating behavior? Are you often the first person finished eating at the table? Do you take time to eat three meals a day in a slow and relaxed manner?

Walking speed: Do you walk faster than most people? Do fellow walkers sometimes ask you to slow down?

Driving: Do you get excessively annoyed in slow traffic? When you are caught behind a slow driver, do you sometimes honk or make rude gestures to try to speed the driver up?

Schedules: Are you addicted to setting and/or maintaining schedules? Do you allot a specific amount of time for each activity? Do you have a fetish about punctuality?

List making: Are you a compulsive list maker? When preparing for a trip, for example, do you make a list of things to do or things to bring?

Nervous energy: Do you have excessive nervous energy? Are you a person who becomes irritable when you sit for an hour without doing something?

Waiting: Do you get more annoyed than most people if you have to wait in line for more than a couple of minutes at the bank, a store, or to be seated in a restaurant? Do you sometimes walk out of these places if you encounter even a short wait?

Alerts: Do others warn you to slow down? How often have you heard your friends or spouse tell you to take it easier, or to become less tense?

Levine, 1997.

Table 10.5   Occupational Tempo in Different Countries

Country	Rank	Country	Rank
Switzerland	1	Canada	17
Ireland	2	South Korea	18
Germany	3	Hungary	19
Japan	4	Czech Republic	20
Italy	5	Greece	21
England	6	Kenya	22
Sweden	7	China	23
Austria	8	Bulgaria	24
Netherlands	9	Romania	25
Hong Kong	10	Jordan	26
France	11	Syria	27
Poland	12	El Salvador	28
Costa Rica	13	Brazil	29
Taiwan	14	Indonesia	30
Singapore	15	Mexico	31
United States	16		

Levine, 1997.

ing an increasing amount of income on leisure equipment, luxury vacations, and home entertainment, placing them in a work-and-spend cycle that is difficult to escape.

People in different parts of the world also live at different tempos. One study measured the tempo of life in 31 countries by collecting data on walking speed, service times in post offices, and the accuracy of public clocks (Levine, 1997, p. 131). The results are shown in Table 10.5, with 1 being fastest and 31 slowest.

Sociotemporal Interventions

The occupational therapist's understanding of the way in which sociotemporality structures our lives is integral to his or her interventions. For example, for a client in an industrial rehabilitation program, the goal may be to reach the work pace required to return to working with certain machines or processes. Other clients may set goals of functional independence in school or work environments that require them to understand and use the calendars, schedules, and clocks so central to success in those settings. As an occupational therapist, you may work with individuals who have actually suffered heart attacks largely as a result of the way they have dealt with work, stress, time pressure, and leisure. This situation will require interventions to help them construct healthier attitudes toward time in their occupational patterns. Sometimes, a therapist is working with an individual who cannot meet the time demands of the environment, such as an elder who needs to cross at a light in his or her neighborhood. In these cases, change in the traffic light setting might be required through the therapist's advocacy efforts to appropriate officials. The sensitivity of the therapist to the ways in which institutions can powerfully influence the temporality of occupational experience is an important safeguard of clients' rights to determine their own life directions (Suto & Frank, 1994). It is especially critical that occupational therapists recognize their own values about the use of time and understand that persons of other cultures may have different attitudes about appointments, pace, and schedules of therapeutic activities.

Subjective Time

Differentiating between Occupational Experience and Activity Idea

An occupation is an occurrence, an event in time (Pierce, 2001). It is a particular person's experience, unique to that moment, place, and makeup of social circumstances. Occupations are not repeatable. They are as unique as snowflakes. Although you may experience a very similar occupation day after day, such as brushing your teeth, it is never really the same. It is morning or night, you are alone or not, you are tired or fresh, you may be in a hotel or at home, or you are thinking about the day of work ahead or excited to be leaving that day on vacation.

For many years, the concept of activity has been entangled with the concept of occupation. An activity, however, is not a person's experience. It is an idea about doing. To return to our example, the idea of tooth brushing is shared with most people in our culture. What tooth brushing means is taught to us when we are young, and we can speak about it to each other. We have had many occupational experiences that included tooth brushing. These experiences contribute to our activity idea about what is included in tooth brushing.

The temporal context of an occupational experience most clearly distinguishes it from an activity idea. The tooth-brushing experience you had this morning had a beginning, a sequence of actions, an end, a time of day, a pace, and a length. The activity of tooth brushing is a global idea, good for communicating with others, but not located in a specific time or experienced by a specific individual. The activity of tooth brushing is a general descriptor of action, a piece of language that refers to a category of occupational experiences. Many activity ideas that we understand and can speak about in general terms, such as bungee jumping or murder, we never experience as actual occupations.

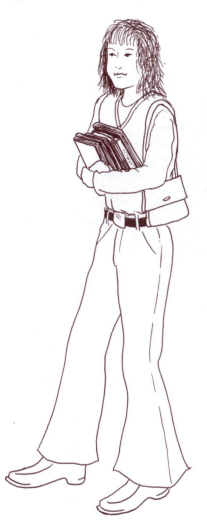

An important point to consider is how activities support and shape occupational experiences. We use activity ideas, combined with memories of past occupational experiences, to guide our engagement in, and completion of, an occupation. For example, a new college student heading into the bookstore the first semester has a general idea about the activity of buying books. She also has past occupational experiences that included buying books. She may have bought books for pleasure reading, books as references for hobbies, magazines at the grocery checkout, books from on-line booksellers, and books as presents for people. She has conversed with people now and then about their book-buying experiences. She has seen television portrayals of people buying books. Also, she has shopped for groceries, clothes, a car, and many other things, contributing to her ideas about how one buys things. Her activity idea about buying books gives her a general expectation of what will occur in her first experience of buying college textbooks. There should be looking for, selecting, carrying, and paying for books. The occupational experience, however, will be unique. Maybe she is surprised at the costs, also has fun looking at college clothing, finds she is in the wrong bookstore, or meets someone who will be in one of her classes. The experience she has at that moment certainly is shaped and supported by her activity idea about buying books, but that idea is quite different from the actual occupation she experienced.

Constructing the Occupational Experience

An occupation is "chunked" (Clark, Parham, Carlson, Frank, Jackson, Pierce, et al., 1991, p 300) in time, or constructed, by the individual as he or she is experiencing it. That is, if you asked the student at the bookstore what she is doing, she might say "shopping for books," "trying to decide whether to get boxers with a university logo on them," or "getting ready to start classes on Wednesday." Humans, with their accurate sense of time, chunk the sequences of their experiences in ways specifically meaningful to them. An individual who has never done a particular activity before, or who has had some disruption to a familiar activity, will chunk experience in shorter segments (Vallacher & Wegner, 1987). So, someone learning to drive may think of what he or she is doing as "starting the car." Then the new driver may turn his or her attention to "pulling out of the driveway." An experienced driver will engage in the same activity, but chunk it as "driving to work," with attention flowing easily between one step and another.

An occupation has several phases. At minimum, it has a beginning, an end, and some action in between (Pierce, 1996). We experience initiating an occupation as the intentional focusing of attention and action to begin some type of activity we have envisioned doing. Initiations take more energy and effort than simply continuing in an occupation that is already occurring. There is a feeling of overcoming inertia. Think of something important you have done lately. Did you experience it in this way—as putting energy into getting started and then it seemed easier to continue? This may be because more attention is required to envision how the occupation is likely to progress, what actions or materials may be needed, and other considerations in beginning an action. Another effort required in initiating an occupation is the effort to screen out the other choices competing for your attention. Once the initiation has been accomplished, the sequence of actions will unfold somewhat one from another, especially if the occupation is familiar. For instance, if you are an experienced cook, your initiation of cooking a meal may include thinking that you really should get dinner started, wondering what to cook, looking in the refrigerator to see what ingredients are available, looking back at what you had been doing before, thinking of just ordering a pizza because you feel tired, and then deciding on what to make. Once you have finished this decision making of committing to and initiating the cooking, the step-by-step preparation follows a loose order that is not too difficult to negotiate.

Occupations can range from brief with few actions in them, to quite complex, multitasked, and lasting for years. An infant probably experiences fairly brief, concrete chunks of occupation: picking up, shaking, and dropping a rattle, perhaps. Adults, with their long-term goals and sophisticated grasp of time, can experience an occupation that is lengthy, complex, and multiphased—such as the occupation of a woman creating a fancy wedding cake for her daughter over several days.

The ending, or discontinuation, of an occupation can also range from simple to complex. The infant simply drops the rattle when the next thing catches her attention. The woman baking the cake will probably end with cleaning up, properly storing the cake, and perhaps taking a moment to admire the finished cake and reflect on her feelings.

Endings, beginnings, and the phases between contain very different sorts of mental attention. Beginnings require disciplined attention, focus, anticipation of action sequence, and choice making. Endings give closure, discontinue action, and may include reflection back on the sequence and the outcome. In the phases between initiation and discontinuation, attention is more in the moment, responsive to the immediately preceding and immediately following steps in the unfolding sequence.

Simultaneity

Within the occurrence of an occupation, from beginning to end, the experience can involve few or many activity ideas. Recall the experienced driver who described his or her activity as "driving to work." On a particular day, this may include several activities: driving the car, listening to the morning news, and planning his or her day. These are general ideas of action that he or she draws on to smoothly engage in his or her occupation of driving to work that day. He or she also draws on experience and routines, but the important point here is that an occupational experience can simultaneously include many activity ideas. Returning to the infant with the rattle, there may be very little activity idea behind such an action. Perhaps the infant just responds quickly to the sight of a shiny rattle by reaching, with a vague activity idea of reaching for and grasping things. Picking up the rattle makes a noise, and so the infant tries moving it again and again, until her or his attention is distracted by something else, and she or he drops the rattle (Piaget, 1952). For adults to experience this moment-to-moment unfolding of an occupation without much use of activity ideas is probably fairly rare.

Pace, Duration, Speed, and Rhythm

We experience occupations as having a certain pace, duration, speed, and rhythm (Fraisse, 1981; Zerubavel, 1981). Occupations that may appear similar from the outside can be experienced quite differently by different people. Consider, for example, two men working across from each other on an assembly line, bolting engines onto car chassis. For one man, new to the job, the work may seem quite challenging, and so feels fast paced, of short length, and without a clear rhythm. For the more experienced worker, who may be rather bored, the work may seem to go slowly, last a long time, and have a clear repeating rhythm.

Often during therapy, clients are learning a new task. Perhaps an injury has taken away previous abilities, or the client is young and learning new things. Regardless of why the person is learning a skill, it is important for the therapist to understand that the person's experience is probably chunked in a brief attentional segment, as each new subpart of a larger task is attempted. Knowing this, the therapist will not try to direct the client's attention beyond the immediate, brief occupational experience in which the client is engaged until the therapist recognizes the ending actions that indicate it is completed.

Working on how occupations are experienced is so broad and central to occupational therapy that it is a dynamic of intervention in all areas. A child with dyspraxia is often especially in need of work in the area of the sequencing and timing of occupations. Sensory integration theory specifically addresses this type of problem (Ayres, 1985). Another example is an occupational therapy program aimed at helping patients post–myocardial infarction to understand and rethink the stressful pace at which they experience the occupations of their lives.

Orchestrating Occupations within the Flow of Time

Humans are unique in their keen abilities to perceive and use the flow of time to plan, enact, and reflect on patterns of occupations. This time sense is due to the neurophysiology that has evolved in humans. The ability to anticipate and plan for coming events, as well as to learn from past experience, must have had a large evolutionary advantage in successfully attracting a desirable mate and raising young to the age of fertility.

Neurology of Memory

Nested in a concentric ring just inside the limbic association cortex is the hippocampus and its efferent pathway, the fornix. Together, they play an important role in short-term memory. Nearly all incoming sensation is entered into short-term memory at the hippocampus. However, it is only through additional attention to short-term memories that they are refreshed and then stored in long-term memory. Edelman (1989) calls the hippocampus the "organ of succession" (p. 119). It records the sequences in perceptual experience through its unique neural structure. The hippocampus, though quite small, is long and laminated with layers of neurons, rather like a jelly roll. The bulk of its neurons are rolled in these layers, but others cross through the layers, recording the relative locations of the sensory information through the roll. Thus the sequence of sensation is perceived (Martin, 1996). Understanding event sequence is particularly important for formulating quick responses (Martin, 1996; Schmidt, 1975).

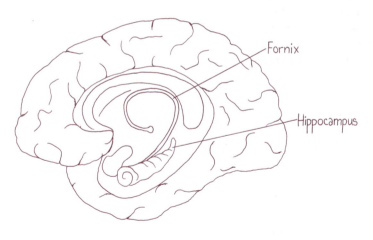

Fornix

Hippocampus

The Temporal Horizon

Out of this ability to perceive and remember temporal sequence emerges human intentionality (Searle, 1995). Seeing our experiences within the flow of time, we learn to draft the sequences we wish to enact well before their occurrences. This is called *temporal horizon* (Cottle & Klineberg, 1974; Fraisse, 1981). Just as we can see a certain distance ahead and behind ourselves in space, we also perceive time in the future and the past to a certain vanishing point, or horizon. Infants have a fairly short temporal horizon, quickly forgetting what has happened and anticipating only what can be expected from visible indicators in the immediate environment. Most adults, however, can plan well into the future and recall many years of their pasts.

Orchestration

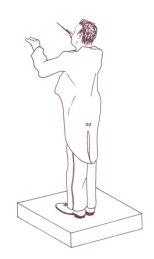

On a day-to-day basis, each person constructs, or *orchestrates,* his or her sequence of occupations (Primeau, 1998). Waking in the morning, we often think of what is ahead in the day, building an expectation of how the day may go. Considering the length of time different things take, we forecast a sequence of where we will be at what times and what we will be doing. Questioning what is most important to get done or worrying over deadlines may also be part of this orchestration effort. Or a person may be entering an activity setting, such as a factory or a fast-paced emergency room, that provides so much external structuring of the sequence of occupational experience that it requires little daily orchestration effort.

Orchestration also happens on a larger scale as we plan the primary goals of our lives and make up the broad occupational patterns that will best result in reaching desired outcomes. Bateson (1990) speaks very eloquently of how we "compose a life" (p. 1), like a quilt, from the materials and opportunities at hand, but work toward a general pattern. Personal projects are the primary accomplishments we are trying to realize in our lives at any one time, thus shaping our choices of occupations (Christiansen, Backman, Little, & Nguyen, 1999). Personal projects are not occupations because they are not actual chunks of experience. They are, however, a part of our thinking and orchestration of occupations. Examples of personal projects are finishing school, building a house, losing weight, and getting well. Progress toward the accomplishment of personal projects increases our sense of well-being.

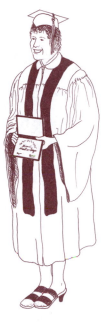

Habit and Routine

One of the ways we reduce the attentional demands of orchestration is through habit and routine (Corbin, 1999; Ludwig, 1998; Strauss, 1993; Zemke, 1994). The brain has only a certain amount of attentional capacity. By using sequences with which we are familiar, we can engage in occupations without having to figure out each step along the way. Activities such as dressing and driving are often experienced by adults as habitual. When engaged in an occupation that uses habit, we often have our mind on other things as well as the routine action in which we are engaging with little conscious attention. Or, sometimes, we engage in several kinds of activity during an occupation, all of which are fairly habitual, such as driving and eating and talking on a cell phone. The concepts of habit and routine are often used interchangeably in occupational therapy. Routine, however, often refers to a larger sequence. An example of a routine might be buying groceries on the Saturday after payday, driving home with them, picking up the dry cleaning on the way, carrying in the groceries and the dry cleaning, putting away the groceries first, and then putting away the dry cleaning.

Narrative

Humans also see their life patterns within a meaning-filled narrative, like a play or a story (Frank, 1996). You can see this most easily as someone relates something that has just happened to him or her. The person makes sense of the pattern that has just occurred by imbuing it with a plot. The story ends with a resolution of the tension that builds in challenges to the unfolding of that plot. Although the person may or may not have been thinking of this narrative during the occupational experience, reflection on the sequence creates the narrative pattern. Reflection on a long span of life can also reveal a narrative pattern, such as "I didn't know that the time we were working together was to end in our getting married, raising a family, and now growing old together. We were so passionately involved in the work we were doing at the time."

Interventions

Working on how individuals orchestrate occupations is frequently a part of intervention with a wide variety of populations. For example, a child with attention deficits may be working with his occupational therapist toward more successfully and independently completing simple classroom routines, such as entering the classroom and beginning the day by putting away coat and backpack and getting out needed books and materials, or filling a tray and completing lunch without leaving the lunch table. Some individuals with brain injuries can have disruptions of memory and time judgment that require intervention. A person with a newly acquired spinal cord injury may need to problem solve how to take care of daily self-care activities on his or her own, and so will work with the therapist to construct and practice a new set of routines to do so. Eleanor Clarke Slagle, a founder of occupational therapy, was a great advocate of the therapeutic effects of habit training, which involves the placing of previously isolated asylum patients in an everyday occupational pattern of dining and working with others. Within those conditions, she facilitated their acquisition of a sense of time, routine, and self-directed occupations.

Broad Temporal Patterns of Occupations

Although this book does not have sufficient space to fully explore them, it is important for the occupational therapist to be grounded in knowledge of broad primate patterns and developmental perspectives on human occupation. Certainly, every individual's life and occupational experiences are completely unique and should be honored as his or her own creation. Still, it is useful to have general maps of aggregated patterns to give the therapist a sense of the types of patterns she or he might expect to see.

Basic Occupational Patterns of Wild-Living Chimpanzees

Studying the occupational patterns of our closest primate relations, the chimpanzees, gives a sense of the template that being a primate lays over human occupational patterns. Chimps, like humans, have routines of daily life, including foraging, eating, traveling, caring

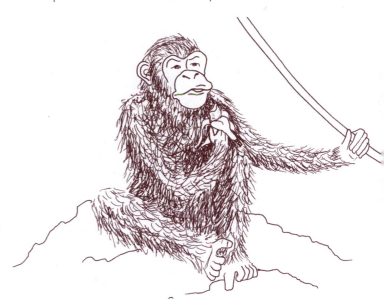

for young, grooming, socializing, courting and mating, competing for status, and sleeping (Goodall, 1986). These are not human patterns, but primate patterns. Pleasure, productivity, and restoration are all in their daily occupations, just as they are in ours. Of course, within the general pattern, the human occupational experience is highly different from the chimpanzee's. Our nervous systems provide us with higher-order reasoning to bring to bear on our occupational efforts. Our culture differs, especially in the structure of a family with a father as well as a mother, and with complex systems of laws, government, and language. Humans, as just discussed in Chapter 9 on the spatial dimensions of occupation, operate within a highly varied and proliferating material culture. Thus, most human occupations include lots of interactions with objects. Despite these differences, we have much to learn about the basic primate pattern from studying the occupational patterns of healthy, wild-living chimpanzees.

Developmental Patterns in Occupation

Typical human development also strongly frames our occupational patterns as individuals (Royeen, 1995). Our life span is, unfortunately, limited. Each phase of life brings certain typical challenges, regardless of our cultural heritage. Infancy and childhood are times of rapid growth, learning, and change in motor and cognitive capacities. Learning to negotiate the physical world, orchestrate one's own occupational patterns, and interact with others within and beyond the family are central interests for the young child. Much of this learning is done through play. School and educational progress are also important aspects of childhood in most modern cultures (Medrich, Roizen, Rubin, & Buckley, 1982).

Adolescents are caught up in the transition into adulthood, busy creating themselves and testing their identities. Bodies continue to change at this stage, blossoming in a flood of hormones that can impact mood and energy levels dramatically. The media seem to prey on adolescents, exerting pressure to live up to an ideal of beauty and behavior that is largely portrayed in media stars through the work of an army of makeup artists, hairdressers, costume designers, choreographers, and marketing specialists. In Western cultures, adolescence is extended by the long periods of high school and college education that many young people complete, keeping them in the dependent and not fully adult role of student. This can be stressful because the young adult is capable of more typical adult patterns of occupation, including employment, committed long-term relationships, and parenting.

The transition to adulthood entails many reconfigurations of occupational patterns to meet new roles and responsibilities. Work and career fill the time previously occupied by school, but often with less flexibility and freedom. Marriage, families, jobs, and reconstructing relationships with extended family to fit the new adult status are typical challenges of this stage. As the adult moves out of young adulthood and into the middle years, occupational patterns are reconfigured because of geographical relocations, career or employment changes, marriage and divorce, the development of children, and changes in the extended family. The adult in middle years is often spoken of as experiencing a "midlife crisis" because developing maturity leads to reflection on occupational patterns and life directions and sometimes to sudden lifestyle changes. Many women at this stage of life take on caregiving for aging parents, often with teenage children still in the home.

Retirement from paid employment brings on another round of occupational adaptation. New sources of satisfaction from productivity must be found. Social worlds previously constructed around colleagues and fellow workers may need to be re-created. Successful planning for retirement needs to include all the financial, emotional, and psychological needs that can emerge when occupational patterns are so drastically altered.

Becoming an elder in Western culture is a mixed blessing. Reflecting on how one has spent the time of one's life can be bittersweet. One may be treated with great respect and love, or feel devalued as a person who is no longer making a productive contribution to the world (McKinnon, 1992). Biological changes set in, often including declining vision and hearing, and sometimes worsening health. The oldest people hold great wisdom, yet in Western culture they are often treated as our least valuable citizens. Creating a gratifying occupational pattern at the end of life is a great challenge.

Using Time

Time is used in many ways in creating effective occupational therapy interventions. We consider circadian rhythms and possible disruptions of the circadian system by neurological insult, irregular schedules, and psychiatric conditions. Sociotemporality must be used to negotiate scheduling client appointments, despite cultural differences in perspectives on time, and to help clients understand the expectations for time use in school and employment settings in which they wish to participate. The degree to which we treat the time of our clients and colleagues with respect demonstrates the degree to which we value them as individuals. A detailed understanding of the temporal dimension in the single occupational experience of a client helps us to deal best with attention span, activity choice, appropriate pace, planning, reflection, and the creation of healthy habits and routines.

Occupational therapists work with individuals of all ages who are dealing with the typical challenges of their life stages. Pediatric occupational therapists make powerful use of developmental forces in assisting children with all sorts of disabilities. At the adolescent phase, occupational therapists see teenagers in psychiatric settings who are reacting to the pressures of culture with anorexia, bulimia, depression, violence, suicidal tendencies, and risk-seeking behaviors. Work with adults runs the gamut of psychiatric and physical diagnoses, including workplace and automobile injuries, and the negative health effects of long-term addictions to alcohol, nicotine, and other substances (Yerxa & Locker, 1990). Later adulthood brings more consequences of long-term unhealthy lifestyles, with increasing frequency of coronary problems. Loss of function in elder years can lead to institutionalization and long-term care, wherein occupational therapists may work on everyday occupational patterns of self-care, feeding, and sleeping. Occupational therapists may be seen working in hospice settings, assisting individuals with reflective and leave-taking occupations important to them and to their families at life's end. Throughout the life span, design of a satisfying and functional occupational pattern involves many typical and atypical challenges. Under conditions that threaten to prevent the individual's construction of his or her desired occupational pattern, an occupational therapist with a deep understanding of those processes and their facilitation can make all the difference in the world.

POWER BUILDERS

Key Concepts for Strengthening Insight into the Temporal Dimension of Occupation

- Biotemporality
- Neurophysiology of time sense
- Circadian rhythms and disorders
- Infant biotemporality
- Elder biotemporality
- Sociotemporality
- Calendars
- Workday-weekend
- Schedules
- Clocks
- Cultural differences in time use
- Economic view of time
- Subjective time
- Occupation differentiated from activity
- Occupation construction
- Subjective differences in temporality
- Pace
- Rhythm
- Orchestration
- Memory
- Temporal horizon
- Habit and routine
- Narrative
- Typical primate patterns of occupations
- Typical developmental patterns of human occupations

Building Insight into the Temporal Dimension of Your Own Occupations

1. Reflect on the following, in discussion with others, as a journal entry, or as a more formal paper or poster presentation:

   - Do you have a very regular circadian pattern, staying roughly the same on weekdays and weekends, or is there a lot of variation?

   - Have you ever experienced a circadian disturbance from jet lag, relocation, time change, shift work, or SAD?

   - Have you lived with a very old or very young person and noticed a difference between your own biotemporal rhythms and theirs?

   - Have you ever tried to live on a schedule different from that of others around you? How well did it work?

POWER BUILDERS

- Have you ever spent time in a place or with a person where time was seen differently because of a cultural difference in perspective? What were the difficulties?
- Do you believe that "time is money"? Why or why not?
- Describe an activity idea you have used in the last 24 hours to guide an occupational experience.
- Describe an occupational experience you have had recently that included multiple activity ideas.
- Describe two experiences you have had of approximately the same length of clock time, one of which passed quickly and one of which passed slowly.
- What techniques do you use to orchestrate your daily occupational pattern (plan in the shower, keep a day-runner schedule, and so forth)?
- What is the most regular and unvarying routine in your life?
- Have you ever tried to change a habit? How successful were you?

2. Put away all clocks and watches in your space for an entire weekend. Try not to talk about, think about, or look for clock time.

3. Figure out your birthday on the French Revolutionary Calendar.

4. Pick someone you know well (who you know will understand and forgive you) and try an experiment in imposing on private time. Pick a time that you would consider private and show up at that person's door, asking if you can come in and talk. After a couple of minutes, explain that it is a class assignment, thank the person, and apologize if you disturbed him or her. Notice how you feel imposing on the person's private time, how he or she reacts, what he or she thinks about you being there at that time.

5. Make a lark-owl lineup by having a group of people line up from the earliest lark at one end to the latest owl at the other. Just start out by heading for the place you think you belong, and then talk to the people there to figure out who is earlier or later in their natural biotemporal pattern, until you agree and can form one long line.

6. Activities are ideas, and thus they exist outside of experienced time. List as many activities as you can think of that you have never experienced as occupations, yet understand what they mean. Can you see how they exist outside of time? Describe this in your own words.

7. Keep a log of your occupations for 1 day or 1 week: note times, places, who was with you, and how you felt. What temporal patterns can you identify? Think of biotemporality, sociotemporality, experience within an occupation, and your efforts to orchestrate your occupational pattern.

8. Do as for exercise 7, for 2 weekdays and 2 weekend days. How are weekday and weekend temporal patterns different?

9. Are you a lark, an owl, or somewhere in between? What about your family members? Make a list of people who are either larks or owls. Have you always been the same in this way, or have you shifted somewhat in your biotemporal pattern?

10. Keep a time log of your occupational patterns for 2 weeks. Note times, places, who was with you, and how you felt for all your occupations. To do this well will require great determination on your part. After the 2 weeks is up, look over your recordings and make a list of the entire pattern you can see there. Use the content of this chapter to suggest to you the patterns you might search for in your recordings. Describe the patterns as a formal written report, supported by the data on your time logs, according to the types of patterns you discovered.

11. Pick something that you do regularly, such as a route you walk everyday or brushing your teeth in the morning. Do it at half the speed you usually complete it as if some type of disability were slowing down your actions. Require yourself to keep to this slow pace until you complete that occupation. How does this feel? How is it different from your usual experience of that same activity? If you were in a public place, did people act differently toward you? Write up or discuss the temporality of this experience with someone.

12. Spend some time writing in your journal about your habits and routines. List your usual daily routines. Have you ever experienced disruption of your routines? What caused this? Did you then reorganize your routines differently? Can you recognize any habits that were taught to you as a child? Are you involved with trying to teach children any daily routines?

Building Insight into the Temporal Dimension of the Occupations of Others

1. As a group or individually, collect clippings of articles or advertisements from magazines or newspapers that relate to some aspect of temporality. Tape them in groupings of biotemporality, sociotemporality, subjective patterns of occupation, orchestration of occupations, and broad developmental patterns of occupation. Discuss together the topics you have found and what the images seem to communicate about the temporality of occupational experience. Why are there more examples of some types of temporality in the media than others? Is temporality well understood in our culture? How much is it influencing our lives?

2. Do an observation of a group of people at some type of governmental services office at a busy time of the month. Call ahead to find out when that might be. Places that might be good to observe include unemployment offices, county health departments, social service agencies, and food stamp offices. Focus your observation on the temporality of the occupations of individuals in the room. Who is moving fast, and who slow? Who is in control of the pace of activity? Whose time appears more and less valued? Are there standard sequences of experience that you can see as part of a routine of operations there? What are the hours? Are there biotemporal rhythms in evidence?

POWER BUILDERS

3. Do a similar observation to the one in the previous exercise but in an occupational therapy clinic. As in previous exercises, consider how the therapist and the client take turns in their actions, who directs the action, who speaks more of the time, and other temporal aspects of the occupations of both client and therapist.

4. Interview someone who works a night or evening shift. What is the quality of his or her sleep? Does this individual have a regular occupational pattern with sleep recurring at the same time every day, or is he or she trying to flex sleep time on different days to fit the rest of the world's schedule? Is the interviewee able to participate in all the social activities at home and out in the community that he or she would like?

5. Select an occupational narrative from Appendix C and read it, keeping notes as you do so on how the temporal dimension is playing out in the narrative. Discuss these temporal patterns with someone, or write a reflection or short paper.

6. Select a case from Appendix A and prepare to discuss any temporal patterns you may be able to discern in the occupations of the person. Are there temporal patterns you would want to assess further in this case, based on your understanding of how this particular disability might create nontypical or disrupted occupational patterns?

7. Read an ethnography of a person with a disability, keeping notes as you do so on the temporal aspects of his or her occupational patterns and experiences. Write up your observations, or discuss them with someone else who has also read that book.

Building Design Skills Using the Temporal Dimension

1. Design for yourself a perfect day, from beginning to end, that you will be able to carry out in the next month or so. Use a simple time/task chart to list what you would like to do on your perfect day; then develop that into a schedule for the day. Once you have completed your perfect day, answer the following questions either in writing or in discussion: How did the implementation of your perfect day have to be adjusted as you carried it out? How did the timing of your day vary from your planned schedule? How did biotemporality, sociotemporality, subjective time, orchestration, and typical patterns of occupation reveal themselves within the temporal dimension of your day?

2. Pick someone you know well, and make the person a calendar of some type, to give as a gift. Personalize the calendar by placing times and dates on it that are especially important to that individual. Try using the following exercises to accomplish this: balloon the possibilities, boil down definitions, brainstorm ideas, rank ideas for selection, time/task chart the steps, construct the calendar, and reflect on the process in writing or in discussion.

3. On your own or in a group, use a seven-step design process to create an experience for a group of people that helps them learn about some aspect(s) of the temporal dimension of occupation.

4. Select a case that shows some biotemporal disturbances and use discussion to design interventions to respond to those disruptions. Try brainstorming to get started and then a simple ranking to decide which intervention you would try first.

5. With a group, select and read a case in Appendix A. Set an intervention goal or select one from the case if they are included. Brainstorm as many possible therapeutic occupational experiences as you could use as interventions. Do a quick ranking together to choose as many as you have people working with you in your group. Round-robin these ideas within the group on paper, each trying to improve the intervention's use of temporal dimension. Use the following steps: (1) Everyone write a very brief description of one of the therapeutic occupations to be used and pass it to the right. (2) Consider the temporal dimensions of occupation and rewrite the intervention briefly, incorporating how you would change the temporality of the intervention, and then pass it to the right. (3) Repeat step 2 until no one can improve the interventions further. (4) Then have each person read one finished and completely revised intervention and lead discussion of it.

6. Imagine that you are working with a 9-month-old infant with failure to thrive and eating problems that appear to be based in an aversion to textures and poor oral motor coordination. How would you use the temporal dimension of occupation to structure a therapeutic eating experience for this infant? What aspects of temporality could you consider? Use the balloon exercise to do this.

References

Adams, J., Folkard, S., & Young, M. (1986). Coping strategies used by nurses on night duty. Ergonomics, 29, 185–196.

Armstrong, S. M., & Redman, J. R. (1993). Melatonin and circadian rhythmicity. In H. Yu & R. Reiter (Eds.), Melatonin: Biosynthesis, physiological effects, and clinical applications (pp. 187–224). Ann Arbor, MI: CRC Press.

Aschoff, J. (1989). Temporal orientation: Circadian clocks in animals and humans. Animal Behavior, 37, 881–896.

Ayres, A. J. (1985). Developmental dyspraxia and adult onset apraxia. Torrance, CA: Sensory Integration International.

Bateson, M. C. (1990). Composing a life. New York: Penguin Books.

Buela, C. G., Caballo, V. E., & Garcia, C. E. (1990). Differences between morning and evening types in performance. Personality and Individual Differences, 11, 447–450.

Christiansen, C., Backman, C., Little, B., & Nguyen, A. (1999). Occupations and well-being: A study of personal projects. American Journal of Occupational Therapy, 53, 91–100.

Clark, F. A., Parham, L. D., Carlson, M. E., Frank, G., Jackson, J., Pierce, D., et al. (1991). Occupational science: Academic innovation in the service of occupational therapy's future. American Journal of Occupational Therapy, 45, 300–310.

Colquhoun, W. P. (1985). Hours of work at sea: Watchkeeping schedules, circadian rhythms and efficiency. Ergonomics, 28, 637–653.

Corbin, J. (1999, January). The role of habits in everyday life. Presented at AOTF Conference on Habits, Asilomar, CA.

Cottle, T., & Klineberg, S. (1974). The present of things future. New York: The Free Press.

Edelman, G. M. (1989). The remembered present: A biological theory of consciousness. New York: Basic Books.

Evans, L. K. (1987). Sundown syndrome in institutionalized elderly. Journal of the American Geriatrics Society, 35, 101–108.

Fraisse, P. (1981). Perception and estimation of time. Annual Review of Psychology, 35, 1–36.

Frank, G. (1996). Life histories in occupational therapy clinical practice. American Journal of Occupational Therapy, 50, 251–265.

Fraser, J. T. (1987). Time, the familiar stranger. Redmond, WA: University of Massachusetts Press.

Giambra, L. M., Rosenberg, E. H., Kasper, S., & Yee, W. (1988). A circadian rhythm in the frequency of spontaneous task-unrelated images and thoughts. Imagination, Cognition, and Personality, 8, 309–314.

Goodall, J. (1986). The chimpanzees of Gombe: Patterns of behavior. Cambridge, MA: Belknap Press.

Hall, E. T. (1983). The dance of life: The other dimension of time. New York: Doubleday Anchor.

Katzman, R., & Terry, R. D. (1983). The neurology of aging. Philadelphia: F. A. Davis.

Levine, R. (1997). A geography of time. New York: Basic Books.

Ludwig, F. (1998). The unpackaging of routine in older women. American Journal of Occupational Therapy, 52, 168–175.

Martin, J. H. (1996). Neuroanatomy: Text and atlas. Stamford, CT: Appleton & Lange.

Mason, D. J. (1989). Circadian rhythms of body temperature and activation and the well-being of older women. Nursing Research, 37, 276–281.

McKinnon, A. (1992). Time use of self care, productivity, and leisure among elderly Canadians. Canadian Journal of Occupational Therapy, 59, 102–110.

Mecacci, L., Zani, A., Rocchetti, G., & Lucioli, R. (1986). The relationship between morningness-eveningness, ageing and personality. Personality and Individual Differences, 7, 911–913.

Medrich, E., Roizen, J., Rubin, V., & Buckley, S. (1982). The serious business of growing up: A study of children's lives outside of school. Los Angeles: University of California Press.

Meyer, A. (1922/1977). The philosophy of occupational therapy. American Journal of Occupational Therapy, 31, 639–642.

Minors, D. S., Rabbitt, P. M., Worthington, H., & Waterhouse, J. M. (1989). Variation in meals and sleep-activity patterns in aged subjects: Its relevance to circadian rhythm studies. Chronobiology International, 6, 139–146.

Moore-Ede, M. C., Sulzman, F. M., & Fuller, C. A. (1982). The clocks that time us. Cambridge: Harvard University Press.

Pierce, D. E. (1996). Infant space, infant time: Development of infant interactions with the physical environment, from 1 to 18 months. Dissertation Abstracts International.

Pierce, D. E. (1997). The neurologic base of primary occupational patterns: Productivity, pleasure, and rest. In C. B. Royeen (Ed.), AOTA clinical course: Neuroscience foundations of occupation. Bethesda, MD: American Occupational Therapy Association.

Pierce, D. E. (2001). Untangling occupation and activity. American Journal of Occupational Therapy, 55, 138–146.

Piaget, J. (1952). The origins of intelligence in children. New York: International Universities Press.

Primeau, L. (1998). Orchestration of work and play within families. American Journal of Occupational Therapy, 52, 188–195.

Raviv, S., & Low, M. (1990). Influence of physical activity on concentration among junior high school students. Perceptual and Motor Skills, 70, 67–74.

Redfern, P. H. (1989). "Jet-lag": Strategies for prevention and cure. Human Psychopharmacology, 4, 159–168.

Rifkin, J. (1987). Time wars. New York: Henry Holt and Company.

Royeen, C. (1995). The human life cycle: Paradigmatic shifts in occupation. In C. Royeen (Ed.), AOTA self-study series—The practice of the future: Putting occupation back into therapy. Bethesda, MD: American Occupational Therapy Association.

Rybczynski, W. (1991). Waiting for the weekend. New York: Penguin Books.

Schmidt, R. F. (1975). Fundamentals of neurophysiology. New York: Springer-Verlag.

Schor, J. (1992). The overworked American. New York: Basic Books.

Searle, J. (1995). The rediscovery of the mind. Cambridge, MA: MIT Press.

Strauss, A. (1993). Continual permutations of action. New York: Aldine de Gruyter.

Suto, M., & Frank, G. (1994). Future time perspective and daily occupations of persons with chronic schizophrenia in a board and care home. American Journal of Occupational Therapy, 48, 7–18.

Swaab, D. F., Fliers, E., & Partiman, T. S. (1985). The suprachiasmatic nucleus of the human brain in relation to sex, age, and senile dementia. Brain Research, 342, 37–44.

Taylor, F. (1911/1967). *The principles of scientific management.* New York: W. W. Norton & Company.

Terman, M. (1994). Light treatment. In M. H. Kryger, T. Roth, & W. C. Dement (Eds.), *Principles and practices of sleep medicine* (pp. 1012–1029). Philadelphia: W. B. Saunders.

Teterina, T. P., Volkov, V. V., & Moldova, L. P. (1989). Dynamics of temporal rhythmic cyclicity of monocular perceptions in the act of binocular vision. *Sensory Systems, 3,* 201–206.

Thalen, B., Kjellman, B., & Wetterberg, L. (1993). Phototherapy and melatonin in relation to seasonal affective disorder and depression. In H. Yu & R. Reiter (Eds.), *Melatonin: Biosynthesis, physiological effects, and clinical applications* (pp. 495–512). Ann Arbor, MI: CRC Press.

Thayer, R. E. (1987). Problem perception, optimism, and related states as a function of time of day (diurnal rhythm) and moderate exercise. *Motivation and Emotion, 11,* 19–36.

Tsujimoto, T., Yamada, N., Shimoda, K., & Hanada, K. (1990). Circadian rhythms in depression: II. Circadian rhythms in inpatients with various mental disorders. *Journal of Affective Disorders, 18,* 199–210.

Vallacher, R., & Wegner, D. (1987). What do people think they're doing ? Action identification and human behavior. *Psychological Review, 94,* 3–15.

Wilson, G. D. (1990). Personality, time of day, and arousal. *Personality and Individual Differences, 11,* 153–168.

Witting, W., Kwa, I. H., Eikelenboom, P., & Mirmiran, M. (1990). Alterations in the circadian rest-activity rhythm in aging and Alzheimer's disease. *Biological Psychiatry, 27,* 563–572.

Yerxa, E., & Locker, S. (1990). Quality of time use by adults with spinal cord injuries. *American Journal of Occupational Therapy, 44,* 318–326.

Zemke, R. (1994). Habits. In C. Royeen (Ed.), *The practice of the future: Putting occupation back into therapy* (pp. 1–24). Bethesda, MD: American Occupational Therapy Association.

Zerubavel, E. (1981). *Hidden rhythms: Schedules and calendars in social life.* Los Angeles: University of California Press.

The Sociocultural Dimension of Occupations

Between Self and Society

Social Ties

Human Culture

Cultures of Service Provision

Sociocultural Aspects of Effective Occupation-
Based Intervention

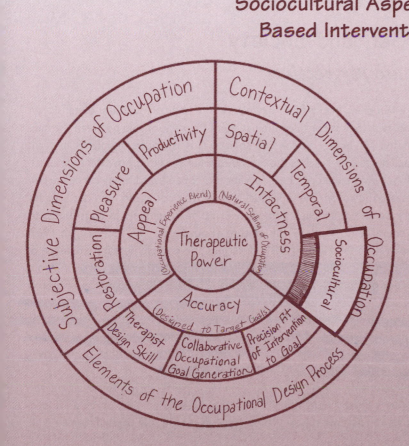

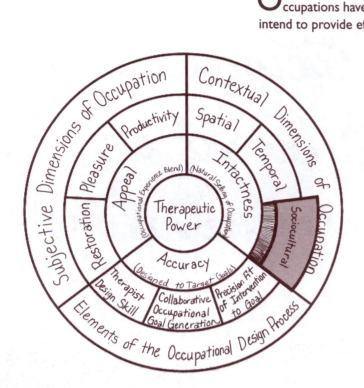

Occupations have a complex sociocultural dimension that cannot be disregarded if you intend to provide effective intervention. This dimension is far better understood in occupational therapy than are the spatial and the temporal dimensions. The term *sociocultural* is a combination of the words *society* and *culture*, which are the primary concepts of the disciplines of sociology and anthropology, respectively.

Mary Reilly (1974) pioneered the importation of social science theories into occupational therapy practice in her creation and development of the occupational behavior approach. Following its roots in occupational behavior, occupational science has continued in this tradition. Occupational science differs significantly from occupational behavior, however, in the degree to which original disciplinary theories are being generated through sophisticated research and imported theories are being subjected to critical examination for a close fit with the values and needs of occupational therapy. Occupational science has often been called a social science. Of all the academic disciplines, occupational science draws most heavily on the discipline of anthropology.

This chapter provides an overview of some of the more outstanding aspects of sociocultural context that flavor our everyday occupational experiences. It is divided into two primary sections, social and cultural. The social aspects of occupational experience discussed here include identity, the continuum of solitary to shared occupations, relationships, and organizations. Key concepts in the cultural aspects of occupational experience covered here are ritual, cross-cultural competence, diversity, gender, and unique professional and client subcultures expressed in intervention settings.

Between Self and Society
Etic and Emic Perspectives

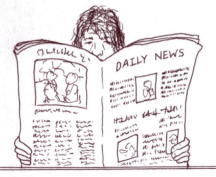

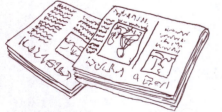

Before launching into a fuller examination of the sociocultural dimension, it is important to first consider the nature of the relationship between the individual and his or her culture or society. This is not as simple as it might appear. The culture teaches the individual what is valued, how things are usually done, what to expect, how families are constructed, what certain activities mean, and so on. The individual may or may not agree with the broader society on all points. Each person's viewpoint is unique and contributes to the general ideas held by the culture (Bourdieux, 1977; Heidegger, 1962; Malinowski, 1944). Harris (1981) describes the complementary existence of *emic* (from phonemic), or individually interpreted, meaning and *etic* (from phonetic) meaning, which is derived from a cultural classification (Pierce & Frank, 1992). Occupational experience is an emic, or personally experienced and interpreted, viewpoint of the meanings for an individual of his or her actions in the world. Activity is the etic, or culturally interpreted, idea of how something is usually done and what it usually means. Both perspectives are essential to occupational therapy practitioners.

Here is an example of the emic and etic perspectives. You see a person sitting in a library holding up a newspaper. Using an etic, or cultural, perspective, you assume this is a library patron reading the paper. From an emic perspective, however, the person looking at the newspaper may be having the experience of a homeless person trying to keep warm in the library by appearing to read the newspaper, although she has lost her reading glasses and cannot actually make out the words. Neither of these perspectives is wrong. They are just different viewpoints. Most important, to provide excellence in intervention, the therapist must be able to work within the individual, emic perspective. Yet, he or she must also depend on a thorough grounding in the sociocultural dynamics and meanings of human activities as a general guide to understanding how clients are situated in their social worlds. It is critical to effective intervention that the therapist knows when he or she is viewing the client from the perspective of the culture, and when from within the life perspective of the individual. It is knowing where you are standing at all times, viewing the client from either an emic or an etic perspective, that will best equip you to intervene within the sociocultural dimension.

Occupation and Identity

Personal identity is a good example of how we negotiate between the emic and etic perspectives in our lives. Occupation is central to the way in which we create our identities, express who we are to others, and conform to expectations for our actions or choose not to conform. Christiansen (1999), in his Eleanor Clarke Slagle Lecture, discussed the interrelations of occupation and identity. We each have a certain experience of the things we do (emic). Simultaneously, we are aware of how what we are doing appears to and is interpreted by others (etic). On some occasions, you may try very hard to appear in a certain way; at other times, you may give it little thought. People with disabilities that result in stigma and exclusion, such as individuals with facial scars or the uncontrollable movements of athetoid cerebral palsy, must work very hard at "impression management" (Christiansen, 1999, p. 554) to minimize the negative social effects of their disabilities. Belonging to certain social groupings, such as a family or a church, also expresses identity. The goals and dreams we hold of things we would like to do in the future, such as fly an airplane or become a therapist, are also a part of our identities. We shape our identities by engaging in certain occupations and not in others. For those of our clients who have suddenly acquired a disrupted occupational pattern, the reconstruction of a personal identity is a pressing, central, and delicate project, to which the occupational therapist must attend. Failing to be aware of the identity work in which a client is engaged will inevitably result in weak interventions.

Solitary, Shared, and Co-Occupations

A primary aspect of how we experience occupations is their social nature. That is, am I engaging in an occupation as part of an interaction with another person, or not? All occupations fall somewhere on a continuum of social involvement from completely interactive to solitary.

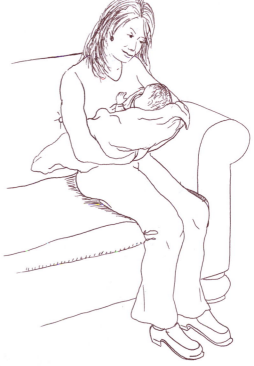

Co-occupations are the most highly interactive types of occupation, in which the occupational experiences of the individuals involved simply could not occur without the interactive responses of the other person or persons with whom the occupations are being experienced. Consider, for example, the likely occupational experiences of a mother and her child during breast-feeding. Another example is the experiences of four people playing a game of tennis. Certain activities are conceptualized as necessarily interactive with others: making love, teaching, caregiving. These highly interactive experiences of doing are called co-occupations. They are a synchronous dance back and forth between the occupational experiences of the individuals involved, the

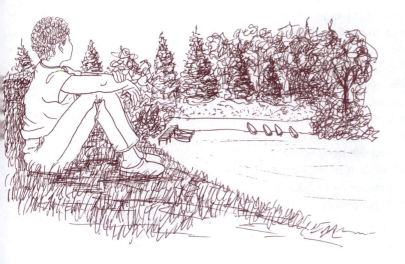

action of one closely shaping the action of the other in a close match.

Solitary occupations are at the other end of the continuum. The person engaged in a solitary occupation perceives his or her experience as completely uninvolved with others. This does not necessarily mean that there are not other people around during the occupation, only that the individual does not perceive them as privy to or participating in the occupation in which he or she is engaged. Activities that we usually think of as solitary are, for example, keeping a journal, taking a bath, worrying, writing, and thinking. Of course, because activities are only general cultural ideas about doing, we can also imagine ways in which these activities might be experienced in nonsolitary ways. Honeymooners might share a romantic bubble bath. One might think out loud, with a friend listening and responding to your expressed thoughts. Whether miles from civilization or in the midst of a crowd, if the individual does not perceive that anyone else is a part of the experience that he or she is having, it is a solitary occupation. For example, a person hiking the Appalachian Trail on his or her own is likely to have a series of solitary occupations. A person flying in a crowded plane full of strangers and composing a poem on a laptop computer is probably also having a solitary occupational experience, unless he or she stops to recite the poem to someone.

In the middle of the continuum of the social nature of occupations are shared occupations. Falling between co-occupations, which require another person, and solitary occupations, which specifically do not include others in the experience, shared occupations are interactive in a more parallel way. A good example of a shared occupation is the experience one is likely to have while eating a family dinner. It is easy to imagine the conversations and passing of food between people as they eat, everyone at the table probably experiencing the meal as interactive with and involving others. Interaction with others at the table is not usually perceived as required or essential to engaging in having dinner as in a co-occupation. Rather, it is just a part of the conditions under which eating is taking place. Another example of a shared occupational experience is watching a football game on television with friends. To the degree that the individual perceives that others are privy to his or her experience of the game, through comments, exchanged glances, and body language, then the occupation is shared.

Social Ties

Relationships

Relationships with others exert a powerful shaping force on our occupational experiences. A relationship is a shared understanding of how two individuals are related to each other within their lives and actions. There are many examples of relationships: coworkers, friends, lovers, the many varieties of family relationships, prisoner and guard, even bus driver and passenger. Relationships vary widely in length, importance to individuals, intimacy, effects on individuals, degree to which they are equal or unequal between individuals, and the types of feelings they evoke. Similar to the way in which the concepts of activity and occupation differ, we all have both cultural ideas about relationships (how a grandmother and grandchild typically relate in our own culture) and real experiences of relationships (how you and your grandmother interacted on a certain day).

Relationships influence occupational experiences in many ways. Adults generally construct a pattern of occupations to include time with those individuals with whom they wish to remain in relationships. Commitments to particular relationships, such as a parent's commitment to a child, can require that certain activities be included in the occupational pattern. Sometimes occupations are engaged in specifically to build relationships: for example, dating or having lunch with a business client. Sharing an activity with a person with whom you have a relationship, rather than engaging in a solitary occupation, can change the occupational experience in many ways. It is difficult to overstate how much primary relationships, such as those that exist between spouses, parents and children, or long-term friends, act on us to shape our lives, our occupational patterns, and our concept of self.

Organizations

The social aspect of occupational experiences and relationships often exists within more formal networks of relationships or organizations. An organization is a group of individuals who share a common goal or effort. These shared goals tend to bring the occupations of individuals within the organization into an interdependent pattern. Consider, for example, a Christian church. Although members of the congregation may have somewhat different goals, they are likely to generally share an aim to engage in religious observations and fellowship to add to the spiritual dimension of their lives. They will take up different forms of participation within the organization, such as choir director, choir member, minister, Sunday school teacher, Sunday school student, church secretary, head of a church service project, or simply a participant in services. Although each person is involved in a different way, the time, place, and social conditions under which individuals experience the occupations of church membership are influenced by the occupational patterns of all the other members and their shared sense of mission. The number of examples of organizations that could be used to illustrate this interwoven pattern of occupations is nearly infinite. A hospital is a healthcare organization. Mothers Against Drunk Driving is a volunteer organization. A university is an educational organization. The United States Air Force is a military organization. The World Trade Organization is a business organization. People in these organizations share a general intent, which brings their occupational patterns into a broadly orchestrated and somewhat synchronous arrangement within time, space, and relationships.

Human Culture

Culture is a broad term for shared meanings about "traditionalized ways of living and working together" (Bruner, 1990, p. 11). Those shared ways of doing include activity ideas, language, symbols, a history of action, values, and typical material objects involved in everyday life. Individuals both acquire culture through their immersion in it and create culture through their actions within a shared life world (Bourdieux, 1977).

Contrasting Primate Cultures

An effective way in which to more clearly understand culture, which is so pervasive in our lives as to make it nearly invisible to us, is to contrast human culture with the culture of

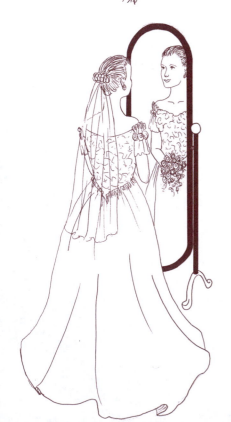

our closest primate cousins, chimpanzees. Chimpanzee culture is different from our own in several primary ways (Goodall, 1986). The structure of the family is quite different because there is no father included, only mother, children, siblings, and other maternal relations. Communities of chimpanzees tend to live in two types of groups: adult males or females with children. Male infants usually stay with their mothers for quite a long time, increasingly spending time with the male troop once they become juveniles. Adult males will socialize with female relatives, especially their mothers, and with other females when they are in estrus. The two groups gather together frequently where food is available or for protection.

Unlike human culture, chimpanzee culture includes very little in the way of material objects and traditions of manufacture. They do not wear clothing, use shelters (beyond nests built for a night's sleep), cultivate crops, raise domestic animals, record language, or create ritual and aesthetic objects. They are nomads traveling to where there is food within a broad home range. The only tools they have been observed to use have been crafted for the moment from available natural materials, such as a stick for fishing for termites, a rock for breaking open nuts, or a crumpled leaf for sponging up water to drink. Still, chimpanzees do have food and activity traditions that differ among communities.

Chimpanzees communicate through sound, eye contact, movement, and gesture, but they do not have the complex written and spoken language of humans. Similarly, although they have a loose hierarchy of leadership and loyalty to which they adhere, they do not have a formal system of laws. Human culture also includes a variety of institutions, which differ somewhat from one culture to the next. Institutions include marriage, law, religion, economy, language, and family. The way in which these structures are enacted within a culture makes up the unique lifestyle typical of being a part of a particular culture. Comparing human and chimpanzee culture in this way makes the unique characteristics of human culture more apparent to us.

Ritual

Rituals are temporal structures of occupations that carry a recognized cultural and personal meaning. That meaning is about the transition of the primary person or persons engaged in the ritual from one status in the culture to another. Examples of culturally recognized rituals are birthdays, religious holidays, and patriotic observances. Rituals are marked by a predictable, seemingly scripted series of symbolic actions and objects. Reenacting annual rituals, such as religious holidays, can bring a flood of feelings, because of the emotional associations of engaging in that same sequence of actions many times before, perhaps with other people or in other places, and always when you were a younger, different self. Sometimes people use the word *ritual* loosely to describe personal routines and habits to which they have become attached. If it does not carry a symbolic cultural meaning, however, it is not actually a ritual.

The most formal rituals are rites of passage. These are rituals with a capital R. Weddings and graduations are good examples of rites of passage, complete with expected sequences of actions, special clothing, particular spaces in which they should occur, and changes in how the person is treated and addressed after the transition. A rite of passage can carry much drama and emotional content for both the primary person involved and the observers. It is often experienced by a person as a sort of test or change. Rites of passage are thought of as one-time events that mark turning points in a person's life.

Diversity

In the industrialized Western culture of the United States, the expressed cultural values emphasize individualism, independence, materialism, mobility, and productivity (Bellah, Madsen, Sullivan, Swidler, & Tipton, 1985; Cross, 1990). To offer strong interventions, therapists must not only understand these Western values in the individuals with whom they work but also recognize when those values are not appropriately used.

How occupations are typically experienced and the patterns they make up differ from one culture to the next. Unfortunately, research into cultural differences in occupation is in its bare beginning. Even if research were plentiful, it would be impossible for an occupational therapist to develop an in-depth understanding of all the cultures and ethnic groups that he or she might work with over an entire career. There are significant differences between cultures in communication styles, gender relations, and how interactions between people of different ages appropriately occur. As well as coming from an identifiable cultural group, individuals are also rooted in family histories of a particular geographical and class background. Persons with whom you work may have backgrounds that are rural, suburban, or urban. They may have recently emigrated or been dislocated from a beloved home. Measures of class are usually translated into socioeconomic status, which considers income, education, and type of employment. The term *class* is often used loosely to refer to upper class (high income; college degree(s); professional and powerful jobs), middle class (middle income; high school to baccalaureate degrees; white collar, higher level service and middle management jobs), and lower or working class (low income; up to high school education; blue collar jobs, lower level service, seasonal work, or unemployed). The working class includes individuals below the poverty line as well as those who are somewhat above that, whether they are working poor or unemployed, homeless or homed, insured or medically indigent. As with geographical diversity, it is worthwhile to gently inquire about family history to gain a picture of the class values your client may bring to intervention.

It is also important to recognize areas of diversity that can be more appropriately termed *lifestyle* diversity, as opposed to cultural, geographical, or class diversity. People live life in all kinds of ways: single, married, gay, lesbian, straight, transsexual, and bisexual. Families are constructed in all kinds of forms: nuclear, extended, grandparents with grandchildren, single parents with children, blended families, gay and lesbian partners with children, and noncustodial parent-child relationships. Among these variations in lifestyle exist individuals who are both able-bodied and disabled.

It is critical to best practice that occupational therapists be able to insightfully identify and describe how their own personal and cultural values shape their perspectives on occupation and occupation-based practice. If the therapist is not able to do so, he or she will inevitably project a set of cultural expectations onto individuals for whom they are not appropriate. This will result in poor goal setting, ineffective intervention, and frustration for both the therapist and the client.

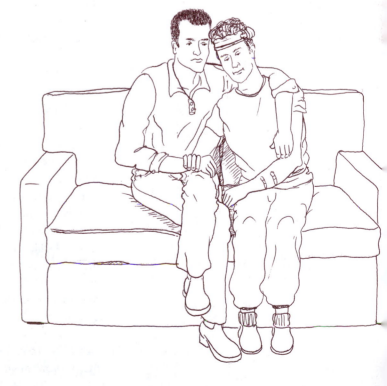

Gender

The way in which gender is constructed is an aspect of culture that places a firm imprint on each person's occupational pattern. Being male or female is likely to result in involvement in certain activities and not in others. It affects the way we see ourselves, the way we see others, our communications and relationships, and the type of work we do. Different cultures, of course, construct gender differently. The following overview primarily addresses how gender is constructed and enacted in modern, industrialized, Western culture.

Understanding gender and how it plays out in terms of the occupational patterns, values, and communication styles of women and men is an invaluable form of insight for the practicing occupational therapist. This requires a scholarly approach, grounded in the understanding that the concept of gender can be both useful in giving a general perspective on typical patterns and dangerous in overdetermining choices and opportunities. The women's movement produced a wave of scholarship that better informs us about the occupational experiences of women, although it is less useful in assisting us to understand how the experiences of men are unique. Gay and lesbian rights movements argue that gender is more of a continuum than a clear black and white dichotomy, graying the differences between the genders.

Our gender is made clear to us through interactions with others from the time we are born (Liben & Signorella, 1987; Maccoby, 1998). From the "pink aisle" of girls' toys at large toy stores to the admonitions of parents regarding proper behavior for girls or for boys, children receive constant messages that influence how they see themselves in terms of gender. Children's time use is significantly different according to gender, with boys spending more time in leisure activities than girls, and less time in personal care and household work (Mauldin & Meeks, 1990).

Socialization to gender results in adults who tend to differ in predictable ways in terms of their thinking, feelings, communication styles, and abilities (Belenky, Clinchy, Goldberger, & Tarule, 1996; Maccoby, 1998; Tannen, 1996). This general notion concerning gender differences between women and men can be a good general guide to understanding someone, as well as a dangerous cultural stereotype that limits life opportunities for persons of both genders. Women are thought of in Western culture as more nurturing, emotional, weak, and defined through relationships with others, whereas men are considered to be more strong, independent, analytical, and defined through their work status. In long-term relationships, the differences between women and men can be thought of not only as bringing complementary skill sets together but also as creating great challenge to communication and a mutually satisfying life (Rubin, 1983).

The work life of women in the United States has undergone especially dramatic changes in the last two centuries, from largely unpaid household work to increasingly equal opportunities to do many of the jobs previously held exclusively by men (Baxandall & Gordon, 1995). Of course, women overall still do not make as much money, control as many assets, or hold as much status and decision-making power as men do. Also, the fact that women bear the children of the culture impacts their participation in paid work. One of the greatest challenges to women in paid employment is what has been called the "second shift" (Hochschild, 1989, p. 4), which refers to the childcare and household work that awaits women when they arrive home after a day on the job. Despite cultural changes in opportunities for women, women and children living in single female-headed households make up the largest percentage of people below the poverty level in the United States.

Household work and caregiving are activities that are often thought of as women's work. The roles that women have played in the home have not changed so much as to make involvement in occupations of caring for the home, family, children, elders, and those who are ill an equal-opportunity event. Women still carry most of the responsibilities in these areas (Primeau, 1992). An additional area of unpaid activity that is commonly associated with women is volunteer work. As more and more women are entering paid employment, however, volunteer contributions to our communities are decreasing (Daniels, 1988). Still, volunteer work can be highly satisfying, and often plays an important part in transitions out of paid work and into retirement, or as the primary community involvement of women who are not employed outside the home (Bird, 1995).

Cultures of Service Provision

Medicine and Rehabilitation

The history of medicine is a long one, charting the rise of doctors from the status of local herbalists working from lore passed from one generation to the next, to the highly specialized, research-oriented, powerful, and wealthy physicians of today. Medicine is not only a profession, but a giant industry that combines service to individuals with the care and feeding of insurance companies, healthcare corporations, manufacturers of medical supplies and equipment, pharmaceutical companies, and governmental support programs. The physician today is viewed as an authority, an expert in a specific area, with nearly God-like capacities to save and restore lives through medical interventions. Foucault (1973) described the physician's powers of observation and diagnosis as "the gaze," an oppressively powerful form of insight and surveillance.

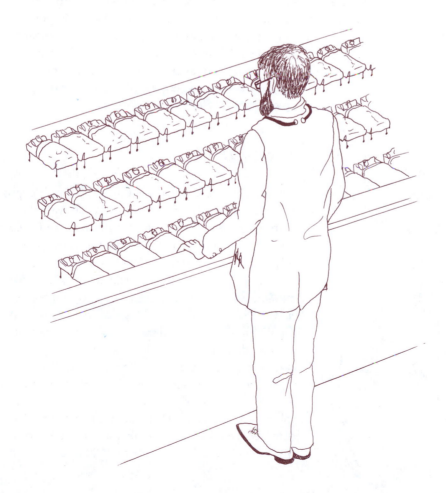

The World Wars created a great demand for medicine to develop the specialty of rehabilitation medicine, to assist returning war veterans with disabilities and help them reclaim function and reintegrate into society. As a specialty, rehabilitation medicine carries a strong emphasis on the importance of technology, surgery, adaptive devices, and interdisciplinary teamwork (Brandt & Pope, 1997; Frank, 2000). It was within the culture of rehabilitation medicine that much of occupational therapy's early growth occurred.

Occupational Therapy

Occupational therapy culture exists in an uneasy relationship with the cultures of medicine and rehabilitation. To be an effective occupational therapist, it is necessary to believe that the client is the final authority and expert on what is needed, valued, and useful in intervention (Yerxa, 1983). Health is judged in occupational therapy not by surgical or technical outcomes, but by the quality of life a person finds in his or her patterns of occupation. This set of humanistic values is in direct opposition to the values of medicine, which place ultimate authority in the hands of the physician and award to the recipient of care a more passive, trusting, and compliant sick role.

Peloquin (1990) characterizes the patient-therapist relationship in occupational therapy as a blend of competence and caring. Emphasizing competence over caring results in a therapist who operates as a technician. Emphasizing caring over competence yields a rather parental, "for their own good," approach that reserves authority for the therapist. More recently, Peloquin (1993) found that the tendency to emphasize competence over caring in the therapeutic relationship was caused by beliefs of both therapists and clients in the effectiveness of technical corrections of medical problems, use of standard procedures, and the profit orientation in health care. The tension of values between medicine and occupational therapy requires therapists, especially those in traditional medical settings such as hospitals, to be constantly reflective regarding the values on which they base therapeutic relationships with their clients. An even balance of competence and caring is the highest quality of therapeutic relationship and resembles friendship.

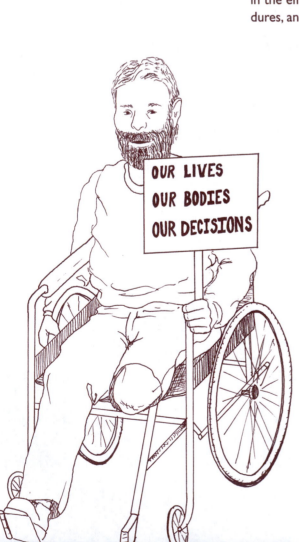

Disability Rights

The disability rights movement arose in direct opposition to the culture and values of medicine. During times rife with social movements, such as protests against the Vietnam War and working for equal rights for women and blacks, people with physical disabilities began protesting their situation as "patients for life" (Frank, 2000, p. 44) within the specialty of rehabilitation medicine (Gritzer & Arluke, 1985; Starr, 1982). The primary tenet of this movement was that disability is not a condition of an individual, but is created by the way in which society excludes, discriminates against, and unfairly treats individuals with disabilities. As consumers of medical services, people with disabilities demanded the opportunity to choose not to live in a medical-care setting or in the homes of caregivers, but to live on their own as free adults. The independent living movement and its landmark legislation, the Rehabilitation Act of 1973, generated the organization of residential centers all over the United States that honored these principles of freedom, self-direction, and the "de-medicalization" of the lives of individuals with lifelong disabling conditions. Within the disability rights movement, people demanded nothing less than the supports and access necessary to be fully functioning members of society. Occupational therapists, using an independent living approach, tend to follow this political voice of consumers by focusing not on the disability and skills of the individual as goals of intervention, but on changes in the environment that can free that individual to engage in the occupational pattern that he or she envisions (Bowen, 1996).

Power is a key issue in the cultures of medicine, rehabilitation, occupational therapy, and the disability rights movement. The question of who has ultimate authority in services to people with disabilities shapes what services are judged most important to provide, who provides them, and where and how they are offered. In some ways, medical practitioners have tried to support people with disabilities by "empowering" them (Neath & Schriner, 1998). Unfortunately, this idea that a service provider can bestow power on a client still seems to rest on the notion that the power is truly in the hands of the healthcare professional. If one listens to the conversations of healthcare teams, the words that indicate a team member's belief that it's not the client who holds the power are easy to hear: "noncompliance," "determination of placement," and "doctor's orders" are all common examples.

Shifting to Community-Based Care

Although occupational therapists have, by and large, negotiated this conflict of values successfully over the years, it has taken its toll on the profession in confusion over what expertise is most important to develop and in the variety of value-shaped modes of service delivery that can be found in different occupational therapy settings. The movement of occupational therapy increasingly into non-medical community settings, where the consumers of service hold more power—such as in schools, independent living centers, and private clinics—has helped to ease this clash of values between medicine and the profession. The most effective occupational therapy is provided in settings in which occupational therapists can operate from their true culture, which values the subjective experience and perspective of the client over their own as experts.

Sociocultural Aspects of Effective Occupation-Based Intervention

Attend to Identity

Questioning the identity issues with which a client may be dealing is a good way to begin intervention. How does this person see himself or herself? To what new identity does the person aspire in the future? Is there a new career, new skills, or new images of the person in the eyes of others that are important? What new occupational patterns and skills will be necessary to reach a desired identity? As you build an increasing rapport with an individual, you may be able to gently raise such sensitive topics. Be careful not to overstep, however, if such a discussion is not welcomed.

Design with Social Context

In the design of treatment, the therapist will consider where on the continuum of solitary occupations to co-occupations an individual will best progress toward his or her goals. There are many examples of this. Very reflective interventions may be better undertaken in solitude with the support of the therapist. A teenager might do better or worse in a peer group, depending on the situation. Significant others may be able to support your client's goals. New occupational patterns that require the involvement of caregivers will best be addressed by including the caregivers in interventions. Re-engaging in a relationship—for example, returning to work relationships or going home to take up parenting again—can be a desired outcome of intervention. Relationship skills can even be a targeted goal of intervention. The relationship between the therapist and the client is also key to the process of intervention, depending on trust, mutual respect, and rapport.

Understanding the interdependent occupational patterns of individuals in organizations is also important to designing interventions. This understanding is especially true when a client is targeting successful entry or re-entry into an organization as an outcome of therapy. For example, occupational therapists involved in the transition of children with disabilities from segregated to more fully integrated school settings or of injured workers back to worksites all depend on a careful understanding of the organizations their clients are entering. Providing intervention within the organization that the client wishes to enter or re-enter, rather than within a separate organization such as a hospital clinic, increases the efficacy of interventions. Helping clients to "read" the organizations within which they wish to be successful and to acquire the skills necessary to contribute to that organization can be a challenging part of community-based occupational therapy.

Cultural Competence

An understanding of the cultural aspects of occupational experience supports skilled interventions. Grasping the basic nature of human culture provides an invaluable foundation for viewing the occupational patterns of your clients. Providing culturally competent intervention for persons with diverse backgrounds is an ability that is required in any setting in which occupational therapists practice. Cultural rituals can be used to frame compelling interventions. Using your connoisseur's insight into occupation, you can effectively explore the occupations of interest to a client from any cultural background, as long as you can find a mode of communication. Ask which occupations are most important, currently problematic, the high point of the year, or predictably a part of every day for that person. Ask for the story of a typical day, or the typical day before and after the event that landed him or her in therapy. Ask for a description of a perfect day to work toward for goal setting. In effective occupational therapy, you can always go back to your core knowledge of occupation as a place to begin, refocus, assess, or bring closure to intervention, regardless of cultural difference.

A basic overview of a specific culture of interest to a therapist can be quickly obtained through some well-selected readings. Of course, these very general descriptions of a culture and its traditions, values, and patterns can be dangerous if applied in any other way than as a sketchy base from which to build an understanding of the unique background each client brings to intervention. If you inquire gently, naturally, and sensitively, individuals with whom you work will be glad to answer questions about the usual activities of their lives, the meaning of occupations they are doing or miss doing, why the goals they have set are of symbolic importance, how health care is traditionally handled in their cultures, and how their communities and families might be involved in supporting intervention goals. Family members and significant others will also be good sources of information. These inquiries can be made as part of an intake interview or assessment, integrated into discussions of progress toward goals, or just included as conversation while the therapist and the client are involved in a therapeutic occupation.

To provide highly effective interventions to clients of different cultures, the therapist's approach must combine a valuing of diversity, a highly developed understanding of occupation, a basic preparation in multiculturalism, a learner's attitude toward inquiry into the culture, and some cultural competency skills. Remember that no matter what culture you may be working with, all cultures have some basic commonalities of occupation. For a culture to survive, individuals must be engaged in the activities of obtaining and preparing food, eating, raising healthy children, working for pay or goods, sleeping, traveling from place to place, and doing many other activities.

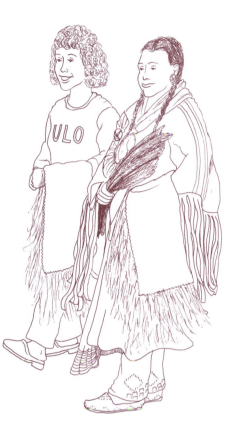

If you are practicing in an area of the country in which a particular ethnic group makes up a significant proportion of your caseload, studying that culture in more depth would be a worthwhile professional development activity. For such exploration, you could read about the culture, take language classes, join some type of activity class (such as cooking) that focuses on that culture, or just join in local events that may be happening in the neighborhoods of the people with whom you work. Or be like an anthropologist on an expedition, and just go see what you can see. You could even record some reflective or observation notes from your experiences to help you gain insight from your adventures.

An important part of increasing your cross-cultural competence is communication skills. Use your understanding of the temporal, spatial, and cultural aspects of occupation to tune your mode of interaction to more closely match that of your client. Consider especially how body language, body space, eye contact, touch, speed of speech, and ways of explaining things are appropriately handled in your client's culture. Think about how gender relations work, especially if you and your client are of different genders. Also take into account how interactions between young and old occur respectfully. Observe the manners of the person. If you are unsure, just ask what is most appropriate.

Communication across cultural differences may also include the use of an interpreter, a skill that requires some practice. If you are expecting to use an interpreter, it may be useful to first observe an interpreter-facilitated session to gain some sense of the rhythms and techniques used by a professional who is quite accustomed to communicating in this way.

In addition to direct intervention across cultural differences, there are also many opportunities for an occupational therapist to make a difference in the way organizations provide care to culturally diverse communities. If you recognize some aspect of care delivery that seems to create a barrier for people of some cultures, actively question that barrier within your team. Consider how the barrier might be removed or minimized, and suggest alternatives ways of operating. Barriers can exist in use of written language, service scheduling, lack of appropriate activities or foods, or not providing spaces for necessary religious observances. Advocating for inclusion of an influential member of a local ethnic community or a traditional healer on advisory boards of your organization can also be effective. Perhaps a person or group of persons from a cultural group to which your organization provides service could suggest ways in which the care provision spaces could be designed to be more comfortable and culturally attuned through arrangement or decoration of space. Informational materials could also be assessed for how well they portray an understandable and welcoming message to people of a prevalent cultural group in your service area. Hiring bilingual staff with diverse backgrounds to help with interpreting and to more closely approximate the makeup of the surrounding community is also helpful.

To grasp the geographical diversity of those you serve, ask yourself these questions:

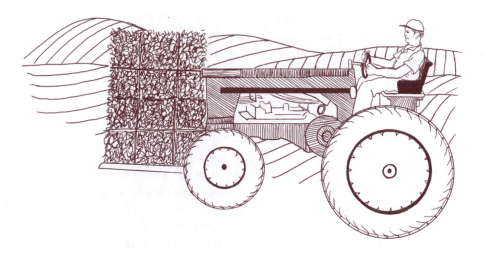

Is the client you are serving living in a rural, suburban, or urban area? Is his or her current location a treasured family tradition, the result of choices to change a way of life, or a result of loss and forced migration? This geographical history will influence the occupational patterns of clients and how they feel about their life opportunities. Exploring this geographical history may uncover highly valued occupations that have been lost to the individual and, therefore, may provide powerful therapeutic experiences. An example is a man who grew up on a farm and is now living in the city and working as a meatpacker. For recovery from a hand injury, he and his therapist might choose community gardening as part of his intervention program.

Working with Diversity

Like working across cultural differences, working with individuals with geographical and class backgrounds different from one's own requires the therapist to carefully focus on conceptualizing occupation from the perspective of that individual. What does the client see, feel, want, and respond to in terms of therapeutic occupations or occupational goals? Care must be taken not to use your own values and background as the primary base for designing intervention that will not provide an adequate guide with those clients who have dissimilar backgrounds from your own.

Parallel to providing care that is sensitive to cultural, geographical, and class backgrounds, the therapist who is committed to excellence may have to work to understand the occupational experiences and traditions of those with very different lifestyles from his or her own. Regardless of your personal beliefs about lifestyle choices, it is unethical to allow your own values to interfere in the quality of care you offer. Services should be offered in ways that are sensitive to lifestyle diversity through open language, inclusion in intervention of any significant others desired by the client, and shaping of interventions to fit the lifestyle and occupational pattern of that unique individual. Competent service provision across differences in lifestyle requires the therapist to value lifestyle diversity, make use of his or her understanding of occupation, acquire a basic understanding of the lifestyle being addressed, take a learner's attitude toward the lifestyle, and use appropriate and effective communication skills.

Gender and Intervention

To understand how a client's gender contributes to his or her past, present, or desired future occupational patterns, it is critical to keep in mind the emic stance of the occupation-based approach. This is especially true as you are interacting with a client of the opposite gender or of a lifestyle other than your own. Always return to that basic grounding in the experience of the individual by inquiring about and observing occupational experiences. Remember that, although the culture's stereotypes of women and men will have an impact, it is your client's own conceptualizations of his or her occupational pattern that is of paramount concern to you, whether those conceptualizations are traditionally mainstream or radically alternative.

Occupational therapists must be knowledgeable about unpaid work in the home for several reasons: to make use of these activities in intervention if they are valued by clients, to effectively set goals addressing a client's abilities to engage in caregiving and household work, and to work successfully with caregivers of clients during intervention. For use of housework in intervention, few examples can outshine the intervention that makes use of a cooking activity. Cooking is a flexible and easily graded activity that many people enjoy. If they do not enjoy cooking, they will usually enjoy eating or offering food to others. An example of an occupational goal in the area of unpaid work is the desire of a young mother who has survived a traumatic auto accident to diaper and dress her infant again. A most common circumstance in home health is the need to work with a spouse or other family member of a client to address the self-care, safety, mobility, and life-quality issues of a client (Abel & Nelson, 1990; Corbin & Strauss, 1988).

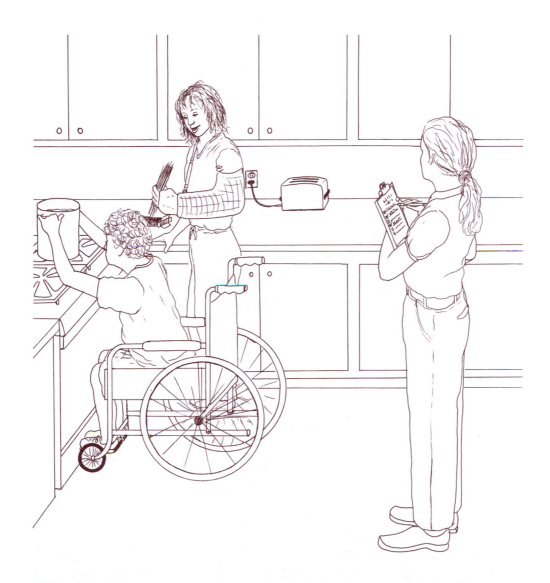

Beware of Social Intuition

Unfortunately, many therapists do not use an informed approach in applying the socio-cultural dimension in interventions. They have good social skills. They use these skills as a form of intuition for reading a client. Because those perceptions, and the interactions of the therapist with the client, are guided only by the therapist's cultural background, he or she often fails to read a client correctly, offends his or her cultural values, or misses the mark in designing appealing and intact interventions because of poor communication or lack of insight into typical cultural patterns of occupation. The impact of the intervention is weakened, although the therapist operating in this style does not realize why. Yes, the sociocultural dimension is complex, but it is also rich in potential for impacting the lives of your clients. Do not be seduced into the easier approach of "intuition." Promise your-self that you will use your understanding of identity, social context, cultural competence, diversity, gender, and the value differences between medicine and occupational therapy to insure that your interventions are powerfully rooted in a connoisseur's appreciation of the sociocultural dimension of occupation.

POWER BUILDERS

Key Concepts for Strengthening Insight into the Sociocultural Dimension of Occupation

- Etic and emic perspectives
- *Occupation and identity*
- *Solitary, shared, and co-occupations*
- Relationships
- Organizations
- Culture
- Ritual
- *Cultural competence*
- *Geographical and class diversity*
- Lifestyle diversity
- *Gender*
- Cultures of medicine, rehabilitation, disability rights, and occupational therapy

Building Insight into the Sociocultural Dimension of Your Own Occupations

1. Reflect on the following, in discussion with others, as a journal entry, or as a more formal paper or poster presentation:

   - Describe an occupational experience you have had in which you would expect that someone watching you would have a completely different idea (etic perspective) about what you were actually experiencing (emic perspective).

   - If you were asked to show who you are by doing something, what would you pick to do? What does this tell you about your occupations and your identity?

   - What do you most like to do alone, in a group, and in an interactive exchange with another person? Why?

   - What are the five most important relationships in your life at this time?

   - Within what organizations do many of your occupations regularly occur?

   - What rituals do you participate in on a yearly basis?

   - What rites of passage have you experienced? What type of transformation of identity did those rites signify?

   - Describe your own cultural background in terms of race, ethnicity, class, geographical history, and lifestyle.

   - Who is the person most culturally different from yourself whom you have known?

POWER BUILDERS

- Who is the person most different from you in lifestyle whom you have known?

- How does your gender shape your identity in terms of how you see yourself, how others see you, and your occupational pattern?

- What experiences have you had in your life with the medical culture? How were the values described here for medical culture expressed, or not, in that experience?

2. In a group, pantomime something you do that absolutely defines who you are and have the other group members guess what it is.

3. Make a list of things that you do that define your identity.

4. Make a list of things you envision doing in the future once you reach a new identity you would like to realize.

5. Find a newspaper clipping about a solitary, a shared, and a co-occupation.

6. Do an activity alone and write down a description of that experience. Do the same activity with one or more other people, and write a description. In as many ways as you can, describe how the experiences were different.

7. Keep track for 2 weeks of all the people with whom you interact by carrying a small notebook with you in a pocket. This will take great determination. After you have finished, analyze the listing for patterns. Do you tend to see people with whom you have a particular kind of relationship at a certain time of week or in a certain place? What other recurring patterns can you find?

8. List the relationships in your life. Compare your list with that of another person. Are there similarities? Differences?

9. Track all the organizations with which you are involved over 1 week.

10. Do an observation of a holiday meal in your family. What is the approved manner of eating a holiday dinner in your culture in terms of traditions, manners, who is included/excluded, place, objects, timing, activities, expected events/steps of the dinner, and interactions with others?

11. Compare the written description of the observation in exercise 10 with someone else's. In how many ways can you say that they are different?

12. If occupational therapy emphasizes working with the emic, or personal, perspective of a client, it requires good empathy, listening and observation skills, and willingness to let the client be in control of the therapy session. Explain to someone what your strengths are in this area, what you would work on to be better, and what you think would be the most difficult part of working in this way.

13. Go out in public with your shirt on inside out. How do you feel? Did people treat you differently? Imagine how it feels to have a physical condition that causes you to look much more different from others than simply having your shirt on wrong.

Building Insight into the Sociocultural Dimension of the Occupations of Others

1. Observe a craftsperson at work (someone who makes his or her living creating some type of material object). Look for clues as to how the sociocultural dimension of occupation is influencing that person's experience. Consider and describe all useful key concepts listed at the beginning of these Power Builders.

2. Do as in exercise 1, observing a parent doing some type of caregiving for his or her child.

3. Do as in exercise 1, observing a person with a disability doing some type of paid or unpaid work.

4. Do as in exercise 1, observing an occupational therapist at work.

5. Interview someone about how his or her paid or unpaid primary work does or does not express identity, or who he or she is as a person.

6. Observe someone over most of a day. How many relationships can you infer exist in this person's life, and what types of relationships are they?

7. Keep your best observation notes on the ritual of a holiday gathering. Summarize your observations. (Even better is to compare the same Power Builder and same holiday with several people to see similarities and differences.)

8. Observe someone who is as different from you as possible on the basis of gender, ethnicity, class, age, lifestyle, and geographical origin. How does he or she differ from you on the key points listed at the beginning of these Power Builders for the sociocultural dimension?

9. Select one of the ethnographies of disability listed in Appendix B. Analyze for key points along the sociocultural dimension.

10. Acquire deafness by wearing earplugs. Do not speak. Do this for 1 day. How did this affect the sociocultural aspects of your occupational experiences?

11. Acquire blindness by wearing a blindfold for 2 hours. Have a friend help you to leave your home and go do something you would usually do: go to a movie, go out to eat, go dancing, or do whatever you choose in a place you have gone before that includes other people. How was your experience different along the sociocultural dimension than your usual occupations in that same place?

12. Select an occupational narrative from Appendix C and analyze its sociocultural factors by describing each one as found in the writer's descriptions of experience.

13. Interview an occupational therapist about how his or her provision of services expresses who he or she is as a person.

14. Observe two client-practitioner interactions—one with a physician and one with an occupational therapist. Reflect on and describe how the values of the two practitioners differed, as expressed in their observed behaviors as they interacted with their clients.

POWER BUILDERS

Building Design Skills Using the Sociocultural Dimension

1. Pick a cultural group that you might be working with as a therapist in the future. Using the first five phases of the design process, create a plan for your own development of insight into this population.

2. In a group or on your own, brainstorm regarding how cultural rituals might be used in intervention. Remember, the more ideas the better, anything goes, no judgement, and tag on.

3. As a group, use the seven-step design process to provide a learning experience for another group that builds insight into an aspect or aspects of the sociocultural dimension.

4. Implement this definition for a group, using the phases of ideation, idea selection, and implementation—"I (or we) will provide a craft activity experience for a group of people from a culture unfamiliar to them that will teach them about the sociocultural aspects of that culture."

5. For a group, make or find a film of a ritual from a culture different from those in the group. Lead a seminar-style discussion of the key points of the sociocultural dimension in the film by posing questions for the group to address.

6. As a group or on your own, and using one of the cases in Appendix A, brainstorm activities that might be effective for intervention, select one using ranking, and develop a description of how the sociocultural aspects of that intervention would best be constructed. Be creative and unconstrained by cost, imagined rules of an intervention setting, or other factors.

7. Design the ultimate party for yourself by creating with the sociocultural aspects of occupation. Use the first four phases of the design process through idea selection. Compare your results with others' when done.

References

Abel, E., & Nelson, M. (1990). *Circles of care: Work and identity in women's lives*. Albany, NY: State University of New York Press.

Baxandall, R., & Gordon, L. (1995). *America's working women: A documentary history, 1600 to the present*. New York: W. W. Norton.

Belenky, M., Clinchy, B., Goldberger, N., & Tarule, J. (1996). *Women's ways of knowing*. New York: HarperCollins.

Bellah , R., Madsen, R., Sullivan, W., Swidler, A., & Tipton, S. (1985). *Habits of the heart: Individualism and commitment in American life*. New York: Harper and Row Perennial.

Bird, C. (1995). *Lives of our own: Secrets of salty old women*. New York: Houghton Mifflin.

Bourdieux, P. (1977). *An outline of a theory of practice*. New York: Cambridge University Press.

Bowen, R. (1996, May). Practicing what we preach: Embracing the independent living movement. *OT Practice*, 17–26.

Brandt, E., & Pope, A. (1997). *Enabling America: Assessing the role of rehabilitation science and engineering*. Washington, DC: National Academy Press.

Bruner, J. (1990). *Acts of meaning*. Cambridge, MA: Harvard University Press.

Christiansen, C. (1999). Defining lives: Occupation as identity: An essay on competence, coherence, and the creation of meaning. *American Journal of Occupational Therapy, 53,* 547–558.

Corbin, J., & Strauss, A. (1988). *Unending work and care: Managing chronic illness at home.* San Francisco: Jossey-Bass.

Cross, G. (1990). *A social history of leisure.* State College, PA: Venture Publishing.

Daniels, A. (1988). *Invisible careers: Women civic leaders from the volunteer world.* Chicago: University of Chicago Press.

Foucault, M. (1973). *The birth of the clinic: An archeology of medical perception.* A. M. Sheridan (Trans.). New York: Pantheon.

Frank, G. (2000). *Venus on wheels: Two decades of dialogue on disability, biography, and being female in America.* Berkeley, CA: University of California Press.

Goodall, J. (1986). *The chimpanzees of Gombe: Patterns of behavior.* Cambridge, MA: Harvard University Press.

Gritzer, A. & Arluke, R. (1985). *The history of rehabilitation.* Berkley, CA: University of California Press.

Harris, M. (1981). *Why nothing works: The anthropology of everyday life.* New York: Simon & Schuster.

Heidegger, M. (1962). *Being and time.* New York: Harper.

Hochscheild, A. (1989). *The second shift: Working parents and the revolution at home.* New York: Penguin Books.

Liben, L., & Signorella, M. (Eds.). *Children's gender schemata.* San Francisco: Jossey-Bass.

Maccoby, E. (1998). *The two sexes: Growing up apart, coming together.* Cambridge, MA: Harvard University Press.

Malinowski, B. (1944). *A scientific theory of culture.* Chapel Hill, NC: University of North Carolina Press.

Mauldin, T., & Meeks, C. (1990). Sex differences in children's time use. *Sex Roles, 22,* 537–54.

Neath, J., & Schriner, K. (1998). Power to people with disabilities: Empowerment issues in employment programming. *Disability and Society, 13,* 217–28.

Peloquin, S. (1990). The patient-therapist relationship in occupational therapy: Understanding visions and images. *American Journal of Occupational Therapy, 44,* 13–1.

Peloquin, S. (1993). The patient-therapist relationship: Beliefs that shape care. *American Journal of Occupational Therapy, 47,* 935–42.

Pierce, D., & Frank, G. (1992). A mother's work: Two levels of feminist analysis. *American Journal of Occupational Therapy, 46,* 972–80.

Primeau, L. (1992). A woman's place: Unpaid work in the home. *American Journal of Occupational Therapy, 46,* 981–988.

Reilly, M. (1974). *Play as exploratory learning.* Beverly Hills, CA: Sage Publications.

Rubin, L. (1983). *Intimate strangers.* New York: Harper & Row.

Starr, P. (1982). *The transformation of American medicine.* New York: Basic Books.

Tannen, D. (1996). *Gender and discourse.* New York: Oxford University Press.

Yerxa, E. J. (1983). Audacious values: The energy source for occupational therapy practice. In G. Kielhofner (Ed.), *Health through occupation: Theory and practice in occupational therapy* (pp. 149–162). Philadelphia: F. A. Davis.

Intactness: Designing with Context

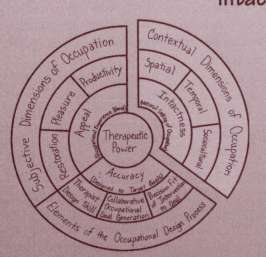

This chapter ends Section III, which has focused on the contextual dimensions of occupation—spatial, temporal, and sociocultural. The primary way in which occupational therapy practitioners use context effectively in treatment is by striving for *intactness*.

> *Intactness is the degree to which a therapeutic occupation occurs in the usual spatial, temporal, and sociocultural conditions in which it would usually occur for that client if it were not being used as intervention. Intactness can also be thought of as the naturalization of therapeutic occupation through the use of typical context. In the client's own settings, the challenges, barriers, adaptations, and potential problem solutions are more clearly evident than they can be in virtual and unfamiliar environments, such as the clinic. In the customary context, the objects, cues, and complete sequences involved in an occupation of concern are physically real to both the therapist and the client. The client is not required to reason from a simulated experience to the real challenge encountered later in full context. The custom-fit nature of an individual's usual settings increases the generalizability and validity of the intervention* (Pierce, 2001, p. 254).

This chapter on intactness parallels the appeal chapter of the previous section, which summarized how the three subjective dimensions of occupation (pleasure, productivity, and restoration) are used to design an appealing intervention.

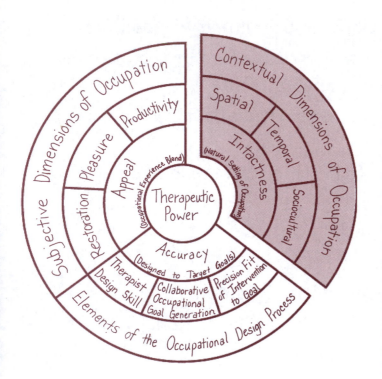

Because occupational therapy is grounded in an individualistic Western culture, designing with subjective appeal is likely to come more easily to practitioners than designing with contextual dimensions. After all, the notions of work, play, and rest have been with us since the inception of the field (Meyer, 1922). Using context to increase intervention power is a newer idea. Perhaps, in some ways, intactness is a more difficult concept than appeal. We tend not to see context. It is so familiar as to be invisible to us. We often do not notice how the context in which a client usually acts offers barriers or potentials for therapeutic change. We tend to think of contextual features as beyond our reach, unchangeable. Also, therapists can easily grow accustomed to the convenience and comfort of working within a standard setting where everything is ready to hand during an intervention. Clinical settings are "home" to therapists: comfortable, familiar, and easy to use. Some clinical settings may offer specific features that are thought to be so effective that they outweigh the usefulness of working within a setting that is more intact for the client. For example, a sensory integration clinic is specifically designed to produce certain therapeutic effects. Claims that clinical settings are more effective than the client's natural setting should be viewed critically, however, and weighed through research. Such statements often disguise the potent motive of increasing profits by reducing the costs of care.

The Profession's Shift to Community-Based Care

Occupational therapy is moving increasingly into more naturalistic, community-based, and intact interventions. Pressures in the healthcare system to reduce costs by getting clients home earlier have supported this movement. Opportunities for occupational therapists to work as integrated providers within natural activity settings, such as in school-based practice, have also moved the profession in this direction. Most important, however, is occupational therapy's discovery that we are less effective in using occupations as a mode of treatment when the occupations are distorted and made artificial. For example, occupations may be undertaken in simulation or selected without relevance for the client's lifestyle just because they can be easily undertaken in a clinical setting. Strengthening intactness is likely to shift intervention toward increased efficacy, greater holism, enhanced understandability for clients, and more community-based interventions.

Providing intervention that is highly integrated into the natural settings of clients is a more challenging mode of occupational therapy than offering service in traditional medical settings. It requires not only insight into the occupational experiences and desired patterns of clients but also an acute eye for the observation and analysis of context. The therapist must be able to negotiate, subtly influence, and clearly use the client's spatial, temporal, and sociocultural contexts to reach goals. A good example of a highly intact intervention is working in a classroom where a student with special needs is fully included in everyday classroom routines. Spatial aspects of the intervention might include removing visually distracting stimuli from the classroom, optimal location of the student's desk within the classroom, seating adaptations, devices and occupations to support handwriting, working on fine motor skills, and goals that address independent negotiation of school buildings and grounds. Just the fact that the therapist enters the child's usual environment instead of pulling the child out to a less natural space is probably the primary spatial intactness in this example. Temporal aspects of intactness might include providing interventions at the student's best time of day for maintaining attention; timing interventions to address challenges that are scheduled into the day, such as lunchtime or playground time; and addressing the circadian disorganization of a child through work with his or her parents. Sociocultural aspects of intactness might include working to insure that the child has the power to speak about his or her own needs; including peers in interventions; supporting partnerships of the special needs student with other children in the classroom; and establishing a strong collaboration with the teacher and the family. Such highly intact intervention is complex but highly effective because of the degree to which it is integrated into the ongoing setting of the child.

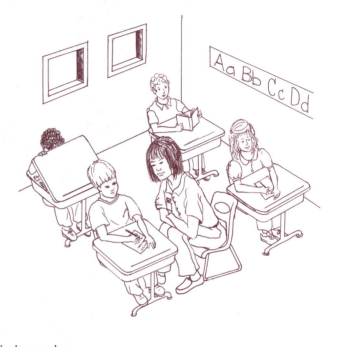

Ethical Imperative to Advocate Use of the Client's Most Therapeutic Environment

In considering how the spatial, temporal, and sociocultural context may or may not support intervention, the needs of the client must supersede all other arguments. Where, when, and with whom a therapeutic intervention should occur should be determined primarily by what would work best for the client. Making and defending such judgments about quality of service is the basis of ethical practice. It is the responsibility and the right of the therapist to advocate for the best possible mode of service provision for each client. If going into the home would be most effective, efforts should be made to do so. Too often, occupational therapy has been judged less than effective, yet other factors may limit the impact of the intervention, such as patient disempowerment and the artificiality of occupation-based interventions in clinical settings. The more that occupational therapy practitioners work within natural intervention contexts, the more powerful will be the

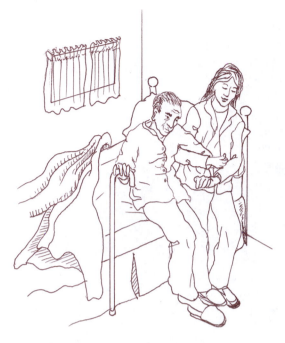

results. Natural, or intact, intervention contexts include the places, times, and sociocultural conditions in which clients would usually undertake the activity being used as treatment.

A good example of successful enhancement of the intactness and effectiveness of interventions is the current movement toward on-site industrial rehabilitation. In this approach, clients with work-related injuries receive occupational therapy at their job sites. This allows the therapist to observe the demands and context of the work; to enlist support from others; to recommend changes to the work context; and to see the client in actual interactions with the spaces, objects, rhythms, people, and culture of the worksite. Barriers preventing the client's full return to his or her job responsibilities are more obvious on-site than they are through the client's report to the therapist at a different location. Gradual recovery can be addressed on-site through a graded re-entry into previous activities. Of course, using an activity or setting with which the therapist is unfamiliar requires some quick study and acute observation skills. Depend on your client to be your best informant as you enter a work setting. This also provides your client with a base for a more equal exchange between client and therapist. Communicating with other workers and supervisors will give you insight into the needs of your client, help to generate problem solutions, and build worksite understanding and support for the client's progress. Recommendations regarding resumption of duties can also be made more safely when the therapist observes the actual performance of the worker under the demands of the machines, materials, and pace of a usual workday.

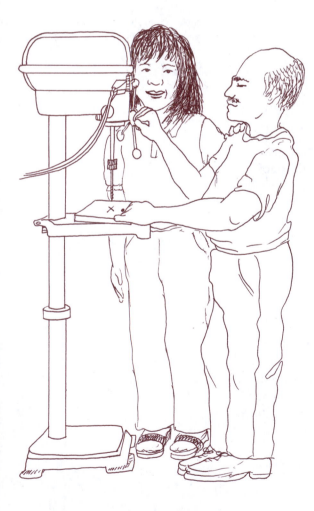

In this example, advocating the use of on-site industrial rehabilitation allows the therapist to combine high appeal (in this case, high productivity) with high intactness (actual workplace context). This will produce much more powerful interventions than would have been possible in a clinical setting less natural to the life and goals of the client. Making efforts to provide intervention for the client in the most therapeutic environment possible is an ethical obligation of service provision. Failure to request and advocate for intact, high-quality interventions is an abandonment of responsibility, whether or not the therapist thinks his or her supervisors will support such a request. Even if the effort fails, it is better than being part of the system, through silence, that prevents clients from receiving effective service.

Four General Modes in the Therapeutic Use of Context

There are four general modes in the therapeutic use of context:

- Therapy occurs in the client's usual life settings.

- Modifications are made to life settings.

- An activity setting new to the client is selected for its therapeutic qualities.

- Changes are made in the traditional clinical setting to more closely approximate intactness for the client.

Of course, a client and a therapist may also select a mixture of these approaches or a gradual transition from one to another, based on needs and progress.

Treating in the Client's Usual Setting

The simplest way to think of intactness is to have the therapist and the client do the therapeutic intervention in the setting in which the client usually does the activity. It is not really as simple as entering a particular place, however. It is important to insure that the temporal and sociocultural conditions for the occupation are kept as close as possible to their natural features when that activity is not being used therapeutically. The therapist's presence will always disrupt the natural context to some degree, of course. It is critical to monitor the balance of power between the therapist and the client, to insure that the client is still the originator of the therapeutic occupational experience, and not simply an actor under the direction of the therapist. If you are doing treatment in the general spatial, temporal, and sociocultural conditions that are usual for the client, you are doing quite well in using an intact, naturalistic approach to intervention.

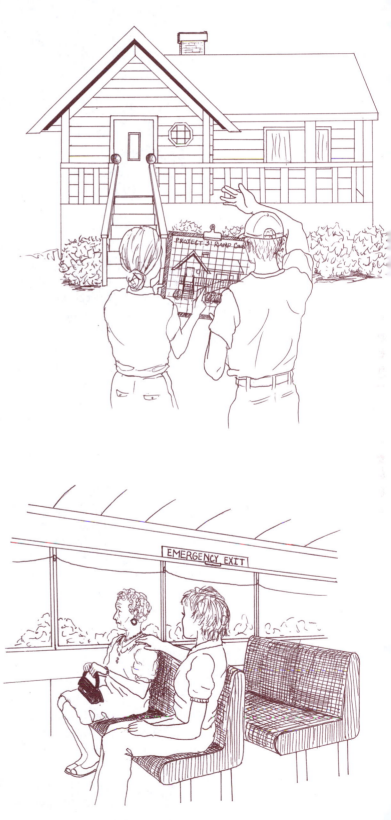

Modifications to Everyday Client Settings

It is sometimes possible to suggest changes in the client's usual settings to support his or her desired occupational patterns. This must be done with care, so as not to introduce the artificiality of a medical approach into homes, schools, or jobs, where they do not belong. You may even be instrumental in accomplishing those adaptations. Consultation on the installation of home modifications is a good example of assisting with changes in the client's everyday life context.

Selecting a Therapeutic Activity Setting

You and your client may choose to use a setting that is novel to the client and which offers some specific therapeutic challenge. This might be a naturally occurring setting in your community that offers a specific challenge, or it might be a setting specifically designed to provide particular therapeutic activities. For example, when an elderly woman is recovering from a stroke and no longer able to drive you might join her in traveling on the bus for the first time to visit a community center for elders.

You may choose a therapeutic activity setting, such as a therapy pool, to work on all or some of a client's goals. Many therapeutic settings are designed around specific activities: therapeutic riding centers, cardiac cooking classes, karate for kids with disabilities, ropes courses, aquatics classes, therapeutic

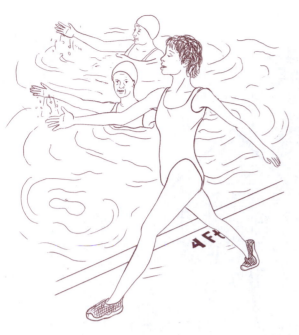

pools, and many others. If you are seeing a population that frequently benefits from a particular activity setting, build a collegial relationship with the managers of that setting through casual contacts, formal consultation, leasing practice space, or other shared practice arrangements.

Productive Dreaming: Approximating Intactness in Traditional Clinical Settings

Dramatic changes in the intactness of interventions may not always be realistic within traditional healthcare settings. In today's medical culture, clients are usually expected to come to the service provider, rather than the service provider going to the client. Cost constraints often reduce quality of service within the healthcare system. More direct, intact, community-based services can take more of the therapist's time, although they usually do reduce the cost of overhead. Even if you find yourself restricted to a traditional clinical setting, such as a hospital, it is still critically important that the vision of a higher-quality, more intact form of service is not lost. Through a little productive dreaming, you can adapt your clinical setting to approximate a more natural client context.

Once a particular activity is being considered for a specific client, reflect on how to enhance the therapeutic context. Ask yourself, "If we could go anywhere, when, where, and with whom would this intervention work best for this client?" The ideal intervention you will envision in answer to this question will give you ideas for smaller changes that may be within your reach within a traditional setting. Talk with other therapists. Perhaps there is some way to provide virtual settings that more closely approximate natural settings. Certainly, this is just what occupational therapy departments in hospitals are well known for: kitchens, workshops, and other daily living areas that are used to simulate the usual environments of clients. Perhaps there are some small, inexpensive ways to make the setting where you provide service more intact, through changes that support typical spatial, temporal, or sociocultural conditions. Shared ideas about more intact interventions may even contribute to the shared creation of a new mode of service or a change in policy that will enhance service.

Another way in which reflecting on ideal, naturalistic intervention can benefit clients within a traditional medical setting is to use it to make programmatic changes that enhance the effectiveness of interventions. Many policies and practices can be considered: involvement of significant others, multidisciplinary sessions, an analysis of the balance of power between service recipients and providers, less clinical and more natural furnishings for intervention spaces, or offering interventions at times more appropriate or convenient for clients. Many small alterations in the way therapists customarily provide services can yield large, positive benefits when extended over a long period of time with, and services to, many clients.

Whether or not such productive dreaming about increasing intactness within traditional clinical settings results in beneficial changes, it is still important that each therapist, regardless of the constraints of his or her setting, retain the ability to envision ideally intact interventions. If you find yourself in a treatment setting in which you are continually frustrated in your attempts to offer high-quality, intact, occupation-based care, remember that moving on to a place where your skills will be more effectively used is always an option.

Therapeutic Use of the Three Dimensions of Context

The four previous chapters of this section addressed the evolutionary basis of occupation and its spatial, temporal, and sociocultural dimensions. A perspective on human occupation that is grounded in evolutionary context supports a masterful insight into why human occupations occur the way they do. Evolution is not, however, a dimension of occupational experience in which one can directly intervene. Evolution is a framework within which humans create a variety of occupational patterns that fit today's cultural template. Some of the evolutionary factors at play here are human adaptability, upright body structure, cortical complexity, sophisticated hand-eye coordination, acute vision, tool use, and various human technologies in stone, basketry, leather, metal, ceramics, and present-day industrial and electronic processes. Being able to imagine the occupations of the human with and without such a framework provides an almost intuitive grasp of what is meant by "the human as an occupational being" (Clark et al, 1991, p. 300).

Following are examples of how spatial, temporal, and sociocultural context might be considered in the structuring of intact interventions. Each dimension is discussed separately for the sake of clarity, although it is understood that all three dimensions of context are, of course, in operation at all times.

Designing with Spatial Context

Of the three dimensions of occupational context, the spatial aspects are perhaps the most easily observable. Spatial context includes the embodiment of our experiences, their physical environment, interactions with material culture, and the social meanings of spaces. In occupational therapy, the spatial dimension of occupation beyond immediate physiology has scarcely been explored, with some exceptions in the areas of tools, adaptive devices, and architectural adaptations (Trombly, 1995; Wilcock, 1998; Zemke & Horger, 1995).

The Body

The physical body and its perceptions and abilities are an inescapable base of occupation-based intervention. The embodiment of your client's experience includes vision, the hand's interface with the physical world, awareness of social stigma due to physical differences, and the variety of activities in which your client engages to care for his or her body. Practice with populations that have sustained physical injuries, such as working with hand injuries, will focus on changes in physical ability as a primary goal area. In other populations, perceptual capacities may require intervention. Visual impairments will especially compromise an individual's ability to use and negotiate the environment. Visual impairments should also be regarded as spatial impairments, thus requiring goals that address spatial skill development and compensation. Disabilities that hinder hand use should be closely observed to determine how they restrict the individual's engagement in desired occupations. Self-care activities, or activities of daily living, may seem mundane, but they are a core set of occupations on which other occupations depend. It is difficult to go out into the world and accomplish great things if one cannot successfully bathe. To effectively use spatial context in designing powerful, intact interventions, the body as the house of the self cannot be dismissed.

Environment and Intervention

In the previous section, I have shared with you the four modes for therapeutic use of context: treating in the client's own spaces, modifying those spaces, choosing to treat in a therapeutic activity setting, and making changes to traditional medical settings to more closely approximate a natural setting for clients. All these modes require a finely honed understanding of the physical environment in which you treat. The qualities of the spatial environment during the intervention include size, lighting, noise, safety factors, object affordances, and opportunities to negotiate space. Consider these as you select or modify an intervention setting, questioning how each would best be configured to suit the needs of your client. Are goals of mapping and negotiating a new environment important? Are there ergonomic or accessibility concerns to be dealt with?

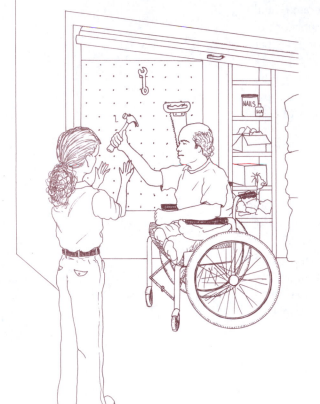

Using Material Culture

Just as material culture is a hallmark of human adaptation, using objects in treatment is central to the efforts of occupational therapists to restore or improve a person's occupational nature and capacities. The material culture of an intact space will offer everyday objects for use in the intervention—spaces dedicated to that activity, highly symbolic objects, spatial routines to which your client is accustomed, and activities focused on manipulations of particular objects. Toys, tools, food, utensils, clothing, vehicles, animals, and many other types of objects are the raw materials of occupation and occupational therapy. Some objects hold great symbolic importance, either in the culture at large or within the life of a particular client. We lay out our occupational routines over familiar spaces, putting the objects in their place to be used when they are needed at each step. All these aspects of material culture must be understood and carefully used in the successful design of intact interventions.

In Social Space

No intervention can occur beyond a space that carries social meaning. To avoid alienating a client, as well as to enhance the success of intervention, the therapist must be sensitive to the social meanings of space in the eyes of each client: public and private space, sacred and profane space, social density of space, indications of social status through space use, and interpersonal body space and eye contact. Violations of any of these understandings of social space can easily result in the client's total or partial rejection of the intervention you offer.

Examples of the Use of Spatial Context

An example of the use of spatial context of intervention as the mode of entering the client's usual setting is a cooking activity in the client's own kitchen, perhaps to address learning to use a new prosthetic limb. In this situation, the interface of the hand and the world is uppermost in the client's mind, and visual cues will be useful in assisting him or her. Before beginning the cooking activity, you may want to discuss with your client arranging the space to optimize its use. You may include room to move around, noise, light, safety, objects of graspable sizes, and space that is free of barriers. Perhaps at this point, you have decided together to postpone issues of self-care and stigma for when your client is feeling more accomplished in using his or her prosthetic. Being in his or her own kitchen will provide lots of familiar cooking tools to use, problems to be solved around use of these tools, a cooking space ready for the therapeutic occupation, symbolic objects that can be discussed or included to enhance the importance of the intervention (for example, filling a thermos with coffee for work), and familiar routines of where things are and where each step is done. Attempting this cooking activity in a less intact setting, such as an occupational therapy department kitchen in a hospital, would be a completely different and much less effective intervention because few of these factors of everyday occupational experience could be used to build skills, test reality, or support the value of the accomplishment.

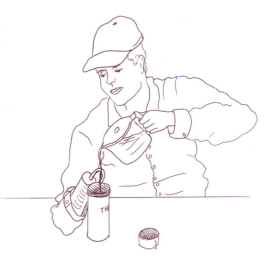

A scenario in which the spatial context of a specifically designed therapeutic environment might be used is a swimming and water-play activity in a therapeutic pool for a child with mild cerebral palsy and attention problems. Here the sensory aspects of the spatial experience would be important—the calming warmth and heavy resistance of the water. Engaging in this activity along with other children might help to ease feelings of difference and stigma. Showering and dressing before and after the pool would also offer opportunities to do self-care activities. The many floats, balls, fins, barbells, and toys common to aquatic approaches should provide many therapeutic challenges not usually available in the everyday life settings of a child.

One instance in which the therapist might be more focused on spatial changes in the life space of a client is in using an ergonomics approach. By creating adaptations, additions, and spatial reorganizations of a work area and its characteristics of light, noise, and other features, the wellness and work-life quality of a person can be significantly improved.

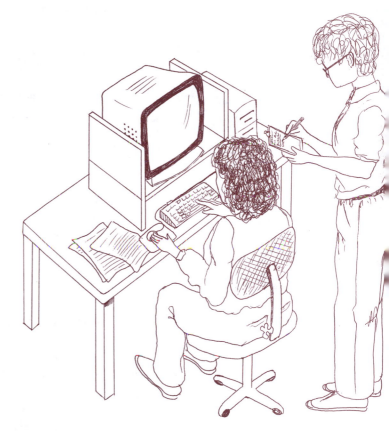

Designing with Temporal Context

Occupational therapists deal constantly with the temporal structures of human occupation in intervention, yet the occupational therapy literature on the temporality of human experience is extremely limited. The key concepts in the use of temporal context are biotemporal rhythms; sociotemporal calendars, schedules, and values; subjective construction of an occupation and its rhythm and speed; orchestration of occupational experiences through memory, temporal horizon, routines, and narratives; and typical human and lifespan patterns in occupation.

Considering Biotemporality in Treatment

The biotemporal rhythms of human occupation cannot be sidestepped in intervention. Providing the most intact and effective therapeutic occupations requires sensitivity to the natural rhythms of the person with whom you are working. When is his or her most energetic time of day? Are there factors, such as shift work, blindness, or brain injury, that might lead you to investigate for circadian disorders? Given your understanding of typical biotemporality in individuals of different ages, what might be some of the expected biotemporal patterns or risks for this person?

Treating on Social Time

Though we may not think of it often, we operate consistently within the social construction of time as we work with a client. We observe the calendar, with its holidays, weekdays, and weekends. We have certain expectations, depending on cultural background, about factors such as pace, length, and punctuality of interventions. If you and your client are from different backgrounds, it is important to understand any divergent values you hold about time as natural, rather than being frustrated and disrespectful because of these dissimilarities. We see our social status reflected in how others use our time, and we can become quite upset if it is wasted because this implies that our time, and thus ourselves, is not important.

The Subjectivity of Time in Intervention

Time moves at a different rate for everyone. You can use this fact to make time fly in treatment, and thus support your client's willingness to engage in working toward his or her goals. Ask about how fast time seems to go in treatment. Ask how to make it move more quickly, or slowly if desired. Think about how many activities to use simultaneously in an occupational experience to better meet goals: several at once, to challenge cognitive complexity? Or just one, to insure focus and success? Consider the pace, duration, speed, and rhythms you can use in intervention to make the therapeutic occupation more intact in its resemblance to other experiences the client has had, or perhaps to add appeal. Games are a good example of an activity that can vary features of the subjective experience of time. Grading along these characteristics of experienced time is also a useful approach to increasing skills.

Interventions in Orchestration of Occupation

Regardless of age or ability, orchestrating our own day, our own life, is something we all must do. Often, with clients who are disorganized by the effects of their disabilities, this is a critical area of need and goal setting. To work in this area, several points must be kept in mind. Are neurological impairments affecting ability to self-orchestrate? How adequate is the client's ability to project into the future and recall the past, along a personal temporal horizon? Perhaps you can use memories or planning in interventions, or relate them to important client goals. Also keep habits and routines in mind as the means or ends of treatment. Consider how narrative is operating in the life of the client or may be used in the construction of a shared view of positive future outcomes.

Examples of the Use of Temporal Context

A particularly poignant example of working within the temporal dimension of an intact intervention is facilitating a life-review process with a woman with end-stage cancer in in-home hospice care. An activity such as scrapbooking, journaling, letter writing, or quilt making might be undertaken as the activity through which the life review can take place.

Consideration would need to be given to her biotemporal rhythms because she might tire easily, have better and worse times to engage in this activity, or have some effects of pain medication. Though she might be quite ill, she would still have preferences as to what days of the week, time of day, pace, and length of project would best fit her goals. She might want to be involved in orchestrating how the activity unfolds step by step, or she might only wish to engage in the activity already structured in a suggested set of steps. Working with memory, reflection back along the temporal horizon into her past, and telling stories of her life, she could construct a unified picture of her life to give closure and a sense of quality in her end-of-life experience, for both herself and her family and friends. In this example, the individual at an end point in her lifespan would be very aware of the temporal meaning and context of her occupational patterns.

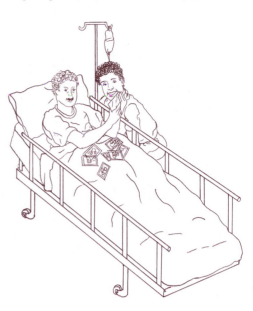

An example of choosing an activity setting that is new to a client for the sake of its therapeutic challenges in the area of temporality is job coaching an adult with mental retardation who is learning to work in a fast-food setting. In this case, temporal aspects of activities of food preparation, serving food, making change, and cleaning may be quite difficult for the client in terms of understanding the temporal expectations of the job, keeping up a rapid pace, accurately timing actions and interactions, being aware of the client's own biotemporal rhythms within the work day, creating routines for getting tasks done, and constructing a personal narrative about experiences as a productive adult worker in society.

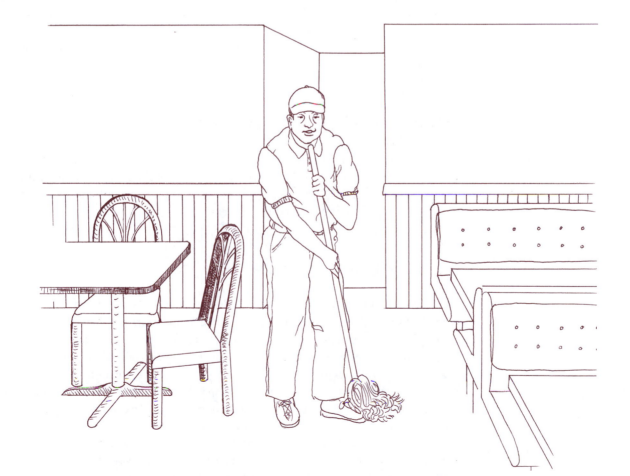

Designing with Sociocultural Context

The sociocultural dimension of occupational context is fairly well understood in occupational therapy in comparison with the temporal and spatial dimensions of occupational context. To use the sociocultural dimension effectively in intact settings for a client, keep several concepts in mind: the differences in viewing an occupation from the emic (subjective) and the etic (cultural) perspectives; personal identity; the continuum of solitary, shared, and co-occupations; relationships and organizations; the culture within which the individual is acting and its rituals and traditions; communicating effectively with persons of diverse backgrounds; gender differences; and the unique cultures of medicine, rehabilitation, the disability rights movement, and occupational therapy.

Working with Identity

Each person to whom you provide service comes with a different identity. Some individuals may be experiencing rapid change in identity caused by unexpected changes in their lives. The most useful approach to identity questions with clients is to keep a dialogue open and let the individual lead. If he or she wants to try out something new or attempt to reclaim former relationships and work duties, you have a responsibility to assist with this. Although from the outside (etic) perspective, it may seem that this person is ill suited for the occupational pattern and identity he or she is considering, it is important to the testing and refinement of personal identity (emic) that it be tried. Although culture does impact the construction of personal identity, the values of occupational therapy call us to support the right of the individual to shape personal identity as he or she envisions.

Using Social Conditions in Treatment

As you design interventions, consider what type of social context would be best: solitary, shared, or co-occupational? Are there specific relationships or organizational ties that should be targeted as goals of intervention, or used to provide therapeutic occupations that are more intact and natural to the client?

Treating Across Differences

As discussed in Chapter 11, successful intervention in today's world of diversity requires the ability to communicate, interact, and provide intervention across differences of gender, age, lifestyle, culture, class, and economics. Never assume that, because you interact well with others of similar background to yourself, those skills will be adequate for intervening with individuals from whom you are significantly different. Learn about cultures and lifestyles of the patients with whom you often interact. Expose yourself to their common rituals, holidays, and activities to use these aspects of occupation to provide more effective treatment. Do not underestimate the importance of gender differences in communication, occupational choices, and social identity. No matter what the source of diversity may be, the best route is to simply ask the individual to tell you about himself or herself, either as a prelude to intervention or while working together.

Examples of the Use of Sociocultural Context

One of my favorite examples of using the sociocultural dimension in intervention is my intervention with Le, a 1-year-old Vietnamese boy whom I saw in his home for about a year. He was referred for feeding problems. I had to work quite hard to envision how he and his family were seeing the intervention, because the mother spoke only limited English, I spoke no Vietnamese except what they taught me, and the father was not involved in the intervention. In fact, I discovered over time that the father considered himself dishonored by having a son who was disabled and that this also was seen as reflecting badly on the mother. For this reason, the mother and child rarely left their small upstairs apartment in central Los Angeles. They had few relationships or ties to local organizations beyond one family member who had come to the States before them. I learned to adopt the quiet and downward-looking interactive style of the mother. We worked with Vietnamese food, utensils, and traditions. The mother was very involved and invested in feeding, and I always tried to work through her as much as possible. I was interested in the cultural differences regarding how independently Vietnamese children were expected to eat. Their parents often fed them with chopsticks until they were 4 or 5 years old. Occasionally we would meet for a session at a grocery store to talk about possible foods for Le, or at a local park to work on visual, motor, and play skills. Eventually, I and other service providers on this little boy's team were able to interest his parents in an early intervention program, in which Le and his family seemed to blossom.

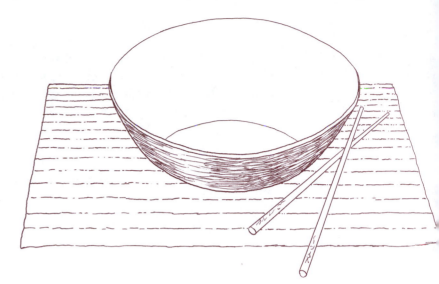

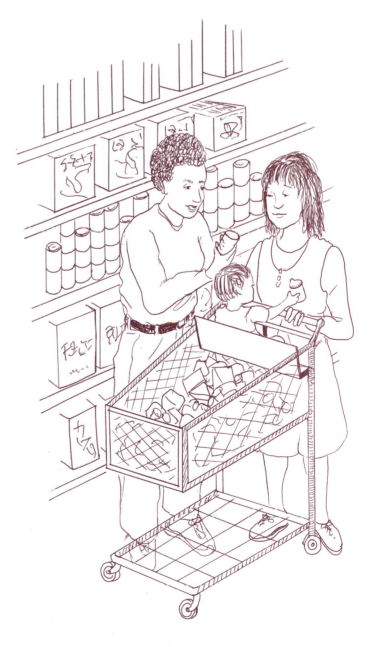

Intactness: Where Means and Ends Run Together

If you are using highly intact interventions by facilitating therapeutic occupations in the usual spatial, temporal, and sociocultural conditions in which that client would normally enact them, you will notice an interesting phenomenon. The means and ends of the intervention will become less clearly distinguishable; that is, by using as intervention a very natural version of an occupation that is an important goal, the intervention and the goal closely resemble each other. Think of the cooking example. The man with a prosthetic arm whose goal was to return to self-care and independent patterns of occupation in his home used cooking as an intervention. Cooking independently is part of the goal of a fully independent pattern of occupation. The goal and the intervention became distinguishable only by a fine line. The more intact your intervention, the more you will see this phenomenon of the means and the ends of intervention approaching and resembling each other.

Increasing therapeutic power through stronger contextual intactness is a relatively new idea for occupational therapy, in comparison with the use of subjective experience to design appealing interventions. Yet this idea holds great promise for supporting effective services to a wide variety of clients. This is especially true as occupational therapy moves increasingly into more community-based, holistic, and naturalistic intervention settings. The simple three-part structure of the contextual dimensions provides a conceptual guide to the therapist's reflections on how to enhance the therapeutic power of occupation-based interventions.

Key Concepts for Strengthening Insight into Designing for Intactness

- Community-based care
- Advocacy for intact interventions
- Intervention in the client's usual settings
- Modifying client life spaces
- Therapeutic activity settings
- Approximating intactness in traditional medical settings
- The body in intervention
- Physical environment
- Material culture
- Social space
- Biotemporality
- Social time
- Subjective time
- Orchestration of occupation
- Identity
- Social conditions in intervention
- Diversity
- The blurring of means and ends in intact intervention

Designing Intact Interventions for Yourself

1. Reflect on the following in discussion with others, as a journal entry, or as a more formal paper or poster presentation:

   - If you were to design a perfect workspace for yourself, what activity space would you choose? What would it be like in terms of spatial, temporal, and sociocultural context?

   - Prepare a statement advocating why you should be allowed to undertake one of your usual activities in a different space, by describing why the alternative space would work better for you.

   - In what setting in your life have you felt most "different" from those around you?

   - Have you ever observed or participated in a setting specifically designed for some type of therapeutic effect? Describe that setting and how it produced that effect on individuals.

   - Select a real space and describe the social expectations that are generally known about that space by those who enter it.

   - When is the best time of day for you to study or read research articles in terms of your biotemporal readiness? Why?

   - Describe when time seemed to move slowest for you in the past week and when it moved fastest, and why.

POWER BUILDERS

- How do you orchestrate your time? Use a planner? Make lists? Depend on daily routines? Just be disorganized? Go with the flow and cues from others?

- When in your life have you had the most experience with cultural, gender, class, and lifestyle diversity?

2. Select a space in which you regularly do a particular activity, such as cooking, sleeping, or showering. Brainstorm as many changes as you can think of to improve the experiences you have in that space. Use a rank and weigh to select the three best modifications to the space from your favorite twenty ideas. Be careful to use realistic and heart-felt criteria for ranking your ideas.

3. Complete previous exercise. Then do a time/task chart for your modifications. Implement the modifications. Do a written reflection on how well your space adaptations turned out, what you learned about your own design strengths and weaknesses, and what you learned that surprised you.

4. To gain an appreciation of what intactness means in your own life, do the following. Identify an activity you enjoy doing and do often. Down one side of a document, list all the key points of the spatial, temporal, and sociocultural contextual dimensions from the introduction to this chapter's Power Builders. Describe for each point the conditions of context in which you usually do that activity. Now, create an experience of the same activity for yourself that is different on every possible contextual point and record the context you are now going to enter to experience that activity in this nonintact way. Afterwards, do a written reflection. How was the experience different?

Building Insight into What Intactness Means in the Occupational Patterns of Others

1. On a note card, list all the key points of contextual intactness from the introduction to this chapter's Power Builders to use as an observation guide. Go to a public place that has lots of people doing the same activity, such as a golf course, mall, dance club, or whatever interests you. Make detailed notes reflecting on the contextual features of the activity.

2. Pick an activity you are interested in or in which you engage frequently. Write a full description of the usual context in which you do the activity, addressing all key points of occupational context. Then, using the same observation guide as Power Builder #1, do a detailed observation of someone as different from you as possible (include age, gender, lifestyle, ethnicity, ability/disability, and class) as he or she engages in the same activity. Write a full, point-by-point analysis of the difference in what is intact context for you on this activity, and what is intact context for the individual you observed.

3. Observe an occupational therapy setting of any kind. Are there portions of the setting that seem to approximate intactness by resembling spaces that might be found in a home? Why do you think these spaces are included in the clinical environment?

Building Therapeutic Design Skills
Using Intactness

1. Using the key concepts from the introduction to this chapter's Power Builders as an observation guide, do observation notes on the context of an occupational therapy intervention.

2. After the preceding Power Builder, write a rationale for what you would change to make the intactness of the intervention more ideal.

3. Select a case from Appendix A. Do a written rationale for the ideally intact setting for working on one goal with that individual. Imagine that you have no constraints on time, money, or travel. Be sure you address all key concepts of spatial, temporal, and sociocultural context listed previously.

4. Select a case from Appendix A for use in a group. Select one goal to address. Use the phases of ideation and idea selection to choose an activity in which to work on that goal.

5. Round-robin an activity idea, perhaps using the preceding Power Builder, until it reaches maximum intactness. To round-robin, pass a written description of the three dimensions of context that you would use from one individual to the next (or from one group to the next), changing the ideas about context to improve them at each stop. Continue until no one can further improve the spatial, temporal, and sociocultural context in which the intervention will occur. If this much creativity makes your brain hurt, then you are really stretching yourself, and that means you are doing it right!

6. Repeat the previous exercise, but round-robin multiple interventions at the same time. To do this, you could use several different activities for the same goal, several different goals (with a designated activity) for the same client, or even different cases. Pass the activity idea and its contextual description along to the next group or person in the circle at designated times on the clock, or when someone rings a bell or says "round-robin now." Push yourself on this one. You cannot expect to be creative without working at it. You must *build* your creative capacities.

7. As a group, in partners, or on your own, use a seven-step design process to create, plan, implement, and evaluate a small pilot of a change in a therapeutic intervention program. Keep maximum intactness uppermost in your mind at all times. This will require access to someone to whom you can provide an intervention. Note: Do not attempt to design and carry out an entire occupational therapy program. Instead, use the idea selection phase to settle on a reasonable portion of the full dream program to implement within the time and resources you have. For example, you may end up creating a sketch and cost estimate for the redesign of a waiting area in a local intervention setting to make it more culturally attuned. Or, you might market a new intervention that a local therapist wishes to offer. Perhaps you will set up a small volunteer program for animal visits to nursing homes. Many exciting opportunities exist to do small, meaningful projects.

References

Clark, F., Parham, D., Carlson, M., Frank, G., Jackson, J., Pierce, D., et al. (1991). Occupational science: Academic innovation in the service of occupational therapy's future. *American Journal of Occupational Therapy, 45*, 300–310.

Meyer, A. (1922). The philosophy of occupation therapy. *Archives of Occupational Therapy, 1*, 1–10.

Pierce, D. (2001). Occupation by design: Dimensions, therapeutic power and creative process. *American Journal of Occupational Therapy, 55*, 249–259.

Trombly, C. A. (1995). Occupation: Purposefulness and meaningfulness as therapeutic mechanisms. *American Journal of Occupational Therapy, 49*, 960–972.

Wilcock, A. (1998). An occupational perspective of health. Thorofare, NJ: SLACK, Inc.

Zemke, R., & Horger, M. (1995). Hands: Tools for crafting human adaptation. In C. Royeen (Ed.), *Hands on: Practical interventions for the hand.* Bethesda, MD: American Occupational Therapy Association.

Designing for Accuracy:
Elements of the Occupational Design Process

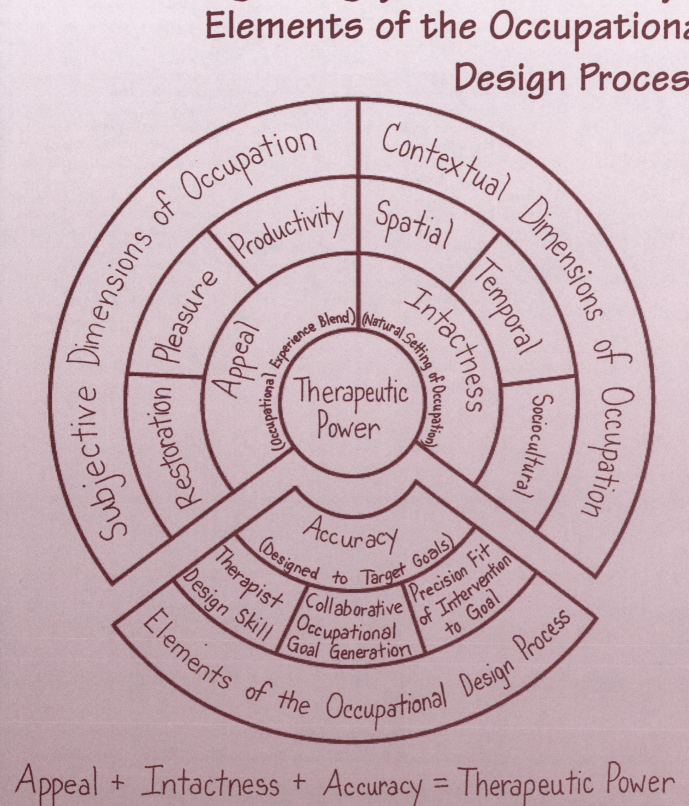

Subjective Dimensions of Occupation

Contextual Dimensions of Occupation

Productivity

Spatial

Pleasure

Temporal

Appeal (Occupational Experience Blend)

Intactness

(Natural Setting of Occupation)

Therapeutic Power

Restoration

Sociocultural

Accuracy
(Designed to Target Goals)

Therapist Design Skill

Collaborative Occupational Goal Generation

Precision Fit of Intervention to Goal

Elements of the Occupational Design Process

Appeal + Intactness + Accuracy = Therapeutic Power

237

This section of *Occupation by Design* builds on your understanding of concepts from previous sections—design from Section I, the experience of occupation from Section II, and the contexts of occupation from Section III—in order to focus more directly on the therapeutic applications of occupation. This section is intended to provide you with a synthesis of current thinking about occupation-based practice, and to contribute to this disciplinary conversation by raising some ideas and questions. The focus of this section is intervention accuracy, or the degree to which an intervention results in progress toward the client's goals.

The concept of accuracy moves beyond the question of how to practice, which is central to the argument of whether an occupation-based approach is most desirable, to the question of how to do high-quality occupation-based practice. Thus we are challenged to examine the relative accuracy of our interventions. To understand accuracy, we must look not only at how treatment unfolds but also at the skills, guiding concepts, values, judgments, and feelings of occupational therapists as they practice.

Because little research exists on occupation-based practice at this time, the first chapter of the section provides a small study of occupation-based practice in an independent- and assisted-living center for elders to ground the section's discussion. The focus of the study is not on the programming itself, but on the thinking of the two therapists involved as they develop an occupation-based program. The remaining chapters use the study as a background for examining how design process, collaborative occupational goal generation, and precision fit of intervention to goal all contribute to the accuracy, and thus the therapeutic power, of the intervention. Because the chapters of this section are somewhat exploratory, they are shorter than those of other sections.

CHAPTER 13

A Study of Occupation-Based Practice

Helene Goldstein-Lohman, Amy Kratz, and Doris Pierce

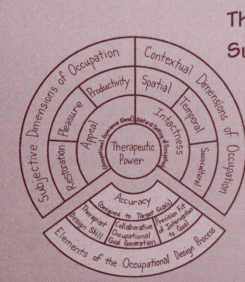

239

A Study of Two Therapists' Experience of Occupation-Based Practice

The focus of the study described here was on the experience of two occupational therapists as they developed and reflected on occupation-based practice in a newly opened center for independent and assisted living for elders (IALC). Because the two therapists were there together, unpaid by the facility, for a 3-month clinical rotation, we had an unusual opportunity to study their thinking about occupation-based practice free of many typical productivity and reimbursement pressures. This chapter does not try to describe a model occupation-based program for elders. It is probably not possible to get to that level of program excellence in 3 months. Rather, we are trying to honestly describe the real process that occurred in one effort to create occupation-based programming, with a particular group of clients, in a particular organizational setting, and through the creativity of two particular therapists. The study explores important concepts, including the meaning of occupation-based practice and high-quality practice, uncovering and reclaiming occupational identity in interventions, use of context in interventions, and the inner tensions therapists experience every day between more traditional medical model approaches to practice and occupation-based practice.

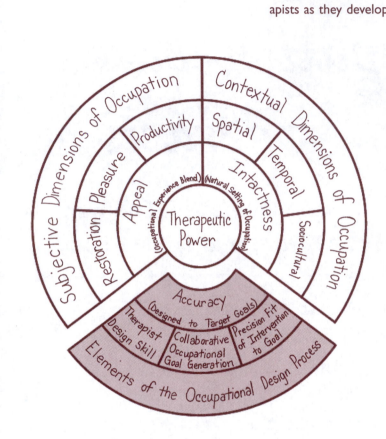

Occupation-based practice is, in some ways, an old and venerable tradition in occupational therapy. To use occupation in intervention is the essence of the field. Today, however, there is a revival of interest in the use of occupation in practice and an increasing discomfort with more traditional, medical model approaches to occupational therapy practice that see the individual in terms of component skills and deficits. The profession requires studies of occupation-based practice to better understand the dynamics of this sophisticated and challenging approach to intervention. Research that focuses on the process of occupation-based practice enables us to learn from and improve the accuracy of our interventions in assisting our clients in reclaiming and creating the patterns of participation in daily life that they desire, despite the disruptions of trauma or illness.

The Researchers

The three authors of this chapter each participated in the study in a slightly different role. The occupation-based program-development project was, for Helene Goldstein-Lohman and Amy Kratz, a 3-month clinical rotation that was part of the postprofessional clinical doctorate program in occupational therapy they completed at Creighton University (Pierce & Peyton, 1999). Rotations are custom designed to respond to the learning goals of the individual student through specific learning objectives and unique experiences at the site. Doris Pierce was their faculty mentor on the rotation.

Helene and Amy were both very interested in geriatric practice. Helene was an experienced and well-published occupational therapist, whereas Amy was an enthusiastic new occupational therapist who chose to go directly into the clinical doctorate program after obtaining her bachelor's degree in occupational therapy. Amy and Helene had both taken two seminars led by Doris: Occupational Science and Advanced Occupation-Based Practice. When they designed their rotations around developing occupation-based programming at the IALC, Doris recognized the research potential of the shared rotation as a study of occupation-based practice.

Study Methods

During their 3-month rotation at the IALC, Amy and Helene collected observational and reflective notes on their experiences. Doris analyzed the notes every 2 weeks. From the concepts that emerged from the analyses, questions were developed for reflection and to explore in intervention. This process continued throughout the 3-month rotation. It was an exciting collaboration, as Amy and Helene worked with the residents in the program they were creating at the site, and in the exciting discussions and discoveries arising from the research meetings as we worked with the data.

Following the rotation, we continued to analyze the data through coding, memoing, and further reflective writing. Results of the analysis are offered here. Initially we expected the study to be primarily about the program itself, and how occupation-based practice with elders might be done, similar to the Well Elderly Study (Jackson, Carlson, Mandel, Zemke, and Clark, 1998; Mandel, Jackson, Zemke, Nelson, and Clark, 1999). As the data and analysis unfolded, however, the study took on its own original direction. It did not seem possible to delve into occupation-based programming without first looking into the thinking of the two therapists. Now, looking back, it does not seem surprising that the highly reflective approach we chose instead produced more concepts regarding the experience of the therapists as they created occupation-based programming for the elderly residents of the IALC.

The Setting

The IALC had been open about 1 year before Amy and Helene arrived and no occupational therapy had been done there previously. The IALC had two sides, an independent-living side and an assisted-living side. The independent-living side was made up of small luxury apartments and offered a range of services for additional cost that included meals; laundry; light housekeeping; wellness programming, consisting of aerobics exercise and water aerobics; and an activities program. The facility provided a bus for group outings and also provided transportation services to and from appointments. Some residents had cars. In addition to residents' individual apartments, there were shared spaces: a dining room, activity room, computer center, wellness center, pool, and meeting rooms. On the independent-living side, residents ranged from those with little physical disability to some impairments caused by loss of energy, depression, balance problems, and sensory deficits. The assisted side looked more like a skilled-nursing facility, with the residents in individual rooms, on hallways accessible to a central nursing station. It included a separate dining room and activity area. Residents did not have kitchens in their rooms, as did the residents on the independent side.

Making the Meaning and Values of Multiple Approaches Explicit

Although Helene and Amy had conceptualized the program as occupation based, they also incorporated other occupational therapy approaches that reflected their vision of excellent geriatric practice. Amy and Helene began at the IALC with a strong background in the literature on occupation-based practice and occupational therapy for elders. Yet initially, as they tried to establish their credibility with the nursing staff and administrators, their practice was more traditional. In their thinking about occupation-based practice, as well as in their review of that literature, there was much graying of boundaries between the meanings of good practice, occupation-based practice, client-centered practice, and evidence-based practice (Baum, 2000; Chisholm, Dolhi, and Schreiber, 2000). There were significant differences in how each approach defined excellence. The research team decided it was essential to begin by identifying all intervention approaches in use, sort out the differences between them, and question whether or not there were any conflicts between the assumptions of the approaches.

The qualitative analysis soon revealed that four identifiable approaches were actually in operation, and each of them included different values about what constituted good practice. The value sets of some approaches fit well together, whereas others did not. The four approaches were:

- occupation-based practice
- client-centered practice
- evidence-based practice
- component-focused practice

As Helene and Amy's understanding of occupation-based practice clarified through reflection and they gained a better sense of the occupational needs of the elders at the IALC, the program became more occupation-based. As both therapists confronted pressures for more medical-model (or component-focused) practice, they were better able to distinguish, reconcile, and balance occupation-based and medical-model practice within the developing program.

Defining and Offering Occupation-Based Practice

Through the analysis, we settled on a minimum definition of occupation-based practice as it was used in the program. The definition was eloquently stated in one of Amy's notes: "Occupation-based practice is using occupation as the framework for intervention." In this study, it appeared that the values of an occupation-based approach locate high-quality intervention in how well occupation was used and how much the resulting occupational pattern is valued by the client. Gray (1998) describes the use of occupation as both the means and the ends of intervention in occupational therapy. By this she means that occupation is both the modality and the goal. At the beginning of the study, this was very much our conceptualization of occupation-based practice. The literature we reviewed on occupation-based (or occupation-centered) practice seemed primarily to emphasize the use of occupation as a modality. Yet we felt that was too restrictive. Helene and Amy felt that component-focused interventions at the IALC, such as their adapting an apartment to prevent falls, was still occupation-based practice. This occurred because the therapist was thinking within an occupational framework of enabling occupations and preventing loss of participation in occupations through a fall injury.

Once the minimum of using occupation as a framework for intervention was established, the meaning of occupation-based practice for Helene and Amy was further explored. It became clear two conditions were required for using occupation in practice: that occupation be viewed from the client's perspective and that it occur within relevant context. Occupation as either the means or the ends of intervention had to be viewed as it was valued and perceived by the individual experiencing it, rather than from the perspective of the therapist, along with assumptions the client might hold about a particular activity. This went beyond activity analysis, or even empathy. Understanding another's experience of doing required highly developed reflective skills and a determination to remain within that perspective. The occupation used or targeted as an outcome also had to be experienced within a real, nonartificial, and familiar context for the client. Developing occupation-based programming at the IALC was greatly supported by the fact that intervention could occur in the everyday life contexts of the residents, rather than in a context that was not usual for them.

Reflection was a key process in Amy and Helene's use of occupation-based practice, because of the importance of insight into the unique occupational nature of each client. To understand individuals as occupational beings and to see their occupational experiences from their viewpoint required thoughtful consideration. Such reflection on clients ranged from a momentary thought regarding the client's perspective to a carefully researched and highly developed insight. Excellence in developing insight into the occupational nature of individual clients also depended on effective top-down assessment (Coster, 1998).

Because the process of occupation-based practice depends very much on the design of individualized programming for each person according to specific occupational needs or goals, reflection regarding the process of intervention design was also essential. As Helene said, "In occupation-based practice, there are no set protocols." Interestingly, Helene and Amy also found that reflection was useful in insuring their adherence to an occupation-based approach through regular examination of the emerging program.

The therapists had to design occupation-based experiences that provided enough external structure to be successful, yet remain focused on the occupational natures of the individuals involved. Here is an example, as Helene reflects on how to provide structure and yet empower the residents.

> *A thought that immediately came to my mind was making cookies with several residents who were functioning at a very low cognitive level. The staff mistakenly believed that these residents were not capable of baking cookies. Yet we knew that they could bake if the activity was structured to their level. There is no way any of them would have been self-directed enough to do this activity without structure. Yet we recognized that for them baking had been an integral occupation in their lives. For example, one had been a home-economics teacher and another valued her role of being a homemaker. You needed to have been there to observe the "joy" both of them felt in reclaiming the occupation of baking. They discussed at length the technique for doing the cookies and criticized us appropriately for not freezing them. However, because of their cognitive deficits most of the conversation was repetitive. To create this joyful interaction and bring them back to an occupation that had been very much part of their lives is, in my opinion, a good example of structuring occupation-based practice to be empowering. (HGL)*

Providing high-quality occupation-based intervention also required attending carefully to the context of occupations. There is a point, although difficult to describe, at which occupations in contexts that are not natural and familiar to the client are not effective. They feel contrived and thus difficult for the client to value. In this setting, Amy and Helene were able to work within the everyday life contexts of the residents, for whom the IALC was home. This greatly supported the quality of the program. Context was addressed in multiple ways, from the creation of new occupational contexts for a resident to the facilitation of social activity groups.

Using Client-Centered Practice

Initially, the three of us had to work to distinguish the differences in meaning between occupation-based practice and client-centered practice. Perhaps because they are so compatible, it was easy to confuse the two. Client-centered practice is "an approach to service which embraces a philosophy of respect for, and partnership with, people receiving services" (Law, Baptiste, and Mills, 1995). Client-centered practice originated in Canada and emphasizes the rights of the consumer to guide intervention. Similar approaches are used by many professions. In the occupational therapy process, locating power with the client in this way is most clearly demonstrated in a participatory style of assessment and goal setting. The client actively engages in determining the priorities to be addressed in intervention.

Amy and Helene concluded that top-down assessment was best done through an informal approach. Top-down assessment begins goal-setting with a discussion of occupational patterns and changes needed in that pattern. Often Helene and Amy would inquire about meaningful objects in the residents' rooms or apartments as a prelude to the more structured assessment. They tried to generate an air of collaboration with the clients in reviewing occupational patterns, de-emphasizing professional authority, and clearly valuing the input of the resident. The top-down assessment often generated reflection on the part of the residents regarding occupational patterns of the past, how they had changed to the present, and what might be missing.

Difficulties in applying a client-centered approach arose in two ways during the study: when the residents were afraid or cognitively unable to assume the direction of their own interventions, and when the therapist and the client disagreed regarding goal priorities. For residents who had impaired cognitive abilities or depression, it was difficult to engage them in a reflective top-down assessment, or expect them to be as much in charge of their interventions as were healthier residents. On the assisted-living side, many of the residents had cognitive impairments, secondary to Alzheimer's disease and other disorders. In this situation, the therapists could not expect the residents to engage in effective priority setting, although attempts were made. On the independent-living side, some residents were afraid to assume responsibility for setting goals. Years of viewing medical professionals as experts made the shift of power toward them in goal setting too surprising, and they were hesitant to assume such a directive role. Over time, with the behavior of the therapists consistently indicating that the clients really were expected to lead their own goal setting, some residents grew more confident and comfortable in suggesting goals and program directions.

In this study, the mark of high-quality intervention in client-centered practice was the effectiveness of the therapist in engaging the client in setting valued goals for intervention. This was best supported by strong top-down assessments designed to elicit the client's perspective on current challenges and desired occupational outcomes. In the program, Amy and Helene used the Comprehensive Occupational Performance Measure, the Kielhofner Occupational History Revised, and an assessment they developed themselves, the Life Pattern Review (shown later in this chapter).

Applying Evidence-Based Practice

Another approach to practice that had to be distinguished from occupation-based and client-centered practice was evidence-based practice. Evidence-based practice is "like a toolbox of methods to aid clinical reasoning, and, furthermore, it is a toolbox consisting primarily of methods designed to integrate research study evidence into the clinical reasoning process. The methods of evidence-based practice help the practitioner select the best assessments and intervention procedures from an array of possibilities" (Tickle-Degnen, 1999). Amy and Helene used an evidence-based approach in developing a depth of expertise in specific areas of need for the population with which they were working, especially cognition and balance in elders.

In an evidence-based approach, excellent intervention is demonstrated by the degree to which published evidence is used in making decisions regarding service provision. The rationale is that judgments based in previous research will enhance the effectiveness of interventions. Amy and Helene further extended the usefulness of the evidence they were reviewing through collaborative review and critique of the literature. They would do "homework assignments" reviewing specific literature and then discuss it together in relation to the developing program at the IALC. Often they used small trials of ideas from the literature on which to base further reflection.

Retaining Component-Focused Practice

As the reflective notes were first analyzed, it was evident that, although the purpose of the project was to create occupation-based programming, a component-focused approach was also in operation. Component-focused practice addresses the problems of clients through intervention in a very specific area of functioning judged to be the primary barrier to a more desirable occupational pattern. It has been the more traditional and most frequently used approach in occupational therapy in the last few decades.

Component-focused practice is often considered to be nearly the opposite of client-centered practice and occupation-based practice. In contrast to occupation-based and client-centered practice, the component-focused approach assumes the therapist can independently identify key limiting skill areas as well as important functional patterns to which the client should return. This approach is often described as the medical model approach because it uses the same rationale as that of medicine, diagnosing and treating very specific areas of dysfunction. This reasoning that reduces the whole of the individual to components that can be separately addressed, assuming this will result in enhanced functioning of the whole individual, has been termed "reductionistic" by critics. A recognized strength of this approach is its excellent fit with the culture, language, reasoning, and reimbursement methods of medicine and other medical professions, such as nursing, which is politically invaluable within healthcare systems. In the right margin is a memo excerpt by Helene that describes why component-focused practice seemed easier than occupation-based practice:

In component-focused intervention, excellence is demonstrated in the therapist's medical knowledge and intervention expertise regarding specific components. For example, a hand specialist using a component-focused approach should be highly knowledgeable about upper-extremity anatomy. Thus, high-quality occupational therapy services in a component-focused approach would be marked by the following factors: accurate and rapid identification by the therapist of component areas in need of intervention, the therapist's ability to explain the disability in sophisticated medical language, protocols for intervention that are highly developed and effective due to years of application and refinement, and rapid change in the component area treated.

> *Medical model practice is simpler because it is based on the model of diagnose, evaluate, and treat. Thus, it involves somewhat linear thinking based on established protocols and requires less deep reflection. Treatment can in some cases become almost rote. For example, with every total hip patient we would [in a previous setting] do the same teaching based on protocol. With clinical pathways, medical model practice becomes even more streamlined.* (HGL)

Compatibility among Practice Approaches

When the research team had distinguished among all of the practice approaches that appeared to be in operation within the program, the next question seemed inevitable. How compatible were all these approaches? How did their values about excellence in practice fit together? The following is a summary listing of the values each approach holds about good practice.

- Occupation-based practice: Excellence is defined as the degree to which occupation is used with reflective insight into how it is experienced by the individual, how it is used in natural contexts for that individual, and how much the resulting changes in occupational patterns are valued by the client.

- Client-centered practice: Excellence is defined by the degree to which goals for intervention are set by the client.

- Evidence-based practice: Excellence is defined by the degree to which published evidence is used in making decisions regarding service provision.

- Component-focused practice: Excellence is defined by the therapist's medical knowledge and intervention expertise regarding specific components addressed.

It was clear to the research team that the values underlying occupation-based and client-centered practice were highly compatible. Both approaches value the perspective of the client, although in slightly different ways, and both make good use of that perspective in assessment. Both attend to a broad, occupational view of human functioning. In fact, the high congruence between the values of the occupation-based and client-centered approaches was probably responsible for the initial blurring between approaches that Amy and Helene experienced, as they worked at creating the program at the IALC.

The values of the evidence-based practice approach did not clearly appear to be either a fit or a mismatch with the three other approaches. Excellence in evidence-based practice emphasized a set of scholarly values that aimed to increase the scientific base, efficacy, and ongoing improvement of intervention by linking it more firmly to current theory and research. In this study, however, the fact that an evidence-based approach requires a significant body of literature on which to base intervention decision-making appeared to pull the program at the IALC toward a more component-focused approach. This resulted because extra-disciplinary research and theory are widely published in regard to different components of occupational experience, but only limited publications either within or beyond occupational therapy have examined occupation or its use in practice.

Finally, the values of component-focused practice appeared to be in fairly direct opposition to those of occupation-based practice and client-centered practice. The client's perspective on goal setting and intervention is the most valued in occupation-based and client-centered practice, and the therapist's perspective is the most valued in the component-focused approach. The opposing sets of values also draw from different types of knowledge—one oriented toward occupational experience, and the other toward medical knowledge of components. Both occupation-based practice and client-centered practice emphasize a fluid design of intervention based on insight into the client, whereas component-focused practice uses more generalizable and standardized intervention protocols that have been developed over years of repeated use and refinement.

Moral Contracts of Intervention

As Helene and Amy worked to create the occupation-based program at the IALC, negotiating among the different practice approaches was most difficult for Helene. She had many years of experience in the component-focused approach. Whereas Amy worked more with the independent-living side, Helene worked more on the assisted-living side, where the residents had more cognitive and physical impairments. Because both therapists were on clinical rotation at no cost to the IALC, they were in the unusual situation of being free of reimbursement constraints. Despite the fact that Helene was so enthusiastic about occupation-based practice and was free to provide intervention according to her own values about excellence, she still "felt guilty." She suspected that it was because she was addressing goals not valued within Medicare and wondered if she had been brainwashed by her years within that reimbursement system. If she was trying to use occupation-based practice and the values it implied, and she was not billing Medicare for her services, why did she still feel this commitment to produce outcomes valued within Medicare? This contradiction of feelings on the part of such an experienced therapist set the research team onto a path of analysis that revealed an interesting intervening factor between the values of a client's approach and the practices of the therapist—moral contracts.

Helene's feeling of guilt was the key to identifying the moral contracts affecting Amy and Helene. In qualitative analysis, such strong feelings, such "stuckness," are indicators of important concepts to be discovered in the data. They call out for analysis. The moral conflict that generated these feelings concerned what was right to address in treatment. It was not about whether Helene was providing good, high-quality treatment, but whether she was providing morally right treatment. Where do therapists find the answer to this question of what is right to provide in treatment? What is their moral contract in service provision? In the reflective data we found as we examined this question, it appeared therapists are making contracts with several entities: reimbursers, employers, other professionals, clients, and themselves.

Moral Contracts with Reimbursers

Helene's reference to being brainwashed by Medicare was an example of a moral contract with reimbursers—a contract to provide treatment that is reimbursable. Here is a portion of a memo from Helene in which she reflects on the strength of the moral contract she had with Medicare.

> *I cannot emphasize strongly enough the moral contract between OT and Medicare. What a love/hate relationship we have had over the years. Our "love" relationship is based on the fact that Medicare has been our number one reimburser so we are tied to Mama Medicare. Our "hate" relationship stems from the confines of this tie. This tie involves carefully following Medicare regulations. Because treatment is closely scrutinized for reimbursement and there have been so many "abuses" in the system, most therapists are very aware of the guidelines and do tend to direct their treatment towards these guidelines. Thus treatment needs to be of a skilled nature (not routine or treatment that can easily be done at the level of an aide), functional addressing basic ADLs, non-diversional (wording is important here if crafts were used to meet a functional goal, although this is never done any more), with a person who has an acute condition, based on physician-ordered treatment, and system specific (psychosocial goals cannot be documented in a skilled nursing facility). Add to this list the time-based restrictions of the prospective payment system and high demands for productivity. Now, from reviewing this list, I am sure that you can imagine how restrictive treatment then becomes in order to get reimbursed. Furthermore, if a therapist decides to go beyond reimbursement regulations there is a high chance of treatment denials. Also other insurers tend to "copy" Medicare as it is the biggest insurer. Therefore, this moral contract runs deep with many therapists. Because I had been a Medicare reviewer, I assumed the moral contract with Medicare very seriously, and that might have been one reason why I was so much in conflict. (HGL)*

An example of how this moral contract with a reimburser can operate with little awareness on the part of the therapist is when medical-model interventions are provided in schools by acute-care therapists who are newly relocated to school settings. They do not see their interventions as morally wrong for the setting, which only values and supports educationally relevant goals and interventions. Rather, they are still honoring a moral contract created to fit a Medicare setting.

Moral Contracts with Employers

Moral contracts with employers can vary, depending on the philosophy of the employing institution. However, in this time of for-profit health care, the concern of the institution is often productivity and income. This is especially true in hospital-based adult care. Thus, the moral contract of the therapist with a for-profit institution is to provide intervention that meets a certain standard of quality in as profitable a way as possible. Helene remarked that the only other time she had felt this freedom to practice in such a holistic and occupation-based fashion had been in a hospice setting. In hospice, the moral contract is not about productivity, but about improving the quality of the end of life for clients. At the IALC, the philosophy was one of maintaining wellness and independence, which was a good fit with occupation-based practice.

Moral Contracts with Other Professionals

The moral contract with other professionals was clearest in the therapists' relationships with physicians and nurses, who are the primary carriers of professional culture in medical settings. When physicians diagnose clients, primary-health problems are framed in a biomedical way rather than in terms of function, quality of life, or re-engagement in lost occupations. The occupational therapist may feel that he or she has been "charged" by the physician in the referral to address a component-level goal, such as full return of finger extension. If the therapist uses the physician's medical diagnosis as a primary orientation to the client, rather than as biomedical information that contributes to a full understanding of the client's occupational pattern, the therapist contracts to primarily address component-level problems.

The moral contract with the nurses is simply to carry out the moral contract with the physicians in an orderly and nondisruptive way. Although physicians set the direction of treatment with individuals, it is the nurses, in their large numbers and medical perspective, who maintain a culture that values the moral rightness of medical goals. Within the interdisciplinary team in medical settings, the therapist is likely to be valued and rewarded to the degree that he or she can speak in terms of medical problems and results. In school-based practice, an important moral contract is with the teachers and administrators and their focus on educational goals.

Moral Contracts with Clients

The moral contract with clients is the whole point of client-centered practice: The clients are the ones who set the goals because, as consumers, they are selecting this intervention as something to which they are entitled as a benefit. There is great variation in the United States regarding the degree to which different settings are consumer-oriented in this way. It seems that in more community-based settings, clients experience more power and control over the direction of intervention, and in acute care, the least. But it also seems to vary according to the economic class of the clientele. The wholehearted adoption of client-centered practice in U.S. occupational therapy is a good fit with understanding occupation as fully owned by the person experiencing it, thus supporting occupation-based practice. Client-centered practice is, however, a creation from the Canadian system of health care and is a much better fit with their consumerist perspective than with that of the U.S. system, which has more of a business perspective.

Moral Contracts with the Profession and Personal Professional Identity

Finally, the occupational therapist has a moral contract to provide quality care that reflects the unique contributions to client service that distinguish occupational therapy from other professions. Occupational therapy literature and educational programs are increasingly identifying a focus on the inherent value of occupation and the commitment to support clients' efforts to reclaim or initiate occupational patterns important in their lives. This clarification of the uniqueness of the field is politically important in distinguishing occupational therapy from other service providers. It also supports the morale and knowledge base of occupational therapists with a focus that is historically essential to the definition of the field.

When the therapist who has a strong moral contract to provide occupation-based intervention is required to provide intervention using a different approach, it can feel frustrating and conflictual. Here is a quote from Amy, while she was working with a sensory-motor group in the rotation following her experiences at IALC.

> *I have found in some of the things I have been doing here that I am very frustrated in the services I am able to provide. I am working with kids (sensory motor group and as a sidewalker in therapeutic horseback riding with visually impaired and/or deaf children) and am not the individual implementing the program, but am expected (at least in the sensory motor group) to use my OT skills. Since I am so occupation-based in my practice, I find it very difficult to provide services for these individuals, because I know nothing about them in the group. At times, I don't even know their names. I would say, that is an example of bad occupation-based practice. Not knowing basics about the individuals. All I do know is their diagnoses and my knowledge of sensory integration. I have to use this along with the setup done by the primary OTR to provide intervention, which I find very difficult. (AK)*

Negotiating among Moral Contracts

The therapists' efforts to negotiate among the moral contracts of care provision continually resulted in difficult choices between conceptualizations of what is "right" to provide, according to reimbursers, employers, other professionals on the team, clients, and the profession. This is where Helene's "guilt" arose, as she attempted to reconcile what is right to provide, with her many years of socialization to the guidelines of Medicare, and her determination to do occupation-based practice. Freed from reimbursement constraints, she was left to examine her values in regard to other moral contracts. For example, Helene struggled to provide intervention to a couple on the independent side, Becky and Jerry. Helene could see that Jerry had a serious balance problem and was at risk of falling, yet he and his wife seemed to be "denying" Jerry's balance problem. For Helene, the conflict about how to proceed with this couple was a struggle between a moral contract to provide a choice of intervention goals to the client and a moral contract with the staff to address balance problems as a part of the program.

This feeling of struggle, this stuckness about what is most right, is all too common in occupational therapy. It comes from changes in the field as we move toward more holistic service provisions centered in occupation and collaboration with clients. Promoting occupation-based practice as the "right" way to treat, that is, as morally correct in terms of a contract with the client and the profession, can create several problems. For instance, those therapists who identify more with component-focused approaches may begin to experience moral discomfort—questioning the moral "rightness" of their current interventions. In some settings, the mismatch between the moral contracts is a significant energy drain for the therapist. Perhaps this questioning and direct examination of the moral contracts of service provision is part and parcel of mature practice.

The Dynamic Tensions between Occupation-Based and Component-Focused Practice

Distinct external forces are at work on both sides of the tug of war that goes on within the therapist's practice, especially between the occupation-based and component-focused approaches. Examining how those forces were expressed, even in the relatively free situation in which Amy and Helene were practicing, illustrates the complex challenges and rewards of occupation-based practice.

Factors That Facilitated Component-Focused Practice at the IALC

On the side that enhanced, or pulled toward, Amy and Helene's use of a component-focused approach, an important factor was the culture of the facility and its staff. The administrators and nursing staff welcomed and understood component-focused practice to a greater degree than they did occupation-based practice. Early in the program, out of the nursing staff's needs and medical thinking, came an official request that the occupational therapists address problems of cognition and memory, as well as balance and safety. This was a time when Amy and Helene were trying to establish their credibility with the site, which made them more vulnerable to external direction. They needed to demonstrate their usefulness to the IALC. A component-focused approach was politically effective, as well as an approach in which Helene had significant expertise.

The policies of the institution that limited resident choices about their own occupations frustrated the therapists' efforts to use an occupation-based approach. In one instance, Helene was working with a patient with memory problems who had been an avid stamp collector before moving to the IALC. He had given away his collection because of rules about limits on the amount of personal belongings a resident could bring to the IALC. He expressed to Helene his regret over not being able to do stamp collecting any longer. When Helene inquired about procedures for taking this resident to the post office to buy some stamps, she was told it was not allowed. In addition, a nurse discussed this with the resident and reported that the resident did not really want to do stamp collecting, effectively preventing Helene from pursuing this lost occupation with the resident. Rather than acting collaboratively with the client, as Helene was trying to do, the nurse was acting protectively, trying to shield the resident from trying something that might be challenging for him.

Another strong pressure toward component-focused practice was the previous training and experience of the therapists. As Helene put it, she had "lost touch with the usage of meaningful occupations in the treatment environment." The therapists not only brought skills in component-focused practice but also had a way of seeing clients that highlighted areas of need in which the therapist had pertinent expertise. As Helene put it, "Old habits die hard."

Amy and Helene concurred that occupation-based practice was also more difficult than component-focused practice. They considered occupation-based practice more complex, requiring more reflection, more collaboration with the client, and more creativity. They found component-focused practice easier because it did not require as much custom design and problem solving. Protocols could be used. One could work fast and "on auto-pilot." Helene stated that although past practice experience could make you more reflective, when you are rushed it can also cause you to drop into old routines of service provision.

Factors That Facilitated Occupation-Based Practice at the IALC

The factors that pulled Helene and Amy toward occupation-based practice were compelling. Of course, at the IALC, they had the unique situation of being free of reimbursement restrictions. They also felt "free" of the medical model. In one of her reflective notes, Helene said, "Life isn't cut and dried like is sometimes thought in the medical model. This is why I like occupational therapy outside of the medical model. You are freer to do what the client needs, not what is diagnosed for you by the physician." This quote seemed to speak to the way occupation-based practice frees the therapist to be creative in collaboration with clients, and to be a more self-directed and autonomous professional. One factor that was a great help to Helene and Amy in establishing an occupation-based program at the IALC was that there was "no precedent" there, no previous occupational therapy program. Not only were the therapists creative in developing the first occupational therapy program at the IALC, but they did not have to deal with a previous occupational therapy approach in trying to use an occupation-based approach.

The collaboration and shared reflection between Helene and Amy were significant supports to the development of the program. With their shared educational background and their differing perspectives on practice, they complemented each other. Their frequent discussions of the program, clients, assessments, and related literature contributed enormously to the development of the occupation-based program at the IALC. They also noticed how talking together helped them keep their occupational focus in programming, despite external pressures.

Amy and Helene made consistent efforts to emphasize to the elders that the program was a partnership with them. It belonged to the residents, and the therapists were there to facilitate the directions in which the residents wished to go concerning changes in the occupational patterns of their lives. At first, the residents were very hesitant to accept the therapists' offer of collaboration. Perhaps the residents were timid about expressing their own views or did not really believe healthcare professionals could act in this way. To create programming that emerged directly from the interests of the elders, Helene and Amy used top-down assessment, individualized interventions, discussion groups, shared reminiscence, life-pattern review comparing what residents used to do with what they were now doing, making lists of activities from which residents could choose, and matching up residents who had identified similar interests to do activities together. The program was grown largely from the identified needs of the residents. It was fluid, responsive, and collaborative with the residents.

Amy and Helene both felt strongly that having the time to develop a reflective, in-depth perspective on each resident was an integral support for the quality of the program. Not only did the top-down assessments and discussions of activity interests help the therapists act in a truly collaborative fashion with the residents; they also gave the therapists a more insightful base from which to develop individual and group interventions.

The strongest factor supporting occupation-based programming at the IALC was the therapists' excitement about the program. They felt that the interventions provided a much higher-quality outcome and were more valued by the clients than they had seen in any other setting. The therapists also saw that, through the program, many of the elders took up more active and fulfilling patterns of occupation. It was a very gratifying way to practice.

> I constantly tried to consider all occupational aspects of the person—a truly holistic perspective. I found that I could no longer just do an assessment and intervention as I had to know the person as an occupational being. Thus all interventions became very individualized. I also developed a love and excitement for doing occupation-based practice, which is evident in my reflective notes. Perhaps one needs that emotional and cognitive investment to do occupation-based practice. (HGL).

Striking the Right Balance in Using Component-Focused Interventions

Here is a reflective note from Doris, who was wondering about the balance between the approaches as she wrote memos on how Helene and Amy were doing top-down assessments.

> It is interesting that this type of assessment rather turns more typical assessment upside down. Instead of doing a component assessment (such as ROM or cognitive function) and collecting info on occupational identity and occupational disruption as a side conversation, the therapist is focusing on assessing occupation and collecting observations and questions about possible component concerns (shoulder pain, visual function, cognitive function) through informal observations and conversation as she does so. It is never one extreme or the other, but both combined, yes? More of a question of emphasis and mindset. . . . Similarly in intervention, the therapist places greater emphasis on participation in desired occupations as the focus and means of intervention, yet will also attend to small component-level interventions to reduce barriers to participation. In creating the inservice on falls, however, it seems more that the therapists have identified an important component need out of prior experience and knowledge, that of safety regarding balance and falls, than of identifying and responding to a goal identified by the elders in terms of desires to engage in occupation. Some of the interventions sound more component-based than occupation-based: cognition/memory, balance/falls. What is the history and rationale of establishing these, although the intent was to create occupation-based practice? (DP)

Although it may seem surprising, the research team concurred that the highest-quality practice combined all the approaches described here. Leaving out the component-focused approach was "not holistic." It has too many effective uses, and fits politically well within the cultures of medical settings. The key to a successful combination of such opposing approaches, however, was to always keep the goal-setting process oriented to the occupational priorities of the client, and to keep assessment and intervention at a broad occupational level. The component-focused approach is useful as subordinate to the occupation-based approach. To keep this balance between the approaches required vigilance and insight about daily practice.

Although most of the program at the IALC emanated from the needs and goals identified by the elders, there were two areas of intervention firmly grounded in a component-focused approach and supported by an evidence-based practice review of pertinent literature: fall prevention and memory enhancement. These areas were identified by the nursing staff and administrators as needed, especially for clients on the assisted-living side of the IALC. The memory group on the independent-living side consisted of weekly modules with the residents. Activities, group discussion, and weekly homework supplemented the didactic parts of the modules. On the assisted-living side a reminiscence group met weekly. The group was oriented to a lower cognitive level and participants were encouraged to reminisce based on an identified theme, such as World War II.

The fall prevention information was addressed in several ways. A general inservice program was provided to interested residents. After the completion of the formal inservice program, residents were invited to participate in an evaluation of an apartment for areas of fall risk. Individual follow-up to the inservice program included apartment safety assessments and standardized balance assessments. In addition, a weekly fall prevention group was organized, addressing fear of falling. Here Amy talks about the inservices that were provided in these areas.

> *We also provided inservices and attempted to do these from an occupation-based perspective. This proved to be more difficult as we didn't know the in-depth occupational history, profile, and patterns of each individual, but we did know that they all had concerns about falling and/or sensory changes that occur with age and how they may accommodate for these. All of the elders we talked with were concerned about losing their independence. They realized that they couldn't always do the things they were able to do and saw friends lose abilities and wanted to understand why and what they could do to alleviate them. I would say we had a "representative sample" from the residents through our interviews to make an informed decision. We were then able to plan the inservices with knowledge gained from residents we interviewed, combined with the knowledge Helene and I have on occupation. (AK)*

Amy and Helene also met with residents to determine what type of intervention would be beneficial to each one. They began with one-on-one interviews targeting occupational history and lifestyle changes brought on by the move to the IALC. This information was used for residents of the independent-living side to modify the Lifestyle Redesign Program (Jackson et al., 1998; Mandel et al., 1999) based on resident input. The group was titled "Empowering Occupations." In these groups, the participants discussed occupation and its impact on their daily lives. They discussed their concerns about memory loss and the effect they had seen it have on others.

In addition to the empowering occupations program, the residents were interested in various educational topics related to aging. Again, Amy and Helene talked with the elders to determine what they wanted to know and determined that there was a great deal of interest in fall prevention. During the fall prevention inservice, residents began asking questions regarding other age-related changes. Amy and Helene created another inservice program focusing on sensory changes with age.

Many of the residents on the assisted-living side had cognitive deficits. The staff had some difficulty adequately working with these residents and engaging them in activities. Amy and Helene met with each of these residents, found out their occupational history as far as they could report, and then developed reminiscence groups based on residents' expressed interests. The reminiscence groups were used to get residents active and engaged in something to help them remember their past. Each group had a theme based on topics discussed in the previous group.

The assisted side one-on-one interviews also brought out common interests, which were used to pair up residents. Amy and Helene determined that there was a strong interest in cooking, yet these residents had difficulty following recipes and gathering ingredients. To make this more contextual, Amy and Helene arranged for residents to bake snacks for an old-fashioned tea party for residents in assisted living. All of Helene's and Amy's programming was designed to emanate in this way from a thorough understanding of the residents and of the needs of the facility.

Uncovering and Reclaiming Occupational Identity

As the program at the IALC evolved, the concept of uncovering and reclaiming occupational identity emerged as a primary organizer of the therapists' thinking, assessment, and intervention. Since the IALC had not been open long, many of the residents had recently experienced significant changes in their daily patterns of activity due to relocation. They had also gone through the reassessment of lifestyle that accompanies the decision to enter an independent- or assisted-living center. The objects and spaces, daily and weekly routines, and people and communities to which they had become accustomed were no longer a part of their lives. Many were dealing with the impact of physical limitations on their occupations and fearfully anticipating futures that included further physical decline. It was apparent in discussions with the residents that many of the activities they had enjoyed, which they considered central to who they were as people, had been lost. In this program, the loss and reclaiming of occupational identity were a central concern.

Uncovering Occupational Identity: The Life Pattern Review

The concept of occupational identity was recognized primarily through Helene and Amy's efforts to settle on a top-down assessment that was a good fit with the needs of the residents at the IALC. They had been pleased with using the Occupational Performance History Interview, Version II (OPHI-II) (Kielhofner et al., 1998), and the Canadian Occupational Performance Measure (COPM) (Law, 1998) in individual assessments as a means of establishing intervention goals for residents. These were, however, difficult to use in a group. They also used observation of an elder engaged in occupation as a mode of assessment, especially with cognitively impaired elders who were less able to participate in the kind of verbal analysis of their own occupational patterns required by top-down assessments.

Helene and Amy developed and used a new self-administered assessment, which they called the Life Pattern Review (LPR). The LPR is used to compare general occupational patterns in the past and present. In the case of the program at the IALC, the past and the present were before and after the move to the assisted-living facility and whatever events or health crises might have precipitated that. The LPR is set up in blocks of a typical morning, afternoon, and evening down the left side, and past and present in two columns down the page. Thus, for example, in the two blocks across the top of the page, the resident would write brief notes on what he or she would typically do in the morning before moving to the IALC, and then what he or she typically does in the morning now that he or she is living at the IALC. This was followed by a section for reflections by residents on which activities were or were not valuable to them, for identifying what they enjoyed previously and are not doing now, and then expressing why they are not doing these things now.

The residents used the LPR in groups or individually with a therapist. After completing the LPR in groups, they would then share whatever they wished with the other

Life Pattern Review

Please write a brief description of your activities in the boxes and note reasons for any changes.

	Usual Past Activities	Usual Activities Now	Why the Difference
Morning			
Afternoon			
Evening			

residents. The first time this was tried, there was a real sense of an "aha!" experience on the part of the residents, as they recognized how much their occupational patterns had changed. As the residents shared about activities they greatly missed, and later requested help in different ways to begin these activities again, Amy and Helene saw that the LPR was uncovering what they came to call occupational identity. Using the LPR as a tool for goal setting worked especially well on the independent-living side where the issues of physical limitation were not as pressing as they were on the assisted-living side, but the issues of occupational loss due to relocation and drastic lifestyle changes were significant. The LPR was a successful way to keep the program on target and address the occupational needs that arose directly from the thinking of the residents themselves. Helene and Amy were very clear in their reflective notes about how critical a historical perspective on the person's occupational pattern was in using an occupation-based approach, rather than using just a snapshot of the person in their present pattern of doing.

Once residents had identified one or more activities of their previous lifestyles that they wished to re-initiate, the therapists would work with them to support that effort. As the research team analyzed how this was occurring, several key strategies of intervention were identified: professional optimism, creating occupational opportunity and community, and delicacy in dealing with loss.

Using Professional Optimism

Examining how occupational identity is reclaimed revealed one interesting aspect of occupation-based practice that may actually be characteristic of occupational therapy in many approaches. We called it "professional optimism": the occupational therapist's encouragement, consistent support, and firm expression of belief that people can make changes in their lives. In the case of the program at the IALC, professional optimism was primarily used to support the reclaiming of lost, valued occupations. At times, it seemed professional optimism was used even when the resident and the occupational therapist, if required to be realistic in their forecast, might have said that reaching a goal was a very difficult challenge that might not be accomplished. By clearly showing that he or she believed reclaiming important occupations was a possibility, the therapist made it possible for the resident to consider whether he or she could believe that also, at least long enough to take a first step. Often the elders seemed overwhelmed by the many factors that came between them and a lost occupation. Instead of working to circumvent barriers, they would just resign themselves to a new lifestyle without those special activities. The professional optimism of the occupational therapists, coupled with their active efforts to remove barriers and facilitate access, gave the residents the support they needed to move toward reclaiming lost portions of occupational identity.

Creating Occupational Opportunity and Community

Amy and Helene also worked to introduce occupational opportunities that one or more of the residents identified as important to them. The more residents showed interest in an activity, the more likely they were to target it. For example, two female residents, one from the independent-living side and one from the assisted-living side, had been avid oil painters. Paintings hung in their apartments. Helene got them started oil painting together. Soon after, another resident joined them, marveling that she had been eating dinner with these ladies all this time and had not even known they were painters. Some opportunities were created specifically for one individual. One resident had always had a habit of going out to her garden to check her plants in the morning and evening. Helene got supplies and helped her to plant some container plants on her patio. After that, she returned to her earlier pattern of beginning and ending the day by going outside to observe her plants. In addition to the new occupational opportunities in which specific residents engaged in the program, a sense of occupational community was developing. Residents increasingly recognized each other in terms of what each other did, or had done, due to sharing of occupational narratives, reflections, and experiences.

The Delicacy of Changing Identity

One aspect of reclaiming occupational identity with these elders was particularly delicate. In some cases, physical changes were a primary factor in the loss of the valued occupation. If the resident chose to attempt re-engagement in the occupation, confronting losses of ability and talent was a poignant part of that re-engagement. At times, although residents would identify particular occupations as sorely missed, they showed resistance when the therapist tried to support re-initiation. In the face of signs of resistance, the therapist maintained her professional optimism and expressions of willingness to assist but did not push, out of concern for the self-image of the resident. It seemed there could be a point at which attempting to reclaim a particularly valued occupation in an area in which one is no longer competent could actually degrade self-concept and should therefore be avoided. Some occupations may be most useful to occupational identity as a part of personal history, rather than as something in which the person is engaged. Thus, for example, the resident remains a great potter or cook, with stories to tell or creations to display, although these occupations are no longer done. In this delicate area of confronting losses of valued occupations, the therapist must be careful to always allow the resident to maintain control of decision making regarding whether or not to re-engage.

Throughout the development and implementation of the program at the IALC, the therapists were constantly reminded by their observations and interactions with the residents that they carried fear about the future. What would their lives be like next year, in 5 years? What abilities and occupations might be lost? Perhaps making the decision to move to the IALC involved enough contemplation of their aging and mortality to make this a fresh issue. The residents on the independent-living side were uncomfortable associating with the residents on the assisted-living side or being identified with them. Some residents were struggling to admit to, and learn to live with, physical limitations and diagnoses that promised declining capacities. The existential challenge to these elders, living the end of life, was one that had to be handled delicately and respectfully by the therapist.

The Subtle Therapist: Working through Context

Amy and Helene had the unique challenge of working completely within the setting in which the residents lived. Through acute observation and subtle action, they found that they could use this close inclusion in the natural life contexts of those they served to support their occupational goals. One of the activities identified by the elders and facilitated by Amy and Helene was an afternoon tea party. The therapists valued this event because they felt it would make the elders feel less isolated, build a feeling of belonging, and give them an opportunity to do something that had been a regular occurrence in their younger days. Some of the residents baked cookies for the event. Everyone who came to the tea was dressed up. It was in the afternoon and all efforts were made to make it a nice event. Staff joined the tea also, socializing with the elders in a way that de-emphasized the differences between their roles at the IALC. Everyone really enjoyed themselves. A tea party may seem like a small thing, but the creation of community by Amy and Helene through a series of events identified by the elders, and occurring in their natural spatial, temporal, and sociocultural contexts, built significantly toward an increase in the quality of life of residents of the IALC.

Using Spatial Context

One of the greatest obstacles and disruptions in the lives of the residents was their recent relocation to the IALC. The spaces in which they lived were unfamiliar and lacked the materials and tools of many treasured occupations. The few objects they did bring with them were precious and expressive. Living within the space of the IALC was a mix of pride of ownership and lack of power over what could be done in the space within institutional rules. Many of the residents did not leave the IALC often because they were new to the community. Many did not have transportation, and most were not comfortable taking the bus.

The therapists used their inclusion in the spatial context to subtly intervene on behalf of the residents. They would use discussions of objects in residents' rooms as an avenue into occupational narrative and assessment. Often they would procure the necessary supplies that prevented residents from engaging in occupations important to them. At times, they would recommend changes in the rooms and apartments of the residents for the sake of safety. Although they did not have enough time to implement this plan, they had hoped to make recommendations regarding changes in the design of the IALC to make it more safe, accessible, and visually interpretable by elders. Helene and Amy were convinced that, if they had had the opportunity to work within the space of the IALC over a longer time, they could have gradually made many subtle changes to the way in which the space supported the occupations of the residents. They also saw an important role for occupational therapy in supporting a transition from the elder's previous home and lifestyle to living at the IALC, in order to reduce the disruption this caused in the elder's occupational patterns.

Using Temporal Context

Time moved differently for the elders at the IALC than it did in the city beyond. They did not wish to rush and liked to think things over before becoming involved. The therapists had to consciously slow their pace to match that of the elders. The residents of the independent-living side had control over their own time and tended to have active social lives, but the elders on the assisted side had few planned activities and a fairly inflexible care routine created for them by the nursing staff. In working with the residents, it was clear to Amy and Helene that it was important for them to offer programming that was flexible, fit easily into the schedules of the residents, and left the residents in control of all choices of how to use their time. Interventions had the flavor of leisure-time activities, in keeping with the therapists' efforts to make them appealing to the elders.

Initiation of new occupations and re-initiation of valued occupations that had been lost were identified by the research team as a primary challenge to the program. Although it is unclear why this is true, the residents found the beginnings of new things difficult. Starting something new was much more stressful than continuing with an activity once it was started. Many fears were expressed about beginning new activities or doing activities that had not been done in a long time. Once the therapists realized this was a common barrier for the residents, they developed some strategies for handling initiations more carefully: insuring that the residents felt in full control of decision-making, providing increased cues and emotional support at beginnings, and taking it as slow as necessary at start-up of new activities.

Using Sociocultural Context

The social and cultural conditions for the residents of the IALC were similar to those in many newly created communities. They were largely isolated from the local community. The range of products and services typically available to individuals were not easily accessible to them, although the IALC did provide a range of on-site services, such as laundry, cleaning, and meals. The spatial layout of the IALC provided few shared spaces where residents might visit and get to know each other. Unlike in most communities, there were only fully public spaces and fully private spaces. As already described, the independent-side and assisted-side residents did not interact very much with each other. The medical culture was much more evident in staff behavior and routines on the assisted-living side.

Working within the sociocultural context of the IALC required care and was impeded by the short time during which Amy and Helene had been building relationships with the residents and staff. Yet they found several successful strategies. Interestingly, outside the constraints of billable service, they found themselves using dyads and triads of shared occupations more often than in previous practice. In some cases, they facilitated social groupings without the presence of the therapist for particular activities in which more capable residents could support those who were functioning less independently. At times they took residents out into the community to get activity supplies, or encouraged them to begin using the bus or to go with others who had cars. Amy and Helene valued the social interaction in the occupational opportunities they created for the residents because many of the residents had expressed a sense of loneliness and disconnection from family and old friends in their new lives at the IALC.

Summary

In this chapter, we have described the experiences and reflections of two therapists as they initiated occupation-based programming in an independent- and assisted-living center for elders. In the analysis of their experiences, the primary themes were clarifying the distinctions among four different practice approaches, the moral contracts of intervention, the dynamic tension between occupation-based and component-focused practice, uncovering and reclaiming occupational identity, and working through context. Until more research is done on occupation-based practice, it is not possible to determine how many of the concepts discovered in this research will also be found in other studies. Certainly, the need to distinguish among the different approaches and the effort to strike an appropriate balance between occupation-based and component-focused approaches may be perhaps inescapable elements. Working through context is also likely to be widely applicable in occupation-based practice. Occupational identity was certainly an important factor for this group of recently relocated elders. But would this be true with all clients? Is occupational identity central to all intervention? Only time will tell.

In the following chapters, this study will serve as an example to illustrate therapist design skills, collaborative occupational goal generation, and the precision fit of interventions to goals. Before moving on, however, try some of the following Power Builders to insure that you have gotten the maximum enhancement of your own skills from this chapter.

POWER BUILDERS

Keep in mind the following primary concepts of this chapter while working with the Power Builders:

- Approaches to practice: occupation-based, client-centered, evidence-based, component-focused
- Moral contracts of intervention with reimbursers, employers, other professionals, clients, and personal professional identity
- Occupational identity
- Working through spatial, temporal, and sociocultural context

1. Imagine you have been required to leave the place where you currently live because you are losing vision and you will now live in an assisted-living setting. Write a fictional journal entry of your first day in the new setting, reflecting on the changes in your lifestyle.

2. Describe your own present occupational identity, either in writing or aloud to a group or another person.

3. Have you had an elderly relative who has lost some degree of independence or some sensory capacities, or has had to give up his or her home to move to a more supported lifestyle? Write a fictional account of his or her experience, as if he or she were writing in a journal, of what life is like with these changes happening.

4. Interview someone who is as unlike you as possible, in terms of gender, ethnicity, age, lifestyle, and ability/disability. Attempt, through your questions, to gain a sense of his or her present occupational identity. Compose a written description of his or her occupational identity.

5. Using the brainstorming exercise, list the different types of occupational therapy in which you are interested. Using a simple ranking, select the most appealing area of practice. Then use the brainstorming exercise again to list as many different creative ideas for occupation-based programming with this population. Remember, do not be constrained by convention. All ideas live in brainstorming exercises, no matter how unrealistic or unusual. The most successful brainstorming is that which generates the largest number of ideas. How many can you come up with?

6. Choose a case from Appendix A. Write a brief description of one occupation-based intervention you could use with this person.

7. Choose a case from Appendix A. Write one goal you can imagine collaboratively generating with this client, in a client-centered approach.

8. Choose a case from Appendix A. What evidence would you seek to support evidence-based interventions with this client?

9. Choose a case from Appendix A. What goals would you set for this client in a component-focused approach?

10. Choose a case from Appendix A. Write a fictional journal entry by this person, describing how pleased he or she is to be returning to a particular occupation because of occupational therapy intervention and why.

References

Baum, C. (2000). Occupation-based practice: Reinventing ourselves for the new millennium. *OT Practice, 5,* 12–15.

Chisholm, D., Dolhi, C., & Schreiber, J. (2000). Creating occupation-based opportunities in a medical model clinical practice setting. *OT Practice, 5,* CE 1–8.

Coster, W. (1998). Occupation-centered assessment of children. *American Journal of Occupational Therapy, 52,* 337–344.

Gray, J. M. (1998). Putting occupation into practice: Occupation as ends, occupation as means. *American Journal of Occupational Therapy, 52,* 354–364.

Jackson, J., Carlson, M., Mandel, D., Zemke, R., & Clark, F. (1998). Occupation in lifestyle redesign: The Well Elderly Study occupational therapy program. *American Journal of Occupational Therapy, 52,* 326–336.

Kielhofner, G., Mallinson, T., Crawford, C., Nowak, M., Rigby, M., Henry, A., et al. (1998). *A user's manual for the occupational performance history interview (Version 2.0).* Chicago: Model of Human Occupation Clearinghouse, University of Illinois at Chicago.

Law, M. (1998). *Client-centered occupational therapy.* Thorofare, NJ: SLACK, Incorporated.

Law, M., Baptiste, S., & Mills, J. (1995). Client-centered practice: What does it mean and does it make a difference? *Canadian Journal of Occupational Therapy, 62,* 250–257.

Mandel, D. R., Jackson, J. M., Zemke, R., Nelson, L., & Clark, F. A. (1999). *Lifestyle redesign: Implementing the Well Elderly program.* Bethesda, MD: American Occupational Therapy Association.

Pierce, D. E., & Peyton, C. (1999). An historical cross-disciplinary perspective on the professional doctorate for occupational therapy. *American Journal of Occupational Therapy, 53,* 64–71.

Tickle-Degnen, L. (1999). Organizing, evaluating, and using evidence in occupational therapy practice. *American Journal of Occupational Therapy, 53,* 537–539.

CHAPTER 14

Therapist Design Skill

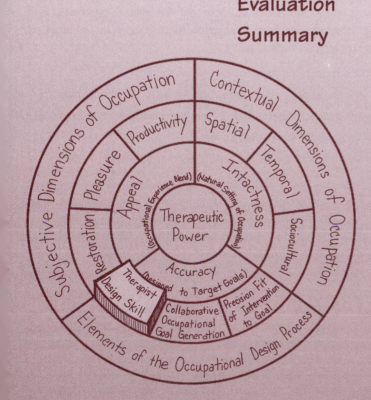

What Is Intervention Accuracy?

The therapist's ability to offer occupational experiences that accurately target the needs of the client, resulting in powerful therapeutic changes, depends on a number of factors: his or her design skills, collaborative generation of goals with clients, and the precision with which interventions fit goals. The next three chapters will use examples from the preceding chapter's occupation-based practice study to illustrate how therapist design skills, collaborative goal generation, and goal fit are used in daily practice. To begin, this chapter will review how the two therapists in the study used design skills in their interventions with residents of an independent- and assisted-living center (IALC).

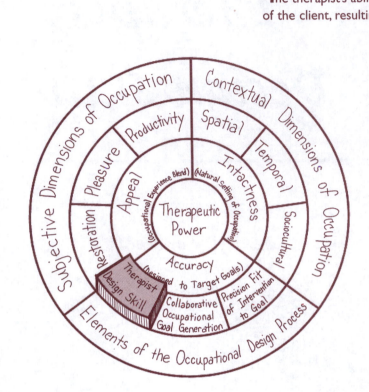

Occupational therapy is a young profession. Consider, for example, how much longer medicine and law have been developing their theories and interventions. Much of occupational therapy's practice theory is still at the stage of describing what works and how it does so. In recent years, the field has begun to turn more attention to assessing the efficacy, or relative success, of interventions. That is, instead of doing research and theory development focused on identifying intervention approaches, we are now beginning to study how well different interventions work and how to provide them more effectively. Questioning what makes an occupation-based intervention more or less accurate, or effective, moves our shared discourse about occupation-based practice from the question of what to do (that is, occupation-based or component-focused) to the question of how to do it best (relative accuracy of occupation-based interventions).

Estimating how accurate and effective one intervention may be in comparison with another is the stuff of daily clinical thinking. Making judgments about intervention accuracy is constant in moment-to-moment practice. Some of the clinical questions with which the therapist using an occupation-based approach must grapple in an effort to increase intervention accuracy include the following.

- What lost occupations are most important for this client to regain?
- How does the client view his or her past, present, and future occupational patterns?
- What activity would work best for this client and how can I facilitate its occurrence?
- In what setting would the activity be most effective?
- How, where, and with whom would the client usually do that activity?

Consistently creative problem-solving and planning skills are required to respond to such questions. The degree to which a therapist can combine his or her connoisseur-level understanding of occupation with the therapeutic abilities of design, collaboration, and precision fit is the degree to which that individual can be expected to facilitate deeply satisfying life changes for his or her clients.

The Demand for Constant Creativity in Practice

No matter what the area of practice, the degree to which the occupational therapist draws on creative skills in a typical day cannot be overstated. The therapist constantly thinks on his or her feet. For instance, when a planned activity for a young child does not appeal, a substitute must quickly be offered. Adjustments to unexpected scheduling or unavailable materials are smoothly made. New programming is planned that is exciting to clients. A quiet caregiver is drawn into a home-based self-care session through a carefully timed comment. A clear explanation helps a team member or reimburser gain an occupational perspective on a client. A way is finally found to gain the trust of a reticent client, uncovering a heartfelt occupational goal. The demand for creativity in occupational therapy is constant.

Design skills are both the art and the vulnerability of occupational therapy. When an occupational therapist has strong design skills, clients and teams find them invaluable. When the therapist's design skills have not been fully developed, however, he or she will be much less effective, feel burned out and overwhelmed by the number and severity of the challenges presented in practice, and resort to a simpler component-focused approach. An occupational therapist without creativity is sad to see. A therapist with poor design skills does great damage to the image of the profession as having valuable and unique contributions to make.

To build creativity, the therapist can self-assess and build skills in the following areas: motivation, investigation, definition, ideation, idea selection, implementation, and evaluation (Koberg & Bagnall, 1981). These are the phases of creativity. All of us have natural strengths and weaknesses in these skills. Once you know your own profile of relative strengths in design, you can invest in your creative potential by developing the areas in which you are not as strong. In Chapter 2, the seven phases of creativity are presented, along with strategies that can be used in each one to accomplish different types of projects. Power Builders are provided at the end of that chapter for skill building in weaker areas.

The skills of the design process can be used with a very direct and structured approach to meet any creative challenge in life. Applied to intervention, therapist design skills result in outcomes that are more effective, more valued by clients, and more accurately targeted to address occupational goals. Whether or not a therapist is aware of the creative process in which he or she is engaged, all projects go through these design phases. In this chapter, the creative challenges that naturally occurred for the two therapists initiating occupation-based programming for the elders of the IALC will be used to illustrate how the creative process can unfold.

Motivation

The motivation phase is the beginning of the creative process and the wellspring of energy that drives a project. It is a convergent thinking phase, identifying why a therapist is investing in a particular effort. By identifying and developing motivation, the therapist can be sure that the projects in which he or she becomes involved are those for which a passion is felt. Doing well at this phase insures that the therapist will be able to sustain enthusiasm and investment in the project from beginning to end, no matter what design difficulties might have to be confronted.

In the IALC project, Amy and Helene did not do any formal assessments of their motivation or plan for its support as they carried out day-to-day involvement with the program's implementation. Still, they did identify and support their motivation. The amount of collaboration and sharing of their thoughts and triumphs as they worked together to implement the program served to keep their investment high. They often returned to discussion of their primary motivation to explore occupation-based practice for elders. The reflective process and research team meetings also gave them opportunities to share excitement over the concepts that were being uncovered in the study.

The motivation phase is often skipped by designers of all types of projects. In my observations, this is true for therapists as well. Assuming they do not need to attend to the personal reasons and energy behind practice, they simply begin new projects that appear important and trust they will find the necessary motivation to do a good job. Unfortunately, neglecting to reflect on why one is engaging in a project can result in difficulties in staying committed to the project, problems in generating multiple creative ideas from which to choose, or an inability to generate effective solutions for barriers to implementation. In this study, the therapists instituted informal methods of maintaining investment in the creative process of therapeutic interventions through collaboration, sharing of treatment experiences and feelings, and reflection. Looking back, it might have been useful for them to spend time specifically reflecting on their motivations for creating new occupation-based programming at the IALC.

A good example of a strong motivation phase is in a current project I am facilitating in the Occupational Therapy Department at Eastern Kentucky University. A faculty group has formed the Occupational Therapy Group for At Risk Youth (OTGARY), interested in research and intervention development for adolescents with and without disabilities in alternative schools and juvenile-justice settings. Seven therapists are in the group, five of whom are faculty, one a postprofessional master's degree candidate, and one a part-time therapist who works for the group and supervises fieldwork students in a rural alternative school. Two of the faculty are experienced and doctorally trained researchers; two are currently working on doctorates. The group initially spent time exploring what they hoped to accomplish together and what each person hoped to gain from involvement in the group. There were differences and similarities, but enough similarity that the group agreed to continue working together, although they might participate to different degrees in projects and publications, according to personal motivation and time availability. Spending time in discussion of our individual motivations for involvement in OTGARY helped to create a working research group that will provide positive, exciting, and collaborative experiences for all members of the group and produce useful outcomes over the long term. We will check again on individual motivations to be involved in each project we do, and as necessary if energy starts to flag. Since that early phase of examining our motivations to participate in the group, we have completed several key steps, including a thorough exploration of the literature (investigation phase), setting goals for the group (definition phase), discussing a variety of possible projects (ideation), initiating an efficacy study of occupation-based programming for grades 6 through 12 in a rural alternative school, and beginning work on an informational Website for occupational therapy for at-risk youth (idea selection and implementation phases).

Investigation

The investigation phase of a project is meant to feed ideas to the creative designer so that he or she can begin to see a project in a new, more expanded, and informed way. Investigation is a divergent phase, an effort to gather as much pertinent information about your potential project as possible. It is the quantity of information gathered that is important, rather than the quality. In investigation, you push your thinking into a new shape. It involves more than just looking for information necessary to accomplish what you have already decided to do. Through investigation, you can explore what the project might include, how others have done similar projects, different ideas that might be incorporated, and anything else. As you search for and try on ideas, your conceptualization of the possibilities in the project you are considering will change.

Remember, information and ideas can be found not only in written resources but also in talking to people with special expertise and unique perspectives. When you get a chance to talk to someone about your project, you can ask specific questions that have been on your mind, or ask him or her to respond to emerging ideas. By talking to an individual, you can get a lot of information in a short amount of time.

Once you have gathered plenty of new, thought-provoking information about your project, it is time to sort through the concepts you have discovered by trying to name the primary topics that came up in your search. There are lots of different ways to do this, as described in Chapter 2: ballooning, sorting into piles, visual modeling, and color coding.

Amy and Helene used an intensive exploration of the literature before and during their implementation of the IALC program. They thought of these repeated reviews of different literature as evidence-based practice. Evidence-based practice feeds the therapist's thinking with an up-to-date review of current interventions and research, resulting in better-informed choices. They also attended presentations of the University of Southern California's Well Elderly Study and discussed their plans with the researchers afterward (Jackson et al., 1998). Helene and Amy also often discussed program ideas and directions with the elders with whom they were partnering. They used formal research methods of reviewing and extracting concepts from their experiences at the IALC, through observational and reflective data.

When I was in private practice in Los Angeles, seeing infants and children in a variety of community-based settings, I would often look for new ideas for intervention by going to toy stores. I would wander up and down the aisles, thinking about the children I was seeing and the goals toward which we were working. By spending an hour just looking at toys, trying out the new ones, imagining how different clients would respond to different activities, I could generate lots of new play ideas to use. It does not matter where you get new practice ideas. It only matters that you do so regularly and to the degree necessary to broaden your thinking.

Definition

The definition phase of a project is the point at which an individual or group works to clarify the intent of the project. Definition is a convergent phase, following the stretching out of the idea in investigation by honing its focus in definition. Again, different ways of doing this are provided in Chapter 2.

For Amy and Helene, not doing a formal clarification of their definition resulted in some problems in implementing the program. Although they intended to do an occupation-based program, their lack of clarity about the differences between high-quality programming for elders and how that would be expressed within the varied approaches of occupation-based, client-centered, evidence-based, and component-focused practice led to some confusion in developing and carrying out the program. This left them easily influenced by the medical culture of the setting, pushing them to focus initially on components, such as cognition, in designing programming.

Because this confusion of definition was an ongoing issue in creating programming at the IALC and in the minds of the therapists, uncovering and understanding exactly what it meant to do occupation-based practice became a focus of the reflective study. Certainly, this exploration of that question contributes a much-needed perspective on how these different approaches are related and in tension with one another. Constantly challenging each other regarding whether or not they were still providing programming consistent with their definition worked well to help Helene and Amy deal with the lack of clarity in the meaning of occupation-based practice.

At one point in my career, I was contracted to develop an early intervention program for a sensory-integration–style occupational therapy practice. I was very excited at the prospect of doing so because my practice was focused on early childhood, I was being well paid, and the program was to be based in developmental, play, and sensory integration theories—my preferred approaches at the time. It sounded like a creative challenge and a nice change from my day-to-day, one-on-one appointments. I did a considerable literature search, interviewed the practice director and a couple of key therapists, and observed other early intervention programs. When it came time for defining exactly what the project was, I had some different ideas on what could be done with the program. After drafting several and not being able to decide which was best, I finally resolved the definition by working with the practice director to choose one that best fit her hopes for the program.

Ideation

Ideation is the generation of multiple ideas and solutions when confronted with an intervention challenge. Often referred to as brainstorming, ideation is the most commonly recognized phase of the creative process (Koberg & Bagnall, 1981). Yet few people can really do it well, on demand, and freely: generating a long list of strong ideas and doing so without getting sidetracked into discussions of the pros and cons of each idea. After the convergent focus provided by definition, the ideation phase again stretches the idea out to encompass a divergent variety of possibilities.

In their occupation-based program, Amy and Helene used several variations on the ideation strategies proposed in Chapter 2. They used shared brainstorming over portions of the program, rather than over the whole of the program. That is, they would brainstorm over the best ways to do evaluation or how to work on cognition. Although they did discuss occupation-based practice together, and question whether they were staying on track with their intent to use this approach, they did not actually brainstorm directly on all the different ways to accomplish their intent to do an occupation-based program. This probably weakened the creativity of their program. Actually, this is a very common problem in design: an unclear definition resulting in a limited ideation phase.

An interesting strategy for ideation that Helene and Amy used was to draw ideas from the elders in group discussions. Involving the elders in generating and choosing activities not only resulted in more creative ideas, but also gave the elders a sense of ownership of the program. Using their ideas insured that the intervention was likely to be something in which the elders would be interested. Similarly, individual evaluations used a client-centered approach, looking to the resident and his or her significant others for intervention goals and ideas.

A simple example of ideation in practice I experienced recently was the effort of the OTGARY to create a name for the intervention program we were creating, providing, and researching in the rural alternative school. We did a simple brainstorm during an OTGARY meeting, producing a list of about 25 possible program names on a white board. We did pretty well at keeping focused on producing lots of choices and not digressing into discussion of pros and cons, except for occasional positive comments. Over the following week, different members added other names to the list on the board. A subgroup tried to move from ideation to idea selection by choosing a name from the list, but had difficulty choosing. After discussing the theory base of the program and the interests of the adolescents at the alternative school, the subgroup picked the five names that seemed like the best fit and decided to offer those choices to the adolescents, giving them the final say.

Idea Selection

Idea selection is a convergent phase. In idea selection, you carefully select the best idea for implementing a project's potential. Selecting the best intervention depends on a clear understanding of your criteria for success. The way in which good criteria for selecting the best idea depend on a clear definition of the desired outcome of the project demonstrates the strong link between convergent design phases as described in Chapter 2.

Because Helene and Amy did not formally brainstorm on the project as a whole, but on different parts, that is also the manner in which they did idea selection. For each particular challenge, they would complete written reflections as well as discussion with each other and with the elders involved. They loosely discussed the pros and cons of different ideas together. If it was in concert with what the elders wanted, they sometimes selected what was used in the literature or what they thought might be well received by the staff of the setting, giving up some degree of creativity for the sake of political outcomes for the program.

A strength of the IALC program was the degree to which Helene and Amy used input from the residents in choosing what activities and services to provide. In an effort to operate in an egalitarian partnership with the residents, they relinquished decision-making power to the elders. At first the residents did not respond by picking up the direction of the program. Once they saw that Helene and Amy really did mean to operate in this way, however, they were glad to be so involved. By encouraging the residents to choose activities for intervention, Amy and Helene were giving over the determination of the criteria for idea selection to the residents.

Although their idea selection strategies were not the careful ranking exercises found in Chapter 2, the collaborative program discussions between the two therapists, their sensitivity to the preferences of their clients, and their written reflection on the program greatly supported their creative choices of ideas to implement. In too many settings, therapists have no one with whom to discuss such decisions, and do no formal reflection on the choices they are making in creating their interventions.

In my experience, idea selection is often a weak phase for occupational therapists, who tend to be stronger divergent thinkers than they are convergent thinkers. There is, of course, a wide range of skills from one individual to the next. Certainly, idea selection is my own weakest phase. In my earlier years of practice, and now as a professor, I always seem to struggle with choosing from among too many ideas and too many projects. As I work with faculty who are attempting to make choices between different scholarly projects and career directions, it is often the same problem: how to select the best idea. In such situations, I often recommend either a simple ranking strategy or, for more complex choices, a rank and weigh grid. At this point in my own career, I am filled with ideas for projects that I feel are important in research, education, and service to the profession. Too many! I find that, if I do not stop and do an idea selection exercise every 6 months or so, I get overcommitted and overwhelmed. I have come to think of this process of reassessment and refocusing as "pruning."

Implementation

Implementation includes both the detailed planning of the selected idea and its actual implementation. By the time that the idea has reached this design phase, it is fairly refined. Yet this phase remains divergent because the details of planning and carrying out the project require adaptability to unexpected conditions that are inevitably uncovered in the real-life operations of any project. This flexibility can be seen in the IALC project in the therapists' willingness to mold their interventions to the preferences of the groups and individuals with whom they were working, their responsiveness to the politics of the setting, and their efforts to use trials of particular aspects of the programming, such as evaluation, before committing to widespread use.

The IALC project can be thought of as one complex and ongoing implementation or as many smaller implementations. It included assessment and intervention with different individuals, conducting groups, experimenting with and developing best practice assessments, and developing and providing inservice programs. Of the formal strategies for implementation described in Chapter 2, the ones most often used by Helene and Amy were reflective journaling and time/task list. As is typical of most interventions, the IALC project had no detailed overall program plan or formal plans for implementing the separate projects of occupation-based programming. Rather, the program emerged somewhat organically from the collaboration between the two therapists and with the staff, from opportunities provided by the context in which they were treating, and from Amy and Helene's responsiveness to the unique needs and talents of the elders of the IALC. As we see more research into occupation-based practice in occupational therapy, I wonder if this responsive growth of new programming to organically fit a setting will be a hallmark of great practice.

In the pilot study of occupational therapy intervention for at-risk youth in the rural alternative high school recently started by the OTGARY at Eastern Kentucky University, we are managing a fairly complex implementation. The study has three main strands of effort: service provision, research, and experiences of entry-level students on site. Service provision includes planning activities, carrying out activities, coordinating with school staff and administrators, administering evaluations, and recording intervention notes. Research includes planning, approval by the University's institutional review board, coordination with school system administrators, obtaining research consents from the students and their parents, recording video/photo/audio/written data, analyzing data, research team meetings, and research write-up. The fieldwork students require some out-of-class instruction about the population and setting, instruction in evaluations, support while involved in interventions, and opportunities for discussion of experiences and feedback from instructors. The three efforts are woven together largely through the strategy of assigning primary responsibility for program development, student fieldwork, and research to three of us who serve as the primary research team.

Evaluation

Evaluation is a careful examination of the relative success of the project in meeting its objectives. Evaluation can also yield unanticipated insights about practice; lessons learned from the experience of doing a new program or intervention approach; or a greater understanding of one's own strengths, style, and learning needs as a practitioner. Like the earliest phase of design process—motivation—the evaluation phase is often neglected. Failure to invest the necessary time to evaluate or reflect on therapeutic efforts and projects stunts the professional growth of many therapists and thus inhibits the efficacy of the profession in serving clients.

As a convergent phase, evaluation is linked with and depends on the clarity of the project definition and the criteria on which idea selection was accomplished. If the project being evaluated has a formal definition and subgoals, a formal evaluation can be developed to assess outcomes via data collected from clients, team members, therapists, or other constituents. Less formal reflections and peer discussions can also be used.

Since Amy and Helene did not use formal definition and idea selection processes in the IALC program, it would have been difficult to use formal program assessments in the evaluation phase. The consistent use of in-depth written reflection for the research, the collaborative work of the two therapists, and the research team meetings did, however, support a constant examination of the project's directions, successes, and difficulties. The formal research analysis produced theoretical insights into occupation-based practice that go beyond those usually expected from program evaluation efforts. And certainly, written reflection and qualitative analysis were especially conducive to the professional growth of both therapists.

A more limited example of evaluation is the use of occupational-therapy assessments to examine a client's progress. This can occur as a basis for a final discharge report or to use as information with which to revise goals and design new intervention. In this type of final evaluation, it is still important to remember to tap a variety of sources of evaluation information: the client's perspective on progress made, appropriate formal assessments, and reflection on your own experience of the intervention.

Summary

In this review of the design process as it naturally occurred in the initiation of occupation-based programming at the IALC, it is clear how central to occupational therapy process the design skills of the therapist can be. Although most therapists are not as cognizant of design skills as they are of the intervention theories they are using, they are clearly applying design process. Since design skills are not routinely taught in occupational therapy curricula, the natural abilities of different therapists vary considerably in taking projects through all phases of the design process. I would not expect most occupational therapists to be able to name multiple strategies for a particular phase of a project, or recognize the personal strengths and weaknesses in design process that we all have. For this reason, they continue to make the same mistakes in different projects: perhaps failing to generate enough self-motivation to remain enthusiastic through completion, settling on their first idea without fully exploring possibilities, being unclear in defining the intent of a project, or using haphazard implementation.

One of the common weaknesses that can be seen in projects that do not use a more informed design process is a general weakness in the linked convergent phases. The convergent phases of the design project include motivation, definition, idea selection, and evaluation. This is evident in the IALC project as well. Perhaps because creativity is more commonly understood to be a divergent skill, the convergent aspects of design process are often neglected. By not spending enough time identifying what was motivating their involvement in the IALC project, Amy and Helene were somewhat unclear on what they wished to accomplish. The project was not clearly defined but emerged from their experiences. This did keep it flexible, allowing the residents to influence and shape the occupation-based programming. However, it also left it flexible to be shaped by the medical perspective of staff, administrators, and the past component-focused practice experiences of the two therapists. Without a clear statement of program intent, it was difficult to select the most valuable ideas according to criteria that reflected that intent. Thus, the therapists spent much time on trial and error, selecting some activities in response to outside pressures, and experimenting with different interventions and approaches. Finally, without clear selection criteria or a project definition, it was difficult to evaluate and reflect on the successes of the program.

Although both therapists in the IALC project were familiar with design process, they did as many therapists do—focused on the process in which their clients were engaged, and neglected to attend to their own. In our efforts to be client-centered, to give clients power over the direction and goals of intervention, it is important that we do not cease attending to our own skills in the interactive dance of intervention. In fact, it is likely that the design skills required to support a client-centered process of occupational therapy are more challenging than those needed in component-focused practice. In occupation-based practice, where design of the intervention relies so much on the therapist's insight into the client's occupational identity, every intervention must be custom designed. Protocols are rare in occupation-based practice. The demands for strong design skills can only be heightened by the profession's increasingly clear determination that, in occupational therapy, best practice is most often occupation-based practice.

POWER BUILDERS

Keep in mind the following primary concepts of this chapter while working with the Power Builders:

- Motivation
- Investigation
- Definition
- Ideation
- Idea selection
- Implementation
- Evaluation

1. Select a strategy from one of the design phases in Chapter 2 and describe that strategy in writing, as you would have carried it out in the IALC program.

2. Select a strategy as in exercise 1, and write a fictional completion of the strategy as best you can with the program information in the preceding chapter.

3. Do as in exercise 1, using a case from Appendix A.

4. Do as in exercise 2, using a case from Appendix A.

5. Describe the phase of intervention design in which you feel you are strongest.

6. Describe the phase of intervention design in which you most need to develop.

7. Using all of the design phases, plan and carry out an intervention to improve your skills in the design phase in which you think that you are weakest. Document your progress.

8. Imagine you have been assigned the development of a new type of intervention program. Write a brief description of the program. Follow this with a brainstormed list of all the personal motivations you might have for developing and running this new program.

9. You are a supervisor of two therapists in a setting similar to the IALC. The three of you have been charged to develop occupation-based programming for the residents. Use design process to create a professional development plan for yourself and your therapists, to prepare you to do occupation-based programming, beginning with the motivation phase and continuing through the plan for implementation.

10. Observe an occupational therapist at work. What phases of the design process do you see in operation?

11. Imagine that you are a therapist who, because of recent under-staffing in your department, has been working so hard and fast that you are feeling completely burned out and lacking in creativity. What will you do to restore your creative potential for strong intervention? Using the design process, from motivation through idea selection, choose the best way to regain your creativity.

12. Choose a case from Appendix A. Use design process to create intervention related to one goal for that individual, from motivation

POWER BUILDERS

through planning for implementation. Document your design efforts and thinking.

13. Using a client-centered approach, it is helpful to engage clients in the design process with you. Describe a population of clients with whom you can see yourself working in the future. Choose one phase of the design process and brainstorm as many ways as possible to involve the creativity of your clients in that phase.

References

Jackson, J., Carlson, M., Mandel, D., Zemke, R., & Clark, F. (1998). Occupation in lifestyle redesign: The Well Elderly Study occupational therapy program. *Americal Journal of Occupational Therapy, 52,* 326–336.

Koberg, D., & Bagnall, R. (1981). *The all new universal traveler: A soft systems guide to creativity, problem-solving, and the process of reaching goals.* Los Altos, CA: William Kaufmann, Inc.

CHAPTER 15

Collaborative Occupational Goal Generation

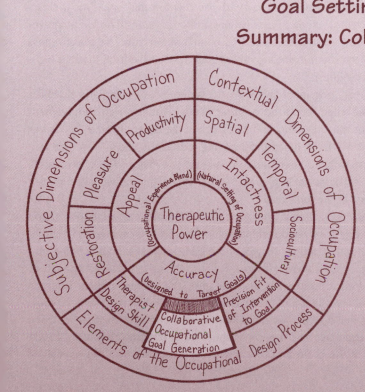

The Contribution of Collaborative Occupational Goal Generation to Intervention Accuracy

Occupation is both the means and the ends in occupational therapy (Cynkin, 1995; Gray, 1998; Trombley, 1995). Occupational goals establish the ends targeted by intervention. By establishing the goals of intervention in collaboration with the client, the therapist ensures that the outcomes will accurately target the changes in the client's occupational pattern that the client most values. Collaborative goal-setting also gives the client more ownership of the intervention process, thereby increasing the consistency and persistence of his or her participation in interventions. In this brief chapter, several key aspects that will ensure strong skills of collaborative occupational goal generation are reviewed.

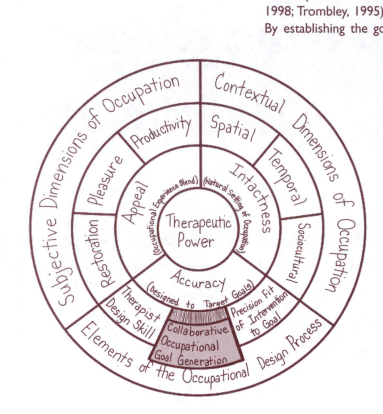

The Interaction Style of Therapist-Client Collaborations in Client-Centered Practice

Client-centered practice is "an approach to service which embraces a philosophy of respect for, and partnership with, people receiving services" (Law, Baptiste, & Mills, 1995). Client-centered practice originated in Canada and emphasizes the rights of the consumer to guide intervention. In the occupational therapy process, locating power with the client in this way is most clearly demonstrated in a participatory style of assessment and goal setting. The client actively engages in determining the priorities to be addressed in intervention. The effectiveness of the therapist in engaging the client in setting valued goals for intervention marks a high-quality, client-centered intervention.

Occupational therapy has long identified with the independent living and disability rights movements. Like the client-centered approach, the disability rights movement requires the therapist to put the judgments and priorities of the client ahead of his or her own. For services provided within an independent living model, the client is viewed as a consumer and the therapist as his or her hired consultant (Bowen, 1996). Often, interventions focus on change in the social and physical barriers in the individual's environment, rather than on change in the individual.

To offer client-centered services, the therapist must cultivate a specific interaction style. In a study of patient-therapist relationships, Peloquin (1990) characterized the different relationship types as dominated by images of the occupational therapist being similar to a technician, parent, or collaborator/friend. For a client to feel secure enough to engage in a collaborative relationship with the therapist, the therapist must offer an unconditional acceptance of the client and his or her lifestyle. Further, the therapist must be secure enough in his or her own professional identity to be open with the client. The relationship between the therapist and the client must be authentic (Matheson, 1998). Although the interactions of the client and therapist remain centered on the needs and goals of the client, the therapist should be able to acknowledge and share his or her personal feelings about the intervention process, such as frustration over barriers or excitement over successes. Clark (1993) refers to this collaborative, egalitarian relationship as being a "therapist-coach" (p.1073).

Assuming such an open, secure approach to interacting with clients can be difficult at times. The therapist must give up power and take risks. We are not all strong all of the time. A novice therapist or one who is working in a new area of practice may not feel secure in his or her understanding of interventions. Or, perhaps the therapist has some familial or health problems that make taking an open stance feel too emotionally demanding. When the therapist finds that he or she is so emotionally depleted or insecure as to be unable to communicate openly and honestly with clients, he or she should immediately seek personal resources and support, in order to return to engaging in secure, open interactions (Matheson, 1998).

It is important to acknowledge that placing power in the hands of the client is a recent shift from the more traditional "expert" approach, which places most goal-setting power in the hands of the therapist and other medical professionals. At this time, therapists vary widely in their abilities to work collaboratively with clients in setting intervention goals. Change in how occupational therapy occurs is slow. Therapists who have been in practice for a long time and who have not been exposed to newer approaches are still using an expertise approach. This can be confusing for students on fieldwork who attempt to work collaboratively while their clinical instructors work more from the expertise stance. Understand that you are in a process of change in the field, one of many that will occur during your career. Keep in mind that the newer, collaborative approach promises greater accuracy. That is, by giving clients a strong voice in setting goals, the intervention is more likely to target goals that have high priority for the client, more likely to motivate the client to work hard in therapy, and more likely to be effective. Client-centered occupational therapy is better occupational therapy.

In the occupation-based practice study at the IALC, the therapists had many successes and struggles in using a client-centered approach. Amy and Helene's efforts to work in partnership with the residents showed the acceptance, respect, and openness of this approach. They made efforts to engage the residents in goal-setting and in generating ideas for interventions. They used group discussions as well as individualized assessments focused on client goal setting. At first the residents did not know what to make of this client-centered approach. They were expecting to take the more passive role they often experienced with other healthcare professionals. As Amy and Helene continued to maintain their collaborative stance, however, the residents began to really believe that the two therapists were not going to become directive and did wish to hear the needs and ideas of the residents. In the groups, once several activities suggested by the residents had been used, the residents became very comfortable and involved in determining the goals and directions of occupational therapy. In individual assessments, remaining client-centered required ongoing negotiations with the client and checking back on how he or she was feeling about the progress and goals of treatment.

For Helene, who had practiced for a long time under an expertise approach, using a client-centered approach was more difficult. Often, she would see needs that the clients did not, and then would struggle in deciding whether intervention was necessary and whether she should allow the clients to set goals in other areas. A good example is the case of Jerry and his wife, Becky, who did not want to address the therapist's concerns about Jerry's standing balance and safety. Helene's struggles to remain client-centered in allowing Jerry and Becky to retain control over the therapeutic goals were evident in her reflective notes. Yet she did not impose on them her own view of which goals were important, beyond explaining her concerns. If Amy and Helene had remained at the IALC for longer than 3 months, it is likely that Jerry and Becky might have gotten past their resistance to working on this area and set goals to address Jerry's balance.

Hearing the Client's Story

In many ways, the effort to provide client-centered intervention depends largely on the therapist's ability to draw out the client's perspective on him or herself in the past, present, and future. Specifically, the therapist aims to engage the client in a review and examination of his or her biography, personal narrative, or, as Amy and Helene termed it, occupational identity. There is great variation in how easily and effectively this is done, depending on the skills and willingness of the client to reflect on life experiences, patterns, disruptions, and aspirations. Clark calls this telling of one's personal tale of doing, and of doing disrupted by illness, "occupational storytelling" (1993, p. 1074). Besides being important to setting collaborative goals, speaking of one's experiences with illness and disability is therapeutic because it begins the process of recognizing and coming to grips with the impact of those experiences on one's life.

Those who have sustained traumatic injuries or other life-altering health conditions need to reconstruct their lives, to envision how to continue on from that point and into the future, and to do what Clark called "occupational storymaking" (1993, p. 1074). Within this process of creating a new life story, clients identify occupational goals. Often spiritual beliefs become woven into the narrative, as clients deal with the difficult question of why the disability has occurred in their lives and at this time (Hammell, 1998). Stories of the future, the aims of intervention, and hoped-for outcomes are co-created by the client, therapist, and significant others together, and are periodically reformulated to integrate new information and experiences (Mattingly & Fleming, 1994).

Interview skills are key to facilitating occupational storymaking in clients. Although interviewing is a key skill in qualitative research methods, it is rarely taught in depth in entry-level occupational therapy programs. Some therapists learn through experience to be highly skilled interviewers. Others do not. Here are a few ideas for doing skilled interviews to support collaborative goal setting.

Interviews can be done in a structured or unstructured format, although the less structured format tends to make the client more comfortable. In initial interactions with a client, interviews are often semistructured, centering on questions of occupational history and goals. A family interview is often effective, especially if the client is young or does not communicate well. Sometimes the interview will require an interpreter. If the interview is the first meeting of therapist and client, it may be difficult to establish a strong rapport to support the interview. It may be helpful to present yourself in a nonthreatening way by wearing casual clothing, offering some limited sharing of personal stories, demonstrating that you are trying to understand the situation from the client's perspective, and making other efforts to gain the trust of the client (Fontana & Frey, 1998). Careful attention to recording the details of the client's narrative, through either note taking or audio recording, requires that written notes or analysis of the interview contents be completed within 2 days of the interview. The quality of initial interviews can be checked by returning to the questions at a later date with the client, seeking input from other key informants, and testing conclusions against other sources of information, such as written records (Gilchrist & Williams, 1999).

One of the difficulties of using a narrative approach to access the occupational identity of clients is that some clients are not willing or able to participate. Storytelling and storymaking require verbal skills, motivation, and cognitive abilities. At the IALC, some of the residents were too depressed or disoriented to engage in the setting of goals via examination of their personal biographies.

Therapeutic Processes of Assessment and Goal Setting

In a client-centered approach, the line can be unclear between facilitating occupational storytelling, which is a reflective review of past occupational patterns and disruptions, and facilitating occupational storymaking, which focuses more on identifying and setting goals for change. In the most effective collaborative goal-setting, client and therapist work together to glean important therapeutic goals from the client's narrative and prioritize them.

Moving from client narrative to client goals can be facilitated through the use of structured assessments. Matheson describes a sequence, from interview to goals, which he calls "the goaling process" (1998, p. 117). The sequence includes:

- A structured interview around desired goals
- Prioritization of the goals with the client
- The client's review of the prioritized list of goals with significant others
- Distribution of the goal list to others

Fearing, Clark, and Stanton (1998) propose a similar process in their Occupational Performance Process Model that continues through the intervention:

- Identify occupational performance issues
- Select potential intervention models
- Identify occupational performance components and environmental conditions
- Identify strengths and resources
- Negotiate targeted outcomes and develop actions plans
- Implement plans through occupation
- Evaluate occupational process outcomes

Top-down assessment is central to client-centered practice (Coster, 1998; Law, 1998). Top-down assessments focus on occupational patterns and problems, addressing components secondarily. At the IALC, Amy and Helene used the Comprehensive Occupational Performance Measure (Law, 1998), the Kielhofner Occupational History Revised (Kielhofner, Mallinson, Crawford, Nowak, Rigby, Henry, & Walens, 1998), and an assessment they developed themselves, the Life Pattern Review (see Chapter 13). The Life Pattern Review was especially effective in bringing out a picture of how the daily-life activities of the residents had changed since their admission to the IALC. Once the residents had discovered and discussed these pattern changes, either in group or just with the therapist, it was easy to consider with them the goals they wanted to set for reclaiming activities important to them.

Keep in mind that the occupational therapist does not serve only an individual client. Clients pass through the process of reconstructing their lives within a circle of significant others. It is important that others who are integrally involved in the lives of clients also be included in the telling of the story and the setting of goals. Primary caregivers are especially important to involve in intervention. This insures their input, their participation, and their support of the efforts clients may wish to make. Caregivers can include parents, adult children, partners, other relatives, and healthcare workers (Abel & Nelson, 1990: Pierce & Frank, 1992; Segal & Frank, 1998). The work of caring for a person with a temporary or chronic disability can hardly be overstated (Corbin & Strauss, 1988). The ability of the caregiver to effectively give care, while maintaining his or her own health, is critical to outcomes for your client. When the client is unable to fully participate in reflection and goal setting, such as when the client is a child or has a cognitive impairment, the therapist should work with the caregiver and others to move through the intervention process. At times, some of the primary goals of intervention may involve the caregiver more than the client. At the IALC, this was seen primarily in the need to work with couples who lived together there, since other family members were not very involved with caregiving for the residents.

Summary: Collaboration and Intervention Accuracy

Collaborative goal-setting is a critical skill for the creation of effective interventions that target outcomes that are deeply valued by your clients. Setting goals for the client without his or her participation may or may not accurately target the outcomes that most concern your client and create the biggest life barriers at the time of interventions. You cannot know a client's goals until you ask. Masterful collaborative goal setting requires an open and egalitarian interaction style, interview skills, effective facilitation of the client's occupational story, and goals that emanate from the client's perspective on the occupational challenges with which he or she is faced. The degree to which you work to develop these skills of collaborative goal-setting will be one predictor of how accurately your interventions will target outcomes that reconstruct the lives of your clients in ways highly significant to them.

POWER BUILDERS

Keep in mind the primary concepts from this chapter while working with the Power Builders:

- Interaction style
- Hearing the client's story
- Therapeutic processes of assessment and goal setting

1. Use a brainstorming exercise to list your own occupational goals for the future. What would you like to accomplish, what skills would you like to acquire, or what changes would you like to make in your daily life? Remember the rules of brainstorming, and that a quantity of ideas is the objective.

2. After completing the previous brainstorming exercise, use a rank and weigh grid to select your top priority occupational goal. Remember to reflect carefully on the criteria you use to rank the options against each other.

3. Practice your interview-recording skills by doing one of the following interviews. Use either note taking that is later fully transcribed, or audio recording that is later fully transcribed. Remember to attempt to elicit as much useful information as possible while saying as little as you can.

   - Interview a person about an activity in which he or she is frequently involved or is particularly interested. Choose an individual as unlike you as possible in terms of gender, age, ethnicity, and experience with the activity.

   - Interview an occupational therapist about his or her area of practice.

   - Interview an occupational therapy consumer about how he or she perceived the strengths and weaknesses of an intervention.

   - Interview a caregiver of an occupational therapy consumer about the experience of providing care.

   - Interview an elder in your family about his or her childhood occupational patterns.

   - Interview an expert worker about his or her experience of the productive, restorative, and pleasurable aspects of the activity in which he or she is an expert.

4. Imagine that you are a therapist who, because of crises in your own life, does not feel able to be open and authentic in interacting with clients. What will you do to restore yourself? Brainstorm and then rank to generate your top choice.

5. Select a case from Appendix A and find a partner to role play the client in that case. Use the role play to try one of the following exercises.

   - Try modeling three different styles of interaction with the client: a technician, a parent, and a friend.

   - Act out to the client the appropriate expression of your own feelings as a therapist about a fictional experience of intervention.

   - Facilitate your client's telling of his or her occupational story.

   - Discuss potential goals of intervention with your client and collaboratively choose the one on which he or she most wishes to work.

POWER BUILDERS

- Use the goaling process to set at least one primary goal of intervention.
- Administer a top-down assessment and write it up as a report.

6. Using the choices from exercise 5, take the part of the client. Write a journal entry on how it felt to be a client.

References

Abel, E. K., & Nelson, M. K. (1990). *Circles of care: Work and identity in women's lives.* Albany, NY: State University of New York Press.

Bowen, R. (1996, March). Practicing what we preach: Embracing the independent living movement. OT Practice 1, 18–20.

Clark, F. (1993). Occupation embedded in a real life: Interweaving occupational science and occupational therapy. *American Journal of Occupational Therapy, 47,* 1067–1078.

Corbin, J. M., & Strauss, A. (1988). *Unending work and care: Managing chronic illness at home.* San Francisco: Jossey Bass.

Coster, W. (1998). Occupation-centered assessment of children. *American Journal of Occupational Therapy, 52,* 337–344.

Cynkin, S. (1995). Activity analysis. In C. Royeen (Ed.), *The practice of the future: Putting occupation back into therapy.* (pp. 7-1–7-52). Bethesda, MD: American Occupational Therapy Association.

Fearing, V. G., Clark, J., & Stanton, S. (1998). The client-centered occupational therapy process. In M. Law (Ed.), *Client-Centered Occupational Therapy* (pp. 67–88). Thorofare, NJ: SLACK, Incorporated.

Fontana, A., & Frey, J. (1998). Interviewing: The art of science. In N. Denzin & Y. Lincoln (Eds.), *Collecting and interpreting qualitative materials* (pp. 47–78). Thousand Oaks, CA: Sage Publications.

Gray, J. M. (1998). Putting occupation into practice: Occupation as ends, occupation as means. *American Journal of Occupational Therapy, 52,* 354–364.

Gilchrist, V., & Willams, R. (1999). Participant observation. In B. Crabtree & W. Miller (Eds.), *Doing qualitative research* (pp. 71–88). Thousand Oaks, CA: Sage Publications.

Hammell, K. W. (1998). Client-centered occupational therapy: Collaborative planning, accountable intervention. In M. Law (Ed.), *Client-Centered Occupational Therapy* (pp. 123–144). Thorofare, NJ: SLACK, Incorporated.

Kielhofner, G., Mallinson, T., Crawford, C., Nowak, M., Rigby, M., Henry, A., & Walens, D. (1998). *A user's manual for the occupational performance history interview (Version 2.0).* Chicago: Model of Human Occupation Clearinghouse, University of Illinois at Chicago.

Law, M. (1998). *Client-centered occupational therapy.* Thorofare, NJ: SLACK, Incorporated.

Law, M., Baptiste, S., & Mills, J. (1995). Client-centered practice: What does it mean and does it make a difference? *Canadian Journal of Occupational Therapy, 62,* 250–257.

Matheson, L. (1998). Engaging the person in the process: Planning together for occupational therapy intervention. In M. Law (Ed.), *Client-Centered Occupational Therapy* (pp. 107–122). Thorofare, NJ: SLACK, Incorporated.

Mattingly, C., & Fleming, M. H. (1994). *Clinical reasoning: Forms of inquiry in a therapeutic practice.* Philadelphia: F. A. Davis.

Peloquin, S. (1990). The patient-therapist relationship in occupational therapy: Understanding visions and images. *American Journal of Occupational Therapy, 46,* 972–980.

Pierce, D., & Frank, G. (1992). A mother's work: Two levels of feminist analysis of family-centered care. *American Journal of Occupational Therapy, 44,* 13–21.

Segal, R., & Frank, G. (1998). The extraordinary construction of ordinary experience: Scheduling daily life in families with children with attention deficit hyperactivity disorder. *Scandinavian Journal of Occupational Therapy, 5,* 141–147.

Trombly, C. (1995). Occupation: Purposefulness and meaningfulness as therapeutic mechanisms, 1995 Eleanor Clarke Slagle Lecture. *American Journal of Occupational Therapy, 49,* 960–972.

CHAPTER 16

Precision Fit of Intervention to Goal

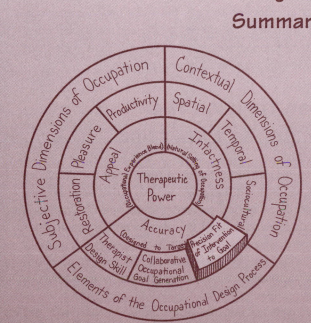

Precision Intervention Design

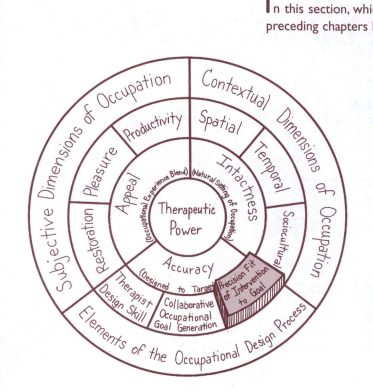

In this section, which focuses on the intervention applications of occupation, the three preceding chapters have presented a study of occupation-based practice, an examination of the therapist's use of design skills in intervention, and an overview of collaboration with clients in the generation of occupational goals. This chapter provides a consideration of the more complex issue of precise intervention design. If occupation-based practice, therapist-design skills, and collaborative goal-setting are desirable approaches in occupational therapy, how can those interventions be made more effective in reaching goals? How do we make the intervention fit the goal more precisely?

To understand the contribution of precision fit to the accuracy of intervention, I often think of experiences I have had in doing group interventions. Of course, in groups, all the clients are slightly different. They have different goals and challenges, but their goals are similar enough to be placed together in a group. No matter what the type of intervention the group may use, it will be more or less effective for each individual in the group, depending on how well it appeals to that person, how the context of that experience is perceived, and what his or her personal goals may be. Although the therapist may try to individualize the group intervention, when he or she sits down to document the group session in each client's chart, it is obvious that the intervention worked better for some individuals than for others. This variation in the degree to which the intervention precisely fits the goals of each client in a group intervention is not unusual.

Variation is also to be expected in how much the intervention precisely fits the goals of the client in individual intervention. From one session to the next, there will be successes and failures, excitement and frustration. Sometimes the therapist will wonder if any progress will ever be possible with a particular client, no matter how carefully he or she has designed interventions and negotiated goals. Other times, a session will go so beautifully that the therapist can hardly wait to tell someone. How do we move all our interventions closer to this precise fit of intervention to goal, and thus toward better outcomes for our clients? Several areas promise this possibility: developing expertise, honing observation skills, using different intervention strategies, reconfiguring client goals, using evidence-based practice, and acknowledging barriers to precise practice.

Increasing Precision through the Continual Development of Expertise

Therapists develop expertise at different rates, depending on the degree to which they invest in themselves. Some have clear plans for developing their expertise: avidly seeking out continuing education, reading resources, and conversations with expert therapists in their areas of practice. Others do not seem to find the time for self-development. Over the years, failure to invest in the growth of expertise results in a widening competency gap between the therapist who is working on self-development and the therapist who is not. This gap in expertise is especially evident in the ability to provide precise, effective interventions.

Another rich source of development for the therapist is reflection on his or her practice. Therapists who value it find plenty of time for this reflection on intervention:

between sessions, while writing notes, talking over lunch, driving to and from work, or in a daily journal. One can ask many questions about daily practice experiences that will contribute to the growth of expertise and ability to provide interventions that precisely fit goals, such as:

- What went well in that session?

- What could have been improved?

- What did the client experience?

- How well did the session move toward established goals?

- What goals are not being well addressed yet?

- Do the goals need revising?

- What did I enjoy most, or least, about the session?

- Was there a better time, place, or social group in which that session would have worked better?

- What would have made the session more appealing for the client?

- What did I learn from this session, if anything?

- What skill do I need to develop further?

Reflecting, evaluating daily practice, and taking the time to think pushes the therapist's development into ever-increasing therapeutic power. For Amy and Helene at the independent- and assisted-living center (IALC), shared reflection was an important part of this process of developing increasingly precise interventions.

Observation Skills

Occupational therapy requires highly sophisticated observation skills. The basics of observation, however, are not as carefully taught in occupational therapy as they are in our sister discipline of anthropology. Honing your observation skills is an excellent way to enhance the precision of your interventions. Observation gives you a more informed perspective on your clients and the contexts in which they live and work. The ability to do accurate, useful observation involves several subskills: gaining entry to settings that provide you with informing observations, establishing rapport with individuals in the setting, and recording accurate and thorough observations (Adler & Adler, 1998; Bogdewic, 1999). Usually, occupational-therapy students receive instruction in activity analysis, environmental assessment, and proper administration of a large number of formal assessment instruments. These are, in a sense, specialized forms of observation.

Observation is fundamentally naturalistic. When doing observation, you want to gain a perspective on the broad patterns and styles of behavior in a setting. Choose your observation to maximize your access to the natural patterns that exist in that setting. Where you choose to do an observation will depend on what you wish to understand. Do you wish to understand the culture of a certain group of people with disabilities, daily life in a particular residential setting, the family world of a particular client with whom you are working, or something else entirely? As you choose a setting, consider the role you should assume in doing your observation. Observation can be done anywhere along a continuum from being purely an observer to being a full participant. What stance will best serve your intention in doing your observation?

Establishing rapport with people in the setting you are observing is a familiar challenge for therapists, as we enter and leave different settings each day. How well your choice of role on the observer-participant continuum fits the expectations of those in the setting will be a part of this rapport-building process. Regular, repeated observations also help build relationships and trust. If you select a role that is more observer than participant, try to be unobtrusive, especially about taking notes. If anyone questions you about what you are doing, always be honest. Be unassuming. Blend in. Be a good, reflective listener. In conversations, be self-revealing within limits, letting the person with whom you are speaking know who you really are as a person, but without giving too many personal details.

Recording your observations can be done in many ways. If it seems unnatural to be writing observation notes in the setting, postpone recording them until immediately after you finish. Do not wait more than 24 hours to record an observation. Although it may seem that you will remember everything, your memories will fade faster than you realize. Consider whether audio or video recordings, or still photography, would be appropriate in the setting. If you can appear natural making some written notes in the setting, such as when sitting at a table in a lunchroom or writing in a client's chart during a home visit, just jot down the most important points, phrases, or words. Later, you can convert these into fully descriptive written observations. Using a computer for full observation notes is very helpful.

While you are doing your observations, it is helpful to have a brief observation guide as a prompt. The guide can be structured in different ways, but is just a short list of cues regarding what questions to consider as you observe. If it is your first time in a setting, you may want to just use an open, unstructured approach to observation. Later, more specific questions to examine will emerge from your observations. Sometimes observers use "who," "what," "when," "where," "why," and "how" as informal prompts to direct initial observations. Whatever the structure you use for observation, be sure to spend adequate time on recording and reflecting on the full descriptive notes. Ask yourself these questions.

- What new information emerged from the observation?
- How did the observation go?
- What might have worked better?
- Are there any points of conflict or confusion to be examined further?
- How was I feeling and thinking as I conducted the observation?

Enhancing your observation skills in this way will increase your ability to provide accurate, effective, occupation-based interventions. By honing your observation skills, you will bring your interventions into a more careful fit with the goals and contexts of your client.

At the IALC, Amy and Helene used a participant-observation method, doing their observations as they went about providing interventions. Later, they would write descriptive notes of the intervention sessions, questions that occurred to them during interventions, and how they felt as they tried to remain occupation based. The research team would analyze the notes and come up with new questions to guide further observations. Through this cycle of repeated observations, they were able to rapidly evolve fairly precise occupation-based interventions in a new area of practice.

Selecting Strategies for Occupational Pattern Change

One way to increase the precision with which interventions fit goals is to be sure that all the basic strategies of intervention have been considered. Strategies should be selected that will best facilitate the changes in occupational pattern desired by the client. Goals, once carefully set, can be reached by two basic strategies: change in the client and change in the client's environments.

Change in the client can take many forms and uses many different theoretical approaches. Changes produced by intervention can be conceptualized as developmental change, skill acquisition, increase in physical capacities, integration of sensory and motor processing, or creating new occupational patterns within the constraints of disability, to name only a few. Often a graded approach to the goal is used in change focused on the individual. Grading is a step-by-step progression along a continuum of ability, starting with the present abilities of the client and gradually advancing to where he or she wishes to be once the goal is reached.

Working on change in an individual requires sensitivity to the subjective experience and perspective of your client, as well as a careful design of occupation-based interventions that are appealing to that person. Consideration of whether interventions could be more effective if provided in a more spatially, temporally, or socioculturally intact setting for your client can also increase the effectiveness of interventions.

Another primary strategy of intervention is to make changes in the environments in which the client wishes to engage in desired occupations. This strategy can take the form of alterations to existing environments, or simply relocating the client to an environment that offers a better fit to his or her goals. Examples of selecting new environments include deciding to move to an assisted-living center, changing jobs, moving to a fully included classroom, and moving from a family setting to a college dorm.

When the client wishes to return to, or remain in, particular environments, changes can be created in any of the three dimensions of context in that setting to make that possible. Possible changes to the spatial context include adaptive devices, splinting, mobility and communication equipment, architectural modifications, environment control technology, visual cues and signage, changes in the tools and devices frequently used, alterations to the furniture and equipment of a frequently used space, restructuring the sensory qualities of a space, and others. Changes to the temporal aspects of context might include redesign of schedules, establishment of routines, changes in expectations regarding time use by the client, and altering the speed and timing demands of the setting. Changes to the sociocultural dimension of environments might include adding or removing specific individuals, changing standards or attitudes, and building relationships between the client and others.

To bring the fit of goals and intervention into a closer alignment, be sure that you have considered all the basic intervention strategies, whether they target change in the individual or change in the setting. Also, remember that the strategies can be combined to provide a stronger, multifaceted approach to the goals. For example, working on a client's job skills could be combined with experiences in a new work setting. Once goals have been established, ask yourself these questions.

- Is this goal best approached through change in the client, change in the client's environments, or both?

- If a selected strategy is change in the client, is the planned intervention appealing to this client?

- If a selected strategy is change in the client, is there a more intact setting within which to address this goal?

- If a selected strategy is to change to new environments for this client, which settings would most precisely support the goals?

- If a selected strategy is to make changes to the client's familiar environments, what spatial, temporal, and sociocultural aspects of those environments might require modification?

At the IALC, Helene and Amy used all the strategies discussed here. An example of working on changes in client ability was trying to decrease one woman's shoulder pain and restricted range of motion so she could return to oil painting, an activity central to her identity. The selected setting was within a group of elderly women at the IALC who were also interested in oil painting, although they had less experience with shoulder problems than the client. To support the goal of one group of elders who wanted to create a more social community at the IALC, a dressy tea party was created. A good example of changes to a setting are the modifications Helene helped to make in the furnishings in one elderly couple's apartment to make it safer and easier to use for the husband, who had some vision and balance limitations.

The Changing Story: Continual Reconfiguration of Client Goals to Increase Precision

One of the common ways in which goals and intervention drift out of a precision fit occurs when changes in the client's perspective on intervention begin to create a new story about where intervention is headed. For example, consider a client with a newly acquired spinal cord injury. Initially, he may wish to focus primarily on goals of physical recovery and self-care. Once he comes to grips with some of the larger questions of living with his disability, however, he may then be concerned with issues of employment, mobility, return to home, and sexual function. As the story the client is living changes, the story the client and the therapist are making together about goals must also change. Skills acquired in intervention may open new challenges. Experiences with new environments and activities may suggest new life directions. No matter how carefully and collaboratively goals are set, they must be continually revisited with the client, and reconfigured as necessary.

Evidence-Based Practice

Evidence-based practice is like a toolbox of methods to aid clinical reasoning, and, furthermore, it is a toolbox consisting primarily of methods designed to integrate research study evidence into the clinical reasoning process. The methods of evidence-based practice help the practitioner select the best assessments and intervention procedures from an array of possibilities (Tickle-Degnen, 1999, p. 537).

In all areas of health care today, research is increasingly being used to examine the effectiveness and outcomes of intervention (Frattali, 1998). Such studies provide important information to guide the work of therapists. Outcomes measurement can document many different types of results from intervention: clinically derived outcomes (for example, grip strength), functional outcomes (ability to dress self), administrative outcomes (number of sessions per day in a particular population), cost outcomes (average length of stay), social outcomes (return to employment), and client-defined outcomes (satisfaction with services).

Three types of research examine the results of intervention: outcomes, efficacy, and effectiveness research. Outcomes research looks at the results of interventions in the lives of actual clients. Efficacy research examines what interventions are most useful in ideal, controlled conditions, such as in randomized clinical trials. Effectiveness research studies the success of interventions in typical conditions, including all clients regardless of variations in their presenting history.

Evidence-based practice serves to increase the effectiveness of a therapist's interventions by providing ways of using research to support clinical decision making. The methods of evidence-based practice can generally be used to accomplish three primary clinical tasks: determine the occupational challenges and risks typical of a particular population, evaluate assessments, and create interventions (Tickle-Degnen, 1999). This is accomplished through five steps (Tickle-Degnen, 2000):

- Create a clinical question.
- Collect evidence.
- Determine what evidence is highest quality.
- Describe the evidence to clients and significant others at points of decision making regarding goals, assessment, or interventions.
- Reflect on the intervention as it occurs, revising as needed for the individual client.

In the occupation-based practice study at the IALC, Helene and Amy used an evidence-based practice approach to identify likely needs of the elders; to guide selection of top-down assessments; and to design interventions to improve balance, prevent falls, and support memory and cognition in residents with Alzheimer's disease.

Barriers to Precise Practice

Practicing with precision is difficult. Some therapists may never experience precise practice. It is important to acknowledge, however, that intervention that fits poorly with the goals of the client often results from barriers encountered by the therapist. A common barrier is reimbursement systems that do not cover important goals or that do not provide enough coverage to last until the client is beyond the acute phase and confronted with the challenges of return to home and work. Another barrier is inflexible institutions that do not allow the occupational therapist to treat in an occupation-based manner appealing to clients, or to treat in settings more intact for the client. In the schools, therapists are often expected to cover too large a caseload to provide high-quality interventions. There are many barriers to precise intervention that accurately targets and accomplishes client goals. Therapists must acknowledge the barriers to good intervention they regularly encounter in their settings. Identifying such barriers helps the therapist and his or her administrators to distinguish between a lack of skills on the part of the occupational therapist and limitations on intervention effectiveness that are created by systemic barriers.

Using Ends as Means

One of the easiest ways to increase the precise fit of the intervention to the goal is to use the occupations targeted for change as the mode of intervention. For example, if return to work following a work-related hand injury is the client's goal, providing intervention at the job site and using graded aspects of the client's work there are likely to accurately target that goal. The demands and materials pertinent to that work are easily available, the occupational therapist can make accurate observations of the occupational pattern being targeted, and coworkers can provide encouragement to the client. At the IALC, an example of the use of ends as means can be seen in the woman who used oil painting to work on shoulder problems to reclaim oil painting as an occupation that was an important part of her identity.

Summary

Once the practitioner, or practitioner-to-be, has reached the point of understanding the dimensions of occupation, he or she is ready to apply them as powerful occupation-based interventions. Once he or she becomes accustomed to the occupation-based approach, the therapist can further develop expertise and accurate targeting of goals important to clients by building skills of design, collaborative goal generation, and precision fit of interventions to goal. Precise intervention design can be accomplished by any practitioner who is willing to work to develop in the areas just described in this chapter: continual development of personal expertise, increasing observation skills, remaining aware of the strategy choices open in all interventions, participating in the reconfiguring of the client's story as needed, using evidence-based practice to ground interventions in current research, and identifying barriers to precise practice.

Keep in mind the following primary concepts of this chapter in working with the Power Builders:

- Continual development of expertise
- Observation skills
- Selecting strategies for change
- Reconfiguration of client goals
- Evidence-based practice
- Barriers to precise practice
- Using ends as means

1. Write a brief description of a type of practice in which you hope to be involved in 5 years. Using the design process, from the motivation phase through implementation planning, create a plan for your own development of expertise in this area of practice.

2. Choose a public place in which many people are engaged in a particular activity. Create an observation guide to cue your observation. Complete a minimum of 4 hours of observation in the setting. Fully transcribe your notes or audio recording of your observation. Write a synthesis of your observation, describing the primary occupational patterns you discovered in your observation.

3. Select a case from Appendix A and do the one of the following exercises.

   - Using one of the case studies and the questions near the beginning of this chapter, write a fictional reflection on how an intervention session went.

   - Describe an observation you could do that would inform your interventions with this individual. Include how you would gain entry to the setting, how you would build rapport or fit in unobtrusively, where you would position yourself on the observer-participant continuum, how you plan to record your observation, and what observation guide you will create to cue your observations.

   - Describe the following for one case: goals you can envision generating in collaboration with the client, changes in the environments of the client that might be beneficial, and settings in which it would be best to work on each goal.

   - Write a fictional reflection, describing why you think the goals you had previously set with this client need to be reconfigured.

   - Using the references for evidence-based practice, complete a review of literature for one clinical question pertinent to the case.

References

Adler, P. A., & Adler, P. (1998). Observational techniques. In N. Denzin & Y. Lincoln (Eds.), *Collecting and interpreting qualitative materials* (pp. 79–109). Thousand Oaks, CA: Sage Publications.

Bogdewic, S. (1999). Participant observation. In B. Crabtree & W. Miller (Eds.), *Doing qualitative research* (pp. 47–69). Thousand Oaks, CA: Sage Publications.

Frattali, C. M. (1998). *Measuring outcomes in speech-language pathology.* New York: Thieme.

Tickle-Degnen, L. (1999). Organizing, evaluating, and using evidence in occupational therapy practice. *American Journal of Occupational Therapy, 53,* 537–539.

Tickle-Degnen, L. (2000). Gathering current research evidence to enhance clinical reasoning. *American Journal of Occupational Therapy, 54,* 102–105.

Accuracy: The Art of Great Therapy

Accuracy and Intervention Power

Therapist Design Skill

Collaborative Occupational Goal Generation

Precision Fit of Intervention to Goal

How Great a Therapist Will You Be?

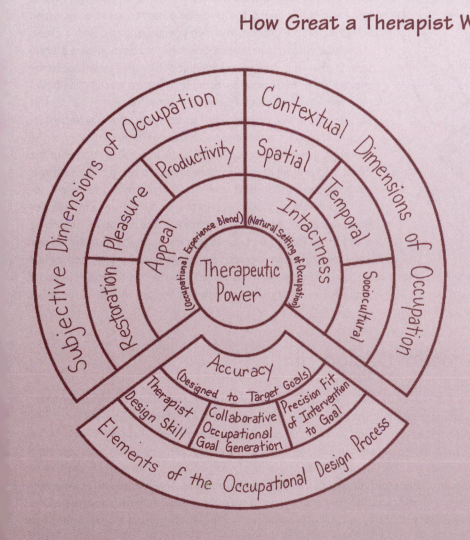

Accuracy and Intervention Power

Accuracy is an ideal value concerning occupation-based practice. In a sense, great therapy is a dream we pursue each time we step into an interaction with a client. We dream that the session will be so perfect it will make significant changes in the exact area of the client's life with which he or she is most concerned. Even small changes, if they are accurately targeted, will advance that person's quality of life—and you will have the satisfaction of having done great therapy that day.

It is a joy to experience highly accurate intervention sessions. Unfortunately, occupation-based intervention is such a complex art that perfect sessions are rare. So many things can happen: the client or the therapist is distracted, the environment is disruptive, judgment or energy fails, the goals desired by the client are unclear, or the therapist's creativity is limited. This is the reality of designing occupational experiences to facilitate change in human beings. It is like hitting a moving target with a melting ball of ice cream—possible, but not probable. Still, even if a session is imperfect, it often results in important changes. You aim for the stars, but you reach the moon. In moving toward the goal, you see better how to move toward the goal. Do not worry about providing perfectly accurate interventions each time. It will be more productive, instead, to envision accurate interventions, to understand how to achieve them, and to reflect on the process in which you are engaged with a client.

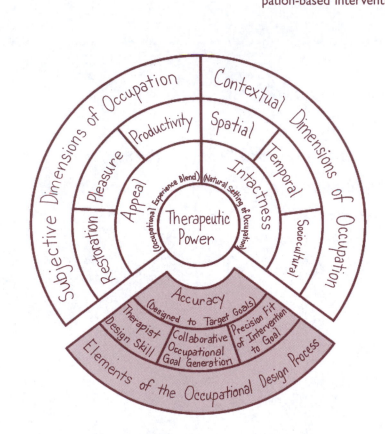

Little research has been done on occupation-based practice. In the next few years, I expect that studies will describe more clearly how best to provide effective occupation-based intervention. Until then, I have attempted to sketch out in this section of the book what seem to be some of the primary factors that support intervention accuracy: the design skills of the therapist, generating occupational goals in collaboration with the client, and precise fit of the intervention to the goal. Since this is relatively new theoretical territory for the field, I have grounded consideration of accuracy in the study of Amy and Helene's experiences at the IALC. I have kept the chapters describing these three factors fairly brief. It is my hope that the limited discussion of effective occupation-based practice provided in this book will incite more research in this area and that discourse on this topic will become richer with time. Here is a quick review of the three primary factors that produce intervention accuracy.

Therapist Design Skill

To meet the demands for practice ideas that accurately and effectively address client goals, occupational therapists must be highly skilled creative thinkers. This requires self-development because all of us have different strengths and weaknesses in the seven phases of the design process. In Chapter 2, the basic phases of design are described along with strategies that can be used in each phase of any project. In Chapter 14, the use of design process in intervention is more specifically discussed. The first phase of intervention design is motivation, in which the therapist identifies his or her own sources of the energy necessary to carry through to completion. The second phase is investigation, in which the therapist gathers and examines information to expand his or her insight into the challenge being addressed. The definition phase is critical to the success of any effort because it helps the therapist to clarify the intent of the design process. Ideation, the most commonly understood phase, develops a wide range of ideas from which to choose. Idea selection uses specific criteria to make that choice. Implementation is the planning and carrying out of the selected idea. The evaluation phase, often neglected, is consideration of the process and outcomes of the project. Therapists depend heavily on skills in all design phases. We must be better-skilled designers than to depend simply on the skills that we happen to have from life experience. To facilitate desired changes in a client's goal area through the design of occupation-based intervention is much more demanding than the creative challenges of everyday life. It is time that occupational therapists become accountable for their creative skills. Do you know where your strengths lie? Do you have plans for the areas in your design skills that need further development?

Collaborative Occupational Goal Generation

Accurate intervention cannot be accomplished unless a strong process of collaborative goal setting with the client is used. Goals must target change in the client's occupations. No matter how skilled the therapist is in other areas, if he or she does not have adequate access to the client's priorities regarding the desired outcomes of intervention, the occupational therapy provided will miss the mark.

To assist the therapist in collaborative goal setting, several specific abilities are helpful. The therapist should take an open, egalitarian, consumer-oriented approach to interactions with the client. This will help the client to see that the therapist truly wishes to give him or her control of the goals of intervention. Interviewing skills are critical to drawing out and understanding the client's story and hopes for the future. Specific methods of goal setting and new top-down assessments also support collaboration with the client. For most therapists today, the new emphasis on collaborative goal setting is a shift from the more traditional approach, in which the therapist's expert judgment qualifies him or her to set the goals for the client. Few therapists are without needs for development in the skills of collaborative goal setting.

Precision Fit of Intervention to Goal

To design interventions that not only are occupation-based but also precisely target goals requires a master therapist. To develop such mastery, occupational therapists would be well served to develop in the following areas. Expertise with populations and diagnoses with which the therapist frequently works is an obvious choice for self-development. Strong observation skills can enhance the therapist's ability to gain insight into clients' perspectives and the settings in which he or she works with them. Intervention can be more accurately targeted if the therapist has a good grasp of the varied potential strategies through which to work on client goals—through changes in the client or changes in environments. Continually reconfiguring client goals as the client's perspective on intervention changes will increase accuracy by keeping the intervention carefully focused on the direction desired by the client. Evidence-based practice methods can assist the therapist in using outcomes research to produce more significant effects of intervention. Finally, using in intervention those occupations that clients have targeted as goals will usually assist in increasing the precise fit of the intervention to the goals desired by the client.

How Great a Therapist Will You Be?

What kind of therapist are you now? What kind of therapist will you be in the future? Will you seek to continually improve your abilities to provide highly accurate intervention or will you try to slide by with the minimum in passable services? Are you ready to tackle the complexity of occupation-based practice, or will you be tempted into simpler approaches by productivity pressures and more traditional practitioners?

In this section of the book, I have provided you with an example of occupation-based practice and brief chapters on therapist design skills, collaborative goal setting, and precision fit of intervention to goal. To what do you aspire in the therapeutic skills described here? Will you choose one that seems important to you and try to practice it? Will you pass these ideas by as "just theory" and practice unprepared in these areas? Or will you aspire to master them all, to be the type of therapist who experiences the joy of accurately targeted and effective interventions on a daily basis? These choices are certainly yours. They will be your choices every day that you practice. No one else will take responsibility for deciding what kind of therapist you will be. The intervention power that you will carry into a session is completely up to you.

Key Concepts for Strengthening Insight into Designing for Accuracy

- Envisioning highly accurate intervention
- Your personal strengths and needs for increased skill across the seven phases of design of therapeutic occupation
- Your commitment to collaborative goal setting
- Strategies for increasing intervention precision
- What kind of therapist will you choose to be?

1. Select a case from Appendix A. Envision highly successful outcomes of occupational therapy for this individual. Write a two-page fictitious reflection on your feelings of accomplishment in helping this client reach his or her goals. Include design challenges you overcame, the client's perspective on goals, and strategies you used successfully to increase precision.

2. Create a fictitious evaluation phase reflection on a highly successful case in your preferred area of practice.

3. Select a case from Appendix A. Describe a fictitious experience you had treating this client when you struggled through the design phase in which you are the least strong.

4. Select a case from Appendix A. Briefly describe each of seven design phases and what occurred within each of them in providing intervention for this client.

5. Use a design process to create a personal development plan to improve your ability to provide accurate intervention. The plan should address a minimum of three skill areas and should be feasible to accomplish while working or studying fulltime. Document your design process in a dated journal format that includes reflection on each phase and all exercises used in the process, from motivation through idea selection.

6. Select one of the skills areas from the previous exercise. Complete the design process for this skill area, including implementation and evaluation. Document your design process in a dated journal format that includes reflection on each phase and all exercises used.

7. Observe an occupational therapist treating a client. Select a design phase you believe would make the greatest contribution to the accuracy of intervention with this client if it were to be completed. Complete the phase, documenting your actions through a reflective note that includes all exercises. Provide the outcome of your work to the therapist if appropriate.

8. Observe an occupational therapist providing intervention in a setting that serves many clients with similar diagnoses. Complete a design process to design a small, additional occupational therapy program or service for this setting, from the motivation phase through the planning portion of the implementation phase. Document your process through a reflective note summarizing each phase. Include all exercises. Provide the outcome of your work to the therapist if appropriate.

POWER BUILDERS

9. Select a case from Appendix A. Write a fictitious script of the interaction between yourself and the client as you work to set collaborative goals. Will you use a structured assessment for setting goals, or a semi-structured interview? Include any documentation completed during the interview.

10. Select a case from Appendix A in which the description includes goals or some description of intervention. Write a brief written analysis of the degree to which the goals of this case appear to have been collaboratively created.

11. Imagine you are providing intervention in an occupational therapy setting that does not use collaborative occupational goal setting. Brainstorm 40 ways in which you might be able to successfully bring collaborative occupational goal setting into this setting. Select the best three ideas according to five weighted criteria.

12. Practice your client-interviewing skills. Role-play one of the cases, with a partner taking the part of the client.

13. Practice your client-interviewing skills. Interview someone who has a decision to make, helping that person to decide, without deciding for him or her.

14. Practice your client-interviewing skills. Administer one of the following assessments, with a partner playing the part of a client from Appendix A: Comprehensive Occupational Performance Measure, Kielhofner Occupational History Revised, or Life Pattern Review.

15. Use a design process to develop a plan to increase your expertise in an area of practice in which you are particularly interested, beginning with the motivation phase and continuing through the planning portion of the implementation phase. Keep the plan within the limits of what you could accomplish while working or studying fulltime. Document your design process in a dated journal format that includes reflection on each phase and all exercises used in the process.

16. Complete the design process described in the previous exercise, through the evaluation phase.

17. Practice your observation skills by observing a client receiving occupational therapy. Use an observation guide that includes the subjective and contextual aspects of the client's occupational experience, the intactness and appeal of the intervention, and any indications of the design skills of the therapist, collaborative occupational goal setting, or precision fit of intervention to goals. Make thorough notes.

18. After completing the previous exercise, write a brief summary of your notes.

19. Following an observation of a client receiving occupational therapy (as in exercise 17), record observation notes on audiotape. Transcribe your notes. Write a brief summary.

20. Complete an evidence-based practice review in an area of practice of interest to you.

21. Select a case from Appendix A. If no goals are included in the case, create one. Create a brief written description of an intervention for this case that uses the ends of therapy as the means.

Conclusion

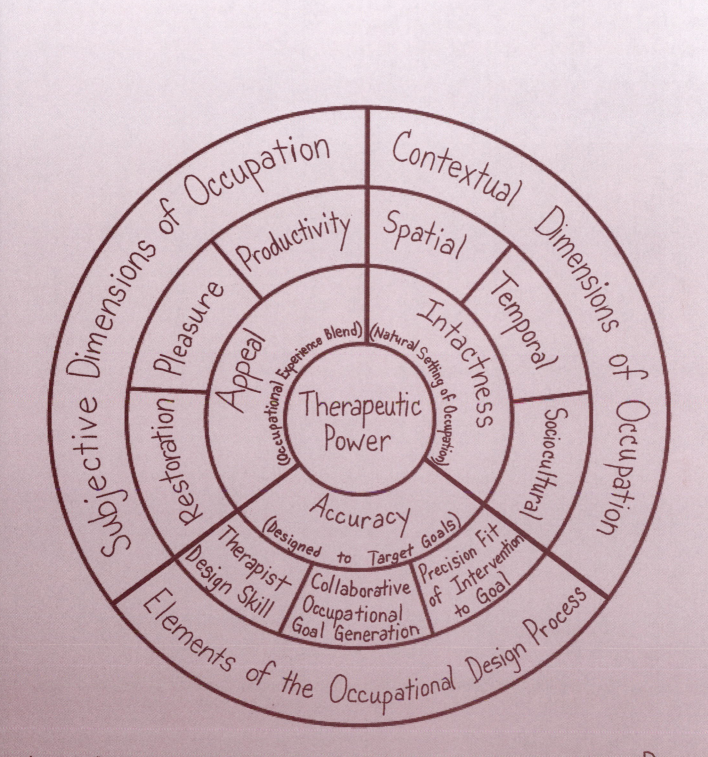

Appeal + Intactness + Accuracy = Therapeutic Power

You Are What You Do

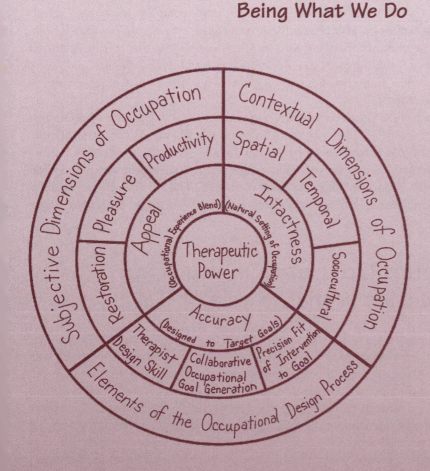

You are what you do.

Occupational therapy has a tiger by the tail. Occupation. Doing. What concept could be more powerful, more central to human life than this? What we do expresses who we are, grounds us in our humanness, demonstrates our desires and hopes, our thoughts and dreams, our values, and what we would change about the world around us. Occupation is such a powerful concept that it is like a tiger whose tail lashes with such natural energy that we are barely able to retain it in our grasp.

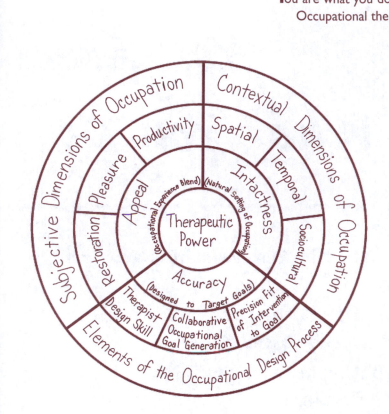

In occupational science and occupational therapy, we are just beginning to understand occupation in a way sophisticated enough to support strong practice. We are a young profession and an even younger discipline. As individual occupational therapists seeking to improve our understanding of occupation, we must take three critical paths. First we must appreciate and learn to shape the subjective and contextual dimensions of occupation in our own lives. Then we must build skills for discerning occupation as it is experienced within these dimensions by others. And finally we must develop expertise in the design of accurate occupation-based interventions.

There is a bittersweetness to journeying down such challenging paths (Pierce, 2001a). We face limits within which we design the occupational patterns of our lives. Our access to the occupational experiences of others will always be imperfect. And though the application of occupation in practice is a powerful force for change, it is agonizingly complex. The master reveals himself within limits, however. It is our ability to therapeutically engage occupation within life limits that makes us master therapists. Persistence in aspiring to such greatness rewards us with incredible growth. Great practice transforms us as individuals, and we are privileged to witness transformations in the lives of our clients as we serve them as agents of those changes.

You have many choices ahead of you. Will you use your understanding of occupation to design your own life? Will you gain the skills to see deeply into the occupational experiences of others? Will you remain committed to becoming a master of occupation-based practice, or succumb to pressures to reduce your practice to a focus on components? Making those choices, you will become what you do. You will become the occupational being and the occupational therapist you produce through your own occupational design process.

Celebrating Occupation in Your Own Life: Dancing in the Stream of Time

Every day we construct a new occupational pattern by making choices: to do one thing instead of another, to do something now instead of later, to try a new activity, to stay with the routine, to change the setting where something is done, to experiment with the pattern or to bring the pattern back into its usual form. You are, right now, an evolving occupational therapist, reading and developing yourself in your understanding of occupation. You are this *doing,* in this moment, the meaning of which within the unique pattern of your life only you can truly know.

You are this occupation you are having now, this experience, this series of thoughts that will unfold in various ways, this commitment, and this desire. You have come down this road, and not another one. You are in this moment, this experience, this growth, this time and place, this set of potentials. And so, moment to moment, we build a life. Some of those moments are exquisitely beautiful, and some are dull, and some are excruciating, and some are wasted, and some are ho-hum, and some are turning points—although we didn't even know it at the time.

The Occupational Pattern That Is You

Over a lifetime, the accumulation of these choices, these moment-to-moment experiences chosen over other experiences, these occupations, create a distinct pattern that can only be you. Think of the choices you have made, the pattern you are weaving with your occupations. This life pattern of yours has a tempo, a music, a beat, colors, partners, movement, shape, tradition, an aesthetic that expresses only you. More than anything you could write or say, this occupational pattern, this moment-to-moment set of movements and choices about doing, express who you are in your life. This is your dance, your dance of self in the world, your dance of doing and being. Your dance of occupation in the stream of time. What pattern could be more beautiful to you, more intriguing, more closely fitted to your own aesthetic, than the pattern of this dance of your own life? Over a week, a month, a year, these daily occupational patterns build to a larger motif that shows who you are, where you are headed, your talents and your challenges. You are what you do.

Each of us creates and lives out a life design so complex that it is best understood only by ourselves. If we are effective in creating the pattern we desire, the design will include the balance of pleasure, restoration, and productivity that is important to us. We experience our occupations in all their spatial, temporal, and sociocultural contexts, though at times we are unaware of their effects. This is the human condition, the human's occupational nature, to be constantly engaged in the experience of doing, from the simple physiological rest of sleep to the focused productivity of work. In the way that a highly trained dancer understands his or her own performances or an orchestra conductor appreciates the music as it flows from his or her orchestra, an occupational therapist well versed in occupational design process understands the patterns of his or her own life as a master appreciates a masterwork.

Dancing Within Limits

We dance, however, within limits. The occupational choices we make, this life dance in which each of us is engaged, is not completely free. This is also the human condition. We do not have endless resources, limitless spaces, or all the time in the world. This pattern we create with our doing occurs within the constraints of each of our lives.

The greatest limit to our occupational pattern, of course, is our own mortality. Regardless of your beliefs regarding an afterlife, our time here in this life is limited. Even more difficult, we cannot know its endpoint. So this pattern we weave, this dance we do, is done within an imagined timeframe, from beginning to end. We dance within the limits of time. Shall we do this, or shall we do that, and what shall we do by the end? Time will run out. The dance will be done. The pattern will be woven, and then set aside. Its beauty, its flaws, its colors, and its movements will all have been made, and the pattern will be done.

We dance too within the limits of skill and talent, and wealth and poverty, and luck and loss, and love and loss, and health and illness, and youth and age. Some dance lightly around the barriers. Others are stopped in their tracks. Life is what you make of it. The exquisite beauty of the occupational pattern is not revealed in how lucky, wealthy, loved, or fun our lives may be. The real beauty of the occupational pattern is in the way we dance our dance within the limits of the space and music we are afforded. We are all gifted with different opportunities, different limits. It is what we make of the materials with which we are presented that reveals the most gifted occupational beings among us and the most beautifully sculpted occupational patterns.

The Master Reveals Himself within Limits

In Alaska, I studied with a potter who had been stationed on a remote island for 6 months over winter, to work in a small school. He had only the native clay and a few bags of chemicals with which to work. No glazes, no colors but what could be found. The ware he created was some of the most beautiful I have ever seen: a dark red clay body covered with a thick glossy white slip, used in a variety of elegant and functional forms. Understanding clay and glazes as he did, and within great limitations, he created great beauty.

The master reveals himself within limits. So it is in our own lives. Presented with limits, does our pattern become more spare, more elegant, more revealing of the character of the dancer who is dancing out these life choices? Does the pattern flow smoothly through change and adaptation to limits, playing and experimenting with how far they can be pushed and what new shapes and lessons they might hold? Or does the pattern become snarled around barriers, stuck in resistance to change, bitter and unmoving, sad and yearning for the dance pattern of earlier days that cannot ever be reclaimed?

The quote in the left margin is from an elderly Kentucky woman, commenting on changes in her involvement in preparing the annual Christmas meal. Those are the words of a master.

> *Well I think it's a wise older person who realizes that things are going to change, because of your physical... ah maybe disabilities or whatever you want to call it and then I think you're wise to realize and accept those things, and work it out as best you can, so that you're still happy with it. That you can enjoy it and not make everybody else have a hard time cause you think you are having one, and I think that is about where I am ([Participant], Nicholas, Pierce, & Shordike, 2001).*

The Bittersweetness of Designing Your Own Occupational Patterns

We are what we do. The bittersweetness of our own occupational pattern is in the limits in which we must dance the best dance that we can create. You can apply your newly developed design skills and appreciation of the dimensions of occupation to your own life: to attain your goals, enrich your daily experiences, and develop new creative directions. In this book, you have completed a study of occupation and design process that is unique in occupational therapy. Will you put this new understanding to work as you create a life for yourself? If you do, you will shape your own life with the appreciation of an artist, and thus you will more consciously shape who you become.

Celebrating Occupation in the Lives of Others: The Limitations of Access to the Other

Understanding the occupations of others can only come through the knowledge that they, and not we, are the authors of their occupational experiences. Whether we are concerned with the lives of our clients, our colleagues, our family, or our friends, it is all the same challenge. We can only understand the occupations of others imperfectly, from the outside of the dance, as observers. If we wish to understand better, we must become very skilled at methods to gain access to the perspective of others. Such methods include empathy, reflection, interview, observation, and rigorous qualitative inquiry.

The Bittersweet Limitations of Access to the Occupations of Others

Clients are the authors of their lives. Clients have the occupational experiences on which we focus in therapy, not the therapists. Our access to their experiences is necessarily imperfect. As people, we think we can know through common sense what is happening with others around us. Surely, our lives and theirs have some parallels. Surely, many of our guesses about what they are experiencing and what it means to them within their larger dance are fairly accurate. But as occupational therapists, as occupational scientists, we must ask more of ourselves than the skills and accuracy of commonsense thinking about occupation.

If you are in some public place now, or the next time you are, just look at the person next to you. Although you might appear to be doing something similar, does that person really understand the experience you are having? Could he or she celebrate what it may mean to you to be here, to be at this time in your life? How well does that individual access your occupation, understand your experience? Can anyone know without asking you?

When we assume we understand the dance we see someone dancing, or the occupation in which we see a person engaged, we cross a dangerous line. Assuming we understand that person's experience, we step away from the potential for real insight into his or her experience and toward the power dynamic of being an "expert" who knows more about the person's experiences than he or she does. People are the authors of their lives, of their occupational experiences. If we do not go cautiously, grounded in carefully crafted methods for gaining access to the perspectives of others, we run the risk, not only of arrogance, but also of failing to obtain the understanding of them that we seek.

We are occupational therapists. Of all these dancers in the world, we have studied the dance of occupation to the greatest degree. We recognize play, work, self-care, rest, adaptation, development, disruption, delay, trauma, narrative, hope, goals, and plans in occupation. In our insight into occupation, we are to other occupational beings as trained dancers are to untrained dancers. But, if we do not proceed with humility, if we do not embrace the bittersweet limitations of access to another's occupational experiences, we will be only clumsy commonsense guessers. To be true connoisseurs of occupation, we must struggle honestly with these limits on our understanding of the occupations of another person.

The Lessons

If we can, with humility and rigor, begin to access and celebrate the occupational experiences, patterns, and insights of others, we will be well rewarded. We could begin to understand, for example, what I call "folk OT." Folk medicine includes traditions for health and illness commonly used by people who are not trained physicians. For example, the Hispanic mothers with whom I worked in Los Angeles would use chamomile tea to sooth an infant's upset stomach. And it worked. That is folk medicine. Folk OT is the common use of occupation to affect health and wellness by people who are not occupational therapists. Maybe you are tired and burned out, so you take a bubble bath. You feel sluggish, you go for a jog. A child is tired and cranky, a parent suggests a story, and the child falls asleep listening. We can learn much in the way everyday people use occupations in therapeutic ways.

If we listened hard enough, we could begin to understand resilience, the ability to pass through difficult life events with limited negative effects. We could study post-traumatic growth: the way in which, following difficult losses such as divorce, death, or trauma, we often experience a spurt of personal growth. I have seen this in my clients. Have you seen this in people you have known? Isn't it amazing when it happens?

Many lessons await us in the occupational patterns of others. By using careful methods to overcome the natural limits on our access to others' experiences, we could begin to understand what it means to live well within the limits of disability by studying those who do. How is it that some people with disabilities successfully craft new, satisfying life patterns, while others are stuck in dissatisfaction or caught in the syndrome of constantly striving to prove ability?

Will You Cultivate Access to the Occupational Experiences of Others?

Accepting the bittersweet limits of our imperfect access to the occupational experiences of others and using appropriate methods to overcome those limits can provide us with much to celebrate. Will you, in your life and in your practice, cultivate this humble openness to seeing through the eyes of others? Will you spend time in reflection, observation, listening? There is much to be discovered in the lives of others, especially those for whom we care so much, or for whom we are the providers of care.

Celebrating Occupation in Practice: Power, Complexity, and Popularity

Providing effective occupational therapy to your clients requires a masterful appreciation of occupation and developed skills of creative design. Whether you are a new student or a highly experienced practitioner, you must have a more reflective, informed, and artful insight into your own occupational pattern than do those who are not occupational therapists. If you do not have a sophisticated grasp of your own occupational experiences, to which you have such ready access, how can you ever assume to understand the occupations of others? To apply occupation as a therapeutic modality requires a level of discernment and design skill far beyond the usual perceptions that individuals have of their daily lives.

The Therapeutic Power of Occupation

Sometimes, when I am working with occupational therapists on their understanding of occupation, they say to me how hard it is to explain the importance of their practice because occupation and activity are so "common sense." Yes, it is true. Occupation is so pervasive, so much a central fact in our everyday lives, that it seems everyone must easily understand it. But do they really? No. All the time, we see people who have a difficult time organizing a day or a life that is satisfying to them. Sure, it may be common sense to have a superficial grasp of activity and experience in human life. Most adults understand how to get a simple meal together or get dressed. But can they help someone to do that same activity in such a way as to regain skills, reconstruct a shattered identity, or overcome cognitive or physical limitations? Probably not. Using occupation as therapy is far beyond common sense.

In the hands of a master clinician, occupation can be powerfully therapeutic. I have experienced those wonderful sessions when everything just clicked. The goals were clear, the activity valued by the client, the progress was rewarding for both the therapist and the patient. I left the session feeling excited, energized, wanting to tell another therapist all about it. In this book, I have theorized that these great sessions come from three factors: appeal, intactness, and accuracy. Appeal is the degree to which the activity used is attractive to the client, in terms of its blend of productivity, pleasure, and restoration. Intactness is the degree to which the session occurs in the usual time, place, and socio-cultural conditions in which that activity would appear in that client's life if it were not being used as therapy. Accuracy is the degree to which the therapist's design skills, collaborative goal generation, and precise fit of activity to goal produced an intervention that was well centered on the needs of the client.

The Bittersweet Complexity of Great Practice

Of course, the bittersweet aspect of these occupation-based interventions is that they are agonizingly complex to pull off! In many ways, understanding great occupation-based practice is understanding the ideals for which we aim more than the realities that we experience in every session. The moral contracts we honor with employers and with reimbursers for levels of productivity and service within coverage can be in conflict with the moral contract with our clients to provide the best possible intervention. The client's frustrations with negotiating life challenges and changes can derail motivation to work in occupational therapy.

The context in which treatment is provided can seem artificial and poorly fitted to what needs to be addressed. Collaboration can be difficult because of family dynamics, patient passivity, or cognitive impairment. The demands for creative solutions to complicated problems are never-ending, leading to burnout and reliance on protocols. Time to reflect on and improve interventions is scarce and sorely needed. Working within all these limits does indeed sort the masters from the novices among us. That is as it should be. To keep in mind these ideals despite difficulties is indeed an experience in the bittersweet satisfactions of great occupation-based practice.

The Bittersweetness of Sudden Popularity

Another factor making our intervention experiences bittersweet is our sudden popularity, or rather, the sudden popularity of occupation, function, and quality-of-life outcomes (Molineux, 2001). After 100 years of occupational therapy carrying this banner of the importance of function, we find that, given the mandates of insurers, many fields have suddenly found that function is exactly what they have been after all along. Work, play, and school outcomes are now important to everyone. The patient's perspective on outcomes is everyone's concern. The World Health Organization is putting the finishing touches on a new classification for studying cross-national differences in health outcomes that use the terms activity, participation, and context. For occupational therapists, rooted in a field long concerned with the study and application of such concepts, the sudden discovery of our key concepts by other fields is unnerving.

This sudden popularity is, indeed, bittersweet. There is nothing to be done for it, however, except to celebrate. The only option for the field of occupational therapy is to move out of the shadows, into the limelight, and dance. We have reached what we always said we wished for, to have care systems recognize the importance of daily function in the provision of services. The time for a focus on occupation and doing is here and now. You had better be able to address function better than anyone else if you wish to remain on the team. Occupational therapists certainly can do this, and do this better than anyone else, when they stay true to their core concern with occupation.

How Will You Practice?

What kind of therapist will you be? Will you cultivate an understanding of the dimensions of your own occupations? Will you consider carefully how best to access the occupational experiences of those for whom you care? Will you strive for creative occupation-based practice even when tempted by simpler protocols and component-focused intervention? As I have said elsewhere, three things will be required to defend our disciplinary concepts and unique professional potentials for clients (Pierce, 2001b).

We must be able to talk the talk of occupation. That is, we must ground our practice in sophisticated theory and research. We must transcend commonsense understandings of daily activity. We must immerse ourselves in our own knowledge base and know it. The talk in our heads during treatment must be this talk. This is an exciting time, in which this knowledge base is going through explosive growth.

We must be able to walk the walk of occupation-based practice. We must commit to providing effective occupation-based interventions and to making them work for clients despite a litany of interfering factors.

And finally, we must be able to talk the talk of occupation-based practice. We must be able to understand its concepts, apply them well and then explain them clearly to others, if we are going to keep them as our unique offering as a field. We must be so grounded in this approach that we can tailor to different audiences explanations of what we are doing, why it works, and what research supports these assertions, and all this while our hands are probably busy elsewhere.

Being What We Do

In this book, I have done my best to describe occupation in its many dimensions, to make acquisition of the skills of creative design both possible and enjoyable, and to provide some insight into how occupational therapists design effective therapeutic occupations. It has been a long and passionate project. I must admit that I am glad to bring its writing to an end so that the book can be used and I can turn to newer and more data-based projects. This has been the longest design project I have ever attempted, unless I were to count the ongoing design processes of creating my own life or parenting a child. Throughout this whole project, I have been fueled by energy rooted in my great respect for, and enjoyment of, occupational therapists and occupational therapy students. They are special people: creative, caring, intelligent, empathic, playful, and humanistic. I am fascinated by seeing occupational therapists become what they do.

The emergence of the discipline of occupational science, and the surge of research on occupation and occupation-based practice that has accompanied it, mark a new era in occupational therapy. Our practice is changing rapidly. We are on our way to becoming a mature profession, with a sophisticated knowledge base and increasingly powerful contributions to society. The future is full of wonderful challenges. Many people will need help in reclaiming or creating occupational patterns within which they can thrive, reach goals, and express the selves that they desire. Occupational therapists will be there, with interventions stronger than ever.

It is a privilege to work with our clients as they experience their struggles and life transformations. They trust us with their feelings and process; share with us their barriers and realizations in designing new occupational patterns. Like the patient who experiences post-traumatic growth when required to undergo a life reorganization, we too, as therapists, can experience much personal growth through our practice if we accept the challenge to do great intervention and to celebrate it. Seeing and operating within the changing dance of the occupational patterns of our clients will give us grace in many different dances. Finding effective access to the true perspectives that our clients have on their lives will increase our insight into our loved ones and others during both joyful and troubled times. Remaining true to our unique disciplinary concepts, despite their complexity and demand on us, will push us toward growth. This growth can be called wisdom, and for that we are truly blessed.

As we seek success in our practice, we learn to dance a new dance with greater grace, making higher leaps, reaping new insights, and even at times, keeping greater faith in what the human spirit can attain. We learn to reconcile the bittersweetness of it all: of life within the limits of mortality and luck, of the difficulty of understanding one another, of the agonizing complexity and unnerving popularity of occupation-based practice. Pushed so far, asked so much of, we grow as dancers, as practitioners, as living beings of our own occupational patterns within limits. It is indeed a beautiful and bittersweet dance. What will you be? You will be what you do—a great designer of therapeutic occupations.

References

Molineux, M. (2001). Occupation: The two sides of popularity. *Australian Occupational Therapy Journal, 48,* 92–95.

[Participant], Nicholas, A., Pierce, D., & Shordike, A. (2001). [*The experience of holiday food preparation in older women of Kentucky*]. Unpublished raw data.

Pierce, D. (2001a). *The bittersweet celebration of occupation in practice.* Keynote, Kentucky Occupational Therapy Association, Richmond, KY.

Pierce, D. (2001b). Occupation by design: Dimensions, creativity, and therapeutic power. *American Journal of Occupational Therapy, 55,* 249–259.

Case Studies

	CLIENT	REPORTING THERAPIST
Case A-1	Mabel	Katy Allen
Case A-2	David	Ashlyn Richardson Cunningham
Case A-3	Mary	Thom Fisher
Case A-4	James	Thom Fisher
Case A-5	Sam	Kathleen Flecky
Case A-6	Tina	Yolanda Griffiths
Case A-7	Bill	Carolyn Hall
Case A-8	Grace	Dana Howell
Case A-9	Jacob	Judy Janson
Case A-10	Mr. McMasters	Scott Johnson
Case A-11	Jeremiah	Jeffery Jones
Case A-12	Alice	Amy Kratz
Case A-13	John	Matthew J. Kraus
Case A-14	Mr. Lowenstein	Curtis Quinn Marti
Case A-15	Alta	Teddy R. Rudder
Case A-16	Donald	Kris Seidner
Case A-17	Lou	Cheryl L. Stewart
Case A-18	Tara	Christy Walloch
Case A-19	Barb	Mary Way

Case A-1 Mabel

Katy Allen

Mrs. Zahn is a well-nourished 85-year-old woman, approximately 5'5" tall and weighing 140 pounds, with the diagnosis of major depressive disorder. She is independent in ambulating. Mrs. Zahn is cooperative but shows little affect. It is obvious she is attuned to her home environment and the people in it. For example, if a topic came up that her sister has told her not to talk about, she would "press her lips" together to indicate she should not talk about it.

Medical History: Mrs. Zahn was initially diagnosed with depression in her mid-twenties at which time she was hospitalized and received electroconvulsive therapy. She has a history of some alcohol abuse throughout her life. Her family feels this was her method of self-medicating for subsequent, but less intense, periods of depression. The county mental health department saw her off and on for several years. Her primary caregiver, one of her sisters, was not cooperative with the agency staff. During the year preceding her recent major depressive episode and hospitalization, her family physician had been treating her for depression. Again, her sister did not carry out the medication routine as prescribed. Mrs. Zahn was found by a niece on the floor of her home in a fetal position. The two sisters living with her at the time reported that she had been acting like this for a while. Mrs. Zahn had been the primary caregiver to these two sisters, who suffered from chronic obstructive pulmonary disease and congestive heart failure.

Mrs. Zahn was hospitalized for approximately 3 weeks. She was diagnosed with Axis I – Major Depression – Recurrent and Axis II – Primary Neurological Dementia. She started a medication routine. She was discharged to her home with follow-up care to be carried out by the county mental heath agency, but her sister would not cooperate with the mental health providers. Approximately 1 month after returning home, Mrs. Zahn fell down a flight of stairs, not at her residence, and sustained a closed-head injury. She was hospitalized, had a craniotomy, and was then discharged to a subacute facility for rehabilitation. She was discharged home with only a few residual deficits, including slight word-finding problems, a visual impairment, and loss of hearing in her right ear.

Family Background: Mrs. Zahn is a widow and the mother of two sons. Both sons live in the same city but have been distant from their mother and each other for several years. Mrs. Zahn is the middle of seven children. Three sisters are alive. Two of the sisters have lived with Mrs. Zahn for several years, and she has provided both physical and financial support to both of them. She appeared to begin declining about the time of the death of her closest sister. One of Mrs. Zahn's nieces became her legal guardian with no resistance from either of her sons. Since that time, her niece has seen to the care of all three sisters in their home. Initially, this involved hiring a home aide to come in during the day to provide meals, self-care assistance, and light housekeeping. After 1 year, one of the sisters living with the client died and the other sister's physical condition worsened. In an attempt to keep them at home, a full-time live-in caregiver was hired. This person was a recent immigrant of Poland who did not speak English. She was employed to provide care to both sisters and maintain the home. She was instructed in Mrs. Zahn's medication routine and encouraged to allow Mrs. Zahn to engage in caring for her sister and home.

Work History: During her adulthood, Mrs. Zahn owned and operated a rooming house for male students from the local university. She later owned and operated rental property and worked part time as a housewares salesperson in a local department store until her early seventies.

Assessment: Mrs. Zahn scores at a 3.2 cognitive level on the Allen Cognitive Level Screening. These are the only formal assessment data available. Other information is from direct observation and family/caregiver report.

Presenting Problems: Cognition. Mrs. Zahn can follow one- or two-step directions. During dressing, for example, frequent cueing is required for her to initiate and sustain the activity until completion. Once an activity is initiated, Mrs. Zahn can perform simple routine activities such as drying dishes. In order to put dishes away, occasional cueing is required to sustain the activity and correctly place items.

Communication: Mrs. Zahn has adequate communication skills both receptive and expressive, but she rarely initiates conversations.

Feeding/Eating: Mrs. Zahn has a good appetite but poor feeding/eating skills. For example, she places more food in her mouth before she has swallowed what is already there. She frequently uses her fingers rather than utensils. Her family reports that feeding etiquette had not been a strength prior to this but has gotten worse.

Rest: Mrs. Zahn has "sundowning" problems. That is, her agitation increases throughout the day and by midafternoon is at its worst. The psychiatric nurse encouraged Mrs. Zahn's caregivers to provide her an opportunity for a nap in the early afternoon to help decrease the agitation. Family members report that Mrs. Zahn has a history of poor sleep patterns such as difficulty falling asleep and waking feeling groggy. Providing a nap is difficult because her sleeping area is in the living room with her sister and has been for several years. In addition, her sister feels that if Mrs. Zahn naps then she will not sleep as well at night.

Goal: Mrs. Zahn's family's goal is to maintain her in her home and provide her with opportunities to perform her regular routine as independently as possible.

Case A-2 David

Ashlyn Richardson Cunningham

David is a 12-year-old boy who is in the seventh grade at a local middle school. He lives with his parents and 13-year-old sister in a two-story home in a semi-urban area. David also has an older brother, who is living away from home finishing his first year of college.

David attends school daily and is enrolled in seven classes. He receives primarily A's and B's and has a strong interest in science and social studies. The subject in which he needs the most improvement is language arts (English). David is vice president of student council and regularly attends council meetings after school. He also engages in Boy Scouts as an extracurricular activity where he currently holds the position as the troop's historian. In addition, David has current interests in collecting cards, playing Game Boy and Playstation, and reading *Harry Potter* books.

David has Becker and Duchenne muscular dystrophies (MD). He was first diagnosed with Becker MD when he was almost 4 years old. His mother described his initial/early symptoms as "falling a lot" and "not catching himself," which resulted in several hematomas on his forehead and other areas. Currently, David's parents have noticed his physician writing "Duchenne" MD on David's medical records, but they have not actually been told that David has Duchenne and no testing has been completed to verify this diagnosis. David's parents are withholding this information from David at this time, stating that they wish to protect him from knowing that he has DMD, which has a very short life expectancy.

David was ambulatory until the fifth grade. At that time, he fell and severely sprained his right foot. He has been using a wheelchair since that time. Last fall, David received a new electric wheelchair to meet his growth needs. He uses his power wheelchair for mobility at home and school. The family has a van equipped with a lift for transportation purposes and David rides an accessible bus to and from school. David has an attendant who is with him at school at all times. This year however, he has not had a consistent person as his attendant, which has been potentially dangerous. Twice this year, David's substitute attendants have dropped him during a transfer. David receives no direct intervention services from related-services personnel (PT, OT, and SLP) at his school.

David's parents are very supportive. They complete the majority of his self-care tasks for him due to David's limited mobility. David can currently perform the following tasks as listed below:

- He is able to wash his face and comb his hair when someone brings the supplies to him.

- He can brush his teeth with setup as well. His mother thinks he is not brushing hard enough.

- The family's bathroom is not accessible. David's father must transfer him from the doorway of the bathroom to the claw-foot bathtub (they do not have a shower) or toilet. David is unable to assist in bathing.

- David is dependent in toileting and cannot assist in transfers. He uses a hand-held urinal, but cannot manage his clothing or position himself.

- David is also dependent on his parents for dressing tasks. He can manipulate buttons, but this takes a lot of time. He cannot don and doff his ankle-foot orthoses.

- David can feed himself if someone else sets things up and cuts his food. He has to lean to one side to feed himself, however, due to limited upper-extremity range of motion. David's parents are trying to monitor his caloric intake due to his high weight (he currently weighs 170 pounds).

Socially, David describes his relationships with others as "good most of the time." He fights with his sister over typical preteen issues. David's parents state that his sister is sometimes required to be the caregiver for David and she does not care for this responsibility, especially when she has to help with his toileting routine. David does not have many friends at school (he has acquaintances through student council and Boy Scouts). His typical peer group consists of his sister and a younger friend. David's parents note that it is difficult for David to go to other people's homes due to accessibility issues. They do, however, attend the muscular dystrophy support group as a family.

As stated earlier, David lives in a two-story home. His bedroom is on the first floor and has an adjoining bathroom. This bathroom is not wide enough for David to have access with his wheelchair. The fixtures are older and include a claw-foot tub that does not allow David to obtain a full long-sitting position. David's entry access into his home is through the front door, where his father has constructed a ramp. David cannot access the doorknob, though, and has to wait on the front porch after school if no one is at home. In addition, David has limited access to the telephone, computer, and other electronics in the home because of his decreased muscle function. These items usually have to be set up or turned on for David before he can use them.

David is usually fatigued by the end of the school day. Because of this, his parents do not require that he complete household chores. Frequently, David's sister is asked to complete chores, and this causes significant animosity towards David. However, David states that he likes to work because it gives him something to do. He has stated that he wants to be a computer-graphics artist when he grows up. He realizes that this would require a college degree and wants to continue his education. David's parents also wish for him to go to college.

Much of David's leisure participation is limited because of his decreased range of motion, strength, and endurance. David's father typically serves as his attendant when participating in leisure activities such as Boy Scouts. This is becoming somewhat frustrating for David because he wishes he could be more like other preteens, who are beginning to experience more independence from their families.

When David is asked what he would like to be able to do, he typically states one or all of the following:

- Play sports like the other guys
- Go to the local amusement parks and ride the rides
- Go hiking, rafting, and camping with his Boy Scout troop and stay in a regular tent
- Be free of his dependence on an assistant/attendant

David's parents have additional goals they would like addressed with David:

- Improve his mobility so that he can reposition himself in the middle of the night (instead of one of them having to get up and do it)
- Improve David's daily living activities, especially toileting procedures
- Improve access in and out of the home as well as allow him to be by himself more (addressing safety concerns)
- Increase his social interactions with peers his own age
- Appropriately address the emerging issues surrounding puberty
- Help David address transition plans in preparation for future vocational options

Case A-3 Mary

Thom Fisher

Mary is 69 years old and lives alone in Lexington, Kentucky. She is a short woman (5'4") weighing approximately 130 pounds. She is serious in nature but does show a sense of humor. Typically she wears slacks and loose-fitting tops. She has had multiple sclerosis for the past 12 years with a significant decline in functioning during the past 2 years. This resulted in her need to stop driving, grocery shopping, and cleaning her home. Mary has been divorced for 20 years. She has one daughter and two grandsons who live in Louisville, Kentucky. Lexington to Louisville is approximately 75 miles.

Mary was employed with the telephone company in a clerical capacity for more than 30 years. She chose to retire at age 60 because of her fatigue and ability to retire with full benefits. There are no cognitive deficits.

Mary has a fixed income from her retirement and social security. She is a Medicare recipient and has a Medicare supplement for her healthcare needs.

Her home is a small one-story, three-bedroom ranch, approximately 1400 square feet. The home also has one and a half bathrooms, kitchen, and living room. The washer and dryer are kept in a small utility room. Three steps lead up to the front door, and the back door from the kitchen has a wooden ramp with no handrail. Mary's trash barrel is at the bottom of the ramp. Rugs were scattered throughout the house the day of the initial evaluation.

Mary uses a cane in her right hand to get around her home while using her left hand to hold onto furniture, walls, and doorways. She ambulates with a wide-based gait because of balance problems. Mary uses a wheelchair for long distances. Her arms and hands are weak and frequently uncoordinated. She reports some problems with vision. During the initial evaluation, she shared with the occupational therapist the disruption in her life roles.

For the past 12 years Mary has been seeing a neurologist who encouraged her to attend a support group, which she found very helpful. According to Mary, attendance at these meetings is unrealistic because she does not drive. During her last physician visit, which was made because of an exacerbation (aggravation of symptoms), she described the difficulty she was having at home and her therapy evaluation and home assessment.

The occupational therapist's evaluation consisted of the Occupational Therapy Home Health Agency Evaluation and interview, the Canadian Occupational Performance Measure, and the Role Checklist, which identified the following:

Physical Limitations: Mary's left hand and both arms were seen to be weak as measured with the dynamometer/pinchometer and manual muscle testing. Mary is dependent on others for housework and grocery shopping. She requires moderate assistance in kitchen skills. She does have a short grab bar attached to the tub. During the evaluation, she shared that her eyes tire easily. Her leisure interests are limited to talking on the phone, watching television, and reading the newspaper. She reports that she did crocheting and sewing before her hands and eyes became impaired. Mary requires moderate to maximum assistance in homemaking activities because of left arm and hand weakness as well as poor coordination in both hands when she is carrying objects from one place to another. Mary reported that she had been dropping things more frequently.

Psychosocial Issues: Isolation from others. Episodes of depression.

Strengths: Mary desires to remain independent. She does have a supportive daughter, even though she is 75 miles away. Mary recognized the decline in her functioning. She does have a support system from her church. A small group of women visit every Sunday afternoon. She has been in the same neighborhood for 30 years. Mary accepts that she needs some adaptive equipment/assistive devices and recognized that home modifications are needed. Mary is articulate and extremely high functioning cognitively. She wants to adapt her home and her daily routine to cope with the progression of her condition. Mary is independent with her basic activities of daily living but concerned about instrumental activities of daily living, safety in the kitchen, and safety with tub transfers.

In the past, Mary engaged in a prayer group one evening a week before she lost energy for extra activities. She is aware of her limitations and strengths. She did attend a multiple sclerosis support group when she was driving. Her daughter visits weekly to do grocery shopping. Mary has a housekeeper who comes weekly for vacuuming, mopping, changing linens, dusting, and scouring bathrooms. Mary did not express awareness of energy-conservation principles or work-simplification techniques during the initial evaluation. She acknowledges episodes of depression but expresses the need to keep pushing forward. Throughout the OT evaluation, she would comment, "I'm not going to give in to this!"

Client's Goals: Mary was asked what she wants to do, needs to do, or is expected to do. The Canadian Occupational Performance Measure was used. Mary identified the following goals, and the occupational therapist asked Mary to prioritize them:

Remain in her home alone and be as independent as possible.

Figure out how to obtain items out of her reach and retrieve newspaper from front porch without falling.

Take out garbage safely.

Be a more active grandmother by spending more time with grandchildren.

Participate more in church activities.

Carry things around the house.

Resume banking and shopping activities.

Move into and out of the bathtub safely.

Resume cooking without becoming tired.

Case A-4 James

Thom Fisher

History: James is 62 years old, married, and has four adult children and five grandchildren. He resides with his wife in Lexington, Kentucky. Three of the four children live in the Lexington area. Their oldest daughter is a registered nurse who works in home health care in Louisville, 75 miles away. James was originally diagnosed with lung cancer. The cancer metastasized to the brain. He then underwent a right craniotomy. After this neurosurgical procedure, James had left hemiplegia, expressive aphasia, and balance problems. As a result, he requires assistance from his wife, Ann, for many activities. He shared that this made him feel less than adequate.

James resides in a large (approximately 2500 square feet) one-story house: four bedrooms, 2.5 bathrooms, living room, kitchen, formal dining room, and family room. The house also has a fully finished basement, but he no longer goes to the basement. The attached garage has one step into the laundry room off the kitchen as you enter the home. The home has carpeting throughout with the exception of the kitchen, bathrooms, and laundry room. These rooms have linoleum.

James retired from the University of Kentucky (UK) 6 months prior to his diagnosis. He had served in an administrative role within the graduate school. He holds a master's degree in statistics. After retirement, he continued to work (part-time) as a research consultant on some projects. He reported enjoying this thoroughly. He tried not to work more than 10 hours a week on those projects. His leisure occupations are golf and collecting antiques. He used to sell his antiques in a small antiques shop in Versailles, Kentucky.

Ann had been employed at UK as well. She retired after her husband became ill. She was 60 years old at the time.

James' insurance is a managed-care product available to state employees. James and Ann are receiving their retirement pension but not their Social Security. James received a modest compensation for consulting.

James uses a quad cane (cane with four prongs) for ambulation (short distances) and a wheelchair for long distances. He has an ankle-foot orthosis for his left lower extremity. This is worn when ambulating. He has a resting hand splint for his left upper extremity, worn at night. He is taking several medications, including an anticonvulsant and an antidepressant. James reports the antidepressants were "actually for sleeping at night." James lost over 40 pounds during the past 6 months and his appetite remains depressed. He has received several radiation treatments but will not receive chemotherapy.

James is alert and oriented and has fair insight and fair judgment. Ann reports occasional impulsivity. His expressive aphasia improved but at times he continues to have word-finding problems.

James and his wife are concerned about use of his left hand, his tolerance for activity, and prognosis. Children and grandchildren visit frequently. The oldest grandson (20 years old) comes and stays with James when Ann leaves the house for long periods of time (for church and errands, for example). The entire family is supportive and interested in his rehabilitation.

James was referred for home-health physical therapy, occupational therapy, and skilled nursing. Physical therapy and occupational therapy were approved by the managed-care organization for a total of 10 shared visits. The physical therapist and the occupational therapist met to discuss how to use these visits efficiently. The therapists decided that since James was terminal and quality of life was central, occupational therapy would use six of the visits and physical therapy would have the remaining four. This would truly reflect the home-health agency's client-centered focus. The physicians felt James had 6 to 18 months to live. The occupational therapist evaluation included the agency's Occupational Therapy Evaluation and interview, the Role Checklist, and the Motor Free Visual Perceptual Test-Vertical. The following is a summary of James' functioning at the time of the evaluation.

Self-Care: James requires moderate assistance for bathing and dressing.

- He uses a quad cane for ambulating short distances and uses a wheelchair for long distances.

- He uses a bedside commode or urinal at night so as not to ambulate far to the master bathroom. He fears falling or having an "accident" (wetting).

- He requires minimal assist from tub and car transfers, mostly verbal prompts.

- James was seen to have dressing apraxia in the past but this is resolving over time.

Work/Productive Activity:

- Poor dynamic standing balance (unsteady)

- Endurance/tolerance for activity limited to about 15 minutes, then becomes tired

- James requires maximum assistance for meal preparation. This is unfortunate because cooking was an activity he enjoyed in the past.

- He thoroughly enjoyed working as a research consultant part time.

Other:

- James' left hand/arm spasticity is moderate (during activity spasticity increased).

- Occasional word-finding difficulty. James finds this embarrassing due to his role as a researcher.

- James has poor insight into his depression and his wife's anxiety but fair insight into his diagnosis and prognosis.

- Many of James' coworkers lost contact due to their discomfort with his diagnosis and deficits. Ann reports that they were "just not comfortable around him."

Leisure:

- Prior to becoming ill, James enjoyed golf, playing bridge, and collecting antiques. He feels these are beyond his skills now that he has become sick. Ann feels that he has unnecessarily withdrawn from many activities (for example, going to church). He had been quite active in the Catholic church.

Strengths:

- James is motivated to resume previous level of independence.
- James has a supportive wife, who is his primary caregiver, and family.
- Cognition remains intact.
- His spasticity decreases with inhibition techniques (neurodevelopmental and proprioceptive neuromuscular facilitation techniques).
- He has an accessible home (large rooms and hallway).
- He remains interested in resuming roles of research consultant and antiques dealer.
- He is receptive to home program and follow-through with instruction from the occupational therapist (especially important with limited visits approved by insurance).
- James and Ann asked about other resources and support services available in the community.

Psychosocial: James is interested in resuming an active life and his prior level of independence but anxious about his balance when walking, and coordination of his hands. He said, "It is just simpler to stay home." He recognized the difficulty and the added responsibility his wife has when he does go out. Ann reports that she is becoming more concerned when she needs to leave him home for short periods of time because of his impulsivity.

Client's Stated Goals: When James was asked by the occupational therapist, "What do you want the occupational therapist to address with you during the home visits?" the following are what James identified (not in order of preference):

Gain control and use of left hand.

Resume independence with toileting, bathing, and dressing.

Drive again.

Continue consulting in research and antique collecting.

Re-engage with friends and church.

Case A-5 Sam

Kathleen Flecky

Sam is a healthy 4-year-old boy who attends a preschool program in which typical children and children with physical deficits are enrolled. Sam is small for his age and appears in constant motion. He is outgoing and talkative and loves to tell stories. His hair is rumpled from his continual twirling and twisting of hair strands, leaving patchy bald areas on his head. Sam frequently adjusts and readjusts his pants up and down and his shirt often comes untucked. He was referred to private occupational therapy by the school physical therapist. The therapist explained that the preschool teachers have concerns with Sam's inability to deal with transitions between activities such as lunch to swimming and gym class to classroom. During classroom time, he continually asks questions of his teacher or classmates and has problems organizing his actions. He refused to cut with scissors and is visibly distressed with sand or glue on his fingers. He is bothered by touch from other classmates and has problems sitting still for more than 1 minute. The physical therapist at the school has concerns about Sam's ability to motor plan gym activities and recognize safety issues. She related that Sam often stumbles and falls during gym activities and seeks out and initiates rough physical contact with other children. Several parents have complained that their children were physically hurt during these interactions.

Sam's mother relates, "Sam is a handful. He was a fussy baby who did not sleep well until 2 years old. He would only eat one kind of baby food and took a long time to switch to solid foods. He won't even try certain foods, like oatmeal—he spits it right out! I have problems getting Sam going in the mornings—he does not like to get dressed, has to wear certain clothes and gets very upset with any changes in routine." She also indicated that Sam was late to begin walking and continues to have trouble kicking a ball and riding his bicycle. Lately, she has noticed that he seems to be so frustrated with learning these and other new skills that he has "given up" and avoids learning new things.

She stated that she was 28 years old at Sam's birth and her pregnancy was unremarkable. She has concerns about Sam's ability to "get along" with other children and adapt to a school routine as he enters preschool. Sam lives with his mother and his grandmother in a small, three-bedroom townhouse in the city. His parents have been divorced for 2 years and he lives with his father during the summer.

Case A-6 Tina

Yolanda Griffiths

Tina is a 38-year-old married woman who works at a local dry-cleaning store in the Midwest. She sustained a closed head injury in a car accident last winter. Tina was too traumatized by the accident to resume driving a car so she takes the bus to work each day. Tina complains of reoccurring pain in her right shoulder since the accident. She has sustained memory lapses and poor concentration. Tina had experienced terrible migraine headaches prior to the accident and she continues to experience these headaches now, especially when feeling stressed or fatigued.

Tina's husband works the night shift in a local dairy and spends much of his leisure time at the local casino. Tina has one daughter aged 17 who ran away from home last year with a 24-year-old boyfriend. Tina feels her daughter is "out of control." Tina is often home alone at night, usually watching television or cleaning the house. Tina reports having trouble going to sleep at night and even her favorite hot tea does not seem to relax her. Tina often finds herself still watching television after 1:00 AM. Prior to the accident, Tina regularly went to bed before 10:00 PM.

Tina was admitted to the mental-health unit when she became extremely irritated and upset with a customer's demand to have a garment recleaned because of a spot. Tina unpredictably threw objects around the store and screamed at the top of her voice until her boss called the police. When her boss tried to calm her down, Tina pushed him. Tina says it felt like "I had no control over my emotions.... Now when I get angry I just keep going until I blow up—then I can't stop crying." Tina's boss reported to the police that he was so surprised at her behavior, as "Tina had always been such a sweet lady and suddenly it was like she someone else. Especially after the accident it seems something changed." Tina's boss indicated to her that unless she could get her anger under control, it was unlikely that she could return to her job. Tina is very concerned about what will happen if she cannot return to her job and contribute to the household financially. Tina also is aware that her job has been a very fulfilling part of her day since she is often lonely at night.

Tina's boss noted to the police that she was always a reliable worker but now frequently mislabels orders from customers or forgets to write down special instructions. Tina argues with her co-workers and customers about the mistakes, saying she could not possibly have made those errors. The police called her husband and Tina was admitted to a local community hospital adult mental health unit.

Tina appears cooperative during her occupational therapy assessment although her affect seems blunted and her mood depressed. The occupational therapist has chosen the "Profile of Occupational Patterns Questionnaire" (Royeen, 1995) to examine any shifts in occupational patterns that have significantly affected Tina's life, and to help to develop postdischarge plans when Tina goes home from the hospital.

A brief summary of the interview follows. Tina has been prescribed Paxil twice a day to help elevate her mood. Because of Tina's closed head injury from the car accident, the staff is observing Tina closely for any side effects of this medication. Tina will be discharged from the hospital in 4 or 5 days and referred to a community-based outpatient program. Tina's primary meaningful activity is work. Her job fulfills her needs for socialization and productivity and enhances her self-esteem. Tina would like to be more independent but feels panicked at the thought of driving since the accident. She lacks physical exercise and her primary leisure activities focus on sedentary television viewing. Tina admits that her diet at home is often junk food, diet cola, and hot tea. Tina worries that her poor sleeping habits may have contributed to her emotional outbursts at work, and that maybe her increasing anxiety over her daughter is keeping her up at night.

Tina was tearful at one point in the interview and said, "I never thought my life would turn out like this. None of this was really my fault. Even the accident was the result of a drunk driver. He died at the scene so I guess I can't blame him now. I guess fate dealt me just an unlucky life."

Tina noted that she has few friends except her coworkers, who always made her job a fun place to go to. Tina said she has no family in the immediate area and her closest relative is her elderly mother, who lives 5 hours away. When asked about her daughter, Tina sighed heavily and said, "She dropped me a note at Christmas and on her birthday asking for money, but I suspect she's on drugs. My husband said that's the way she wants it, so let her go."

The occupational therapist asked what specific goals Tina would like to pursue or which specific activities she would especially like to engage in when she returns home. Tina rubbed the side of her head and requested to continue the interview later as she felt a migraine headache coming on and needed to lie down.

As a result of the initial assessment, the occupational therapist identified the following shifts in occupational patterns:

- From worker to hospital patient
- From independent driver to bus rider
- From mother to unwanted empty nester
- From competent worker to person with disabilities
- From sweet personality to person with unpredictable outbursts
- From reliable worker to person who makes mistakes at work
- From happy person to depressed, angry, and anxious person
- From restful sleeper to insomniac
- From satisfied employee to possibly unemployed

The driving accident that resulted in the physical injuries was a major incident and this was compounded by the outburst at her job leading to the current hospitalization. The shifts in Tina's occupational roles have significantly impacted her life and the activities associated with those role changes. Work is a very meaningful activity in Tina's life. Few activities bring the same sense of productivity or pleasure for Tina. The disruption in Tina's regular sleep pattern, whether caused by her diet or by anxiety, has shifted her normal rhythms and restoration habits. The occupational therapist noted that Tina has an external locus of control in her perspective and her self-esteem seems very low. Tina's emotions are affected by her closed head injury and by the demand of adapting to her major shifts in occupational patterns.

Royeen, C. (1995). The human life cycle: Paradigmatic shifts in occupation. In C. Royeen (Ed.), AOTA self-study series—The practice of the future: putting occupation back into therapy, 5–24.

Case A-7 Bill

Carolyn Hall

Bill became an electrical journeyman at age 30. He established his own business, called Bill's Electrical Company. Initially he was the only employee (for the first 5 years), and he had a strong work ethic. As his reputation grew, so did his business.

When he retired 5 years ago, he stepped down from being the commanding executive and appointed his son to the position. The company now employs 26 people. Bill's Electrical Company's primary source of income is from the bigger commercial accounts in the area.

After retiring, Bill has had more time for his hobbies. He likes to garden, read, golf, and travel. His pension, investments, and income from his business allow him and his wife to travel. They travel two to three times a year for approximately 4 weeks at a time, both within the United States and to other countries.

After returning home in the late evening from one of their trips, Bill was unable to sleep in the next day. The sun was shining brightly and it promised to be another warm spring day. Bill decided it was time to get the garden ready for planting. He went outside to his tool shed and took his rototiller out to the garden. He had been running the rototiller for at least 45 minutes when he decided to rest on a nearby bench.

As he sat there, he began to feel pain in his right arm and pressure in his chest area and began to gasp for air. He tried to call for help, but he was unable to vocalize. Luckily his wife, Betty, had been watching out the kitchen window and saw the signs of distress that her husband was having. She ran out of the house to see what was happening. She attempted to talk to Bill, but he was not responding. She went back into the house and dialed 911.

Later that same day she waited patiently in the emergency waiting room area at the local hospital. Finally, their family physician came out of the emergency room to talk to her. She was advised that her husband had suffered a severe cerebrovascular accident (CVA).

She and the doctor went into the room to see Bill. The doctor began to describe to Betty his assessment of her husband. The doctor stated that Bill had a problem with breathing on his own, and they connected him to a ventilator. The doctor went on to inform Betty that the right side of Bill's body was experiencing hemiparesis affecting both upper and lower extremities. Betty touched his right hand and felt the coolness of his skin. His arm felt strange to her and the doctor explained that his arm was flaccid and hyporesponsive. The doctor also stated Bill's right arm and leg were not showing any signs of independent movements.

The doctor stated that Bill would not be able to walk at the present time or use his dominant hand. The doctor advised that his level of consciousness appeared to fluctuate, and it was too early to tell if Bill's memory had been affected.

Betty also noticed the right side of his mouth was lower than the left side. She was concerned about his eating. The doctor stated that Bill was in no condition to eat by himself and a gastrostomy tube would be put in place for future stomach feeding. As they were talking, Bill opened his eyes and smiled. His wife thought he had recognized her until she realized that his left eye appeared to be more in focus than his right eye. The doctor advised Betty that vision was frequently impaired from CVAs. The doctor also stated that they were going to keep Bill in the intensive care unit until he showed signs of medical stabilization.

Betty was at Bill's side continuously and would only leave for a brief time when their son, Roger, was there. Roger came to see his father every night. He tried to persuade his mother to go home and to get some rest. Her son and her friends offered to stay with Bill, but Betty would not leave the hospital.

She would leave the room only when their son came to visit; then she would go to the hospital's cafeteria, for short walks through the halls, or to the hospital chapel. The chapel was a place for Betty to pray and to give thanks. She didn't even want to think what life would be like without her husband. In 3 more months, they would have been married for 52 years.

She recalled how both her mother and father-in-law had had heart problems. Until the last week, Bill had not complained of health problems. He was the one who never would get the flu or seasonal colds. Suddenly, her thoughts were interrupted by the doctor's presence.

For 4 long days she was at her husband's side. The doctor always kept Betty informed. He finally told Betty that her husband had improved enough to be transferred to another floor in the hospital. The doctor also said that he was going to begin having the rehabilitation team begin their evaluations.

He explained to her that he was going to recommend physical therapy, occupational therapy, and speech therapy to assess Bill. Betty gave a sigh of relief; she knew this was a step toward recovery.

When her son arrived that night, she told him the good news. She also let him drive her home that night. She was exhausted and didn't realize how much until she lay down in her own bed.

Case A-8 Grace

Dana Howell

Grace is a 52-year-old Native American woman who just arrived at the Adobe Rehabilitation Hospital. She had been hospitalized following the onset of Guillain-Barré syndrome.

Her medical history began when an emergency medical team was called to her home because of her symptoms of severe weakness and respiratory distress. She was airlifted from her remote house on a Navajo reservation and taken to the nearest hospital equipped to handle ventilation, which was a 4-hour drive from her home. Upon arrival at the hospital, she was placed on mechanical ventilation and exhibited full body paralysis. She remained in the hospital for 6 weeks and began to slowly improve during that time. Ultimately, she was removed from respiratory support and regained slight use of her shoulder and neck muscles. At that time, she was thought to be past the critical stages of the disease and was expected to begin a gradual recovery. With this in mind, she was transferred to the Adobe Rehabilitation Hospital to begin occupational, physical, and speech therapy.

Upon evaluation, Grace is fully dependent for all self-care including feeding, dressing, toileting, and bathing. She is unable to sit unsupported because of the continued paralysis of her trunk muscles. Both legs also remain paralyzed, although she is able to move both arms slightly. Her arm movement, however, is minimal and ineffective for functional use in activities of daily living. Passively moving her extremities causes her considerable pain. Since the ventilator has been removed and she has regained much of her face and neck movement, she is able to speak and to eat a diet of soft foods. Cognition is intact, but is difficult to assess because Grace has only fair English skills and appears uncomfortable with speaking during the evaluation.

Grace's husband and one daughter are present during the initial assessment and offer a wealth of additional information. They report that the first time Grace had ever left the reservation was the day she was airlifted to the hospital. The family also provided information about their home on the reservation. While the house has water and electricity, it does not contain many other modern amenities, such as a television, dishwasher, or washing machine. The house is surrounded by fairly rugged terrain, and it is doubtful that a wheelchair could access the house or the surrounding area easily.

Grace reports that her typical day includes cooking traditional Navajo foods and cleaning the house. In addition to household management, Grace is responsible for some of the livestock care, including feeding and watering the sheep. She is an avid gardener and spends as much of her time outside as possible. In the winter, she enjoys painting intricate designs on the pottery made by her sister, who lives nearby.

Grace has two daughters who attend college in other states. The family is very supportive but limited by time, distance, and resources. Grace reveals that she would very much like to return home, even if she is not fully recovered. She is willing to participate in therapy to get home as soon as possible.

Case A-9 Jacob

Judy Janson

Jacob was referred for a comprehensive evaluation by the school team. He is a 9-year-old boy in the fourth grade who moved into the school district 3 months ago. Jacob's appearance is often disheveled with his short brown hair uncombed, clothes mismatched, and shoestrings dragging behind. It is not uncommon for Jacob to stop the line progression of his class to look at a wall poster in the hall. His teacher often finds herself redirecting Jacob's attention to catch up with the class in line or to line up when the whistle blows at recess. The teacher describes Jacob as having a short attention span, often forgetting to write down assignments, not remembering to take home books for his homework, and losing his papers between school and home and between classes. Jacob's desk area and locker are disorganized. Jacob has difficulty following two- or three-step instructions. When his pencil needs sharpening, Jacob will not initiate going to the pencil sharpener until directed by the teacher. Jacob gets lost if he is sent to the office or library, down the hall to another fourth-grade room, or to the lunchroom. Jacob will raise his hand to answer a question but is unable to answer when called upon. The physical education teacher reports Jacob reacts more slowly than his peers when a ball is thrown to him, when attempting to hit a ball with a bat, or when dodging a ball in games. Socially, Jacob has not been able to make new friends. He is easygoing but shows sudden irritability for insignificant reasons.

Medical records transferred from his previous school do not indicate any significant injuries or deficits. The parents moved from a small town in a rural setting. They described the school as an early 1900s building that comprised grades kindergarten through 12. The kitchen and cafeteria were located in the basement. The office and elementary classrooms for grades kindergarten through 6 were arranged in the front of the building on the main floor. The gym was set up in the rear half of the main floor. The counselor's office and grades 7 through 12 encompassed the second floor.

Jacob was evaluated by an occupational therapist during two 90-minute sessions and during observations in physical education and the classroom. The Bruininks-Oseretsky Test of Motor Proficiency notes below age-level performance on response speed and within 5 months of his age level with all other subtests. The Test of Visual-Perceptual Skills (nonmotor) noted below age-level performance on the subtest categories of visual memory and visual sequential memory. An area of weakness at the lower end of his age range was visual-spatial relationships. The Wold Sentence Copy test was used to determine if Jacob had the ability to rapidly and accurately copy a 110-letter sentence from the top to the bottom of a page. Letters per minute are calculated and compared to the Ayres letters-per-minute grade equivalence. Jacob's copy speed is at the third-grade level for cursive writing. Observation during the test noted that Jacob required two fixations (looking back to the sentence) for each word. His cursive letters are legible. However, words are difficult to read because of crowding on the line. A short break was necessary during the assessment period for Jacob to move about the room. Attention span was maintained for 5 minutes if active-gross and fine-motor testing was interspersed between less active subtests. Jacob began to change positions in his chair, looked around, and asked unrelated questions after 10 minutes. Instructions during the test had to be repeated and/or demonstrated when possible.

Jacob was independent with the daily living tasks of putting on/removing a jacket, shoes/boots, gloves, and hat. He was independent with self-care in the bathroom, lunch line, and eating in the cafeteria. Problems became evident when executive functions were required in Jacob's daily routine. He was unable to follow a sequence of two instructions without cues, and could not follow verbal directions to simple destinations. His concept of time is very poor. An outburst of anger was observed in the classroom when papers were passed forward, stacking up on his desk. Jacob was unaware of what he was supposed to do with the papers or why they ended up on his desk.

The individualized educational plan (IEP) meeting was scheduled with the team and parents to review the assessment information. The psychologist noted an academic performance scale on the borderline of his age level. The same attentional difficulties were noted during the psychologist's assessment. The social worker's social adjustment rating noted areas of concern with peer relationships, attention, follow-through of tasks, immediate memory, organizational skills, and noticeable fatigue during his daily routine, as well as periodic irritability.

The parents stated that teachers in the past had not noticed any of these problems. The school nurse questioned if there were any injuries, for example, concussions, in Jacob's history. His mother stated he had been knocked down several times the previous year in soccer and basketball, bumping his head. During the last injury, Jacob lost consciousness momentarily. The doctor checked him and told the parents to watch for dizziness, drowsiness, or headache. Jacob never had any other physical complaints.

The IEP team qualified Jacob for 2 hours of aide assistance in the least restrictive environment of the classroom. The aide would receive input from the team to train Jacob in appropriate adaptations and accommodations for his deficit areas. Occupational therapy will provide an integrated service delivery model including direct and/or consultative intervention for 30 minutes per week.

The parents asked why the problems seemed to show up now, in the fourth grade. The team suggested that these problems could have been exacerbated by stress from the move, forcing him to adapt to new people, routines, and an unfamiliar environment. The psychologist explained that executive functions of the student are expected at a higher degree in fourth grade. Prior to that, students are guided and supervised in their subjects more. In the lower grades there is only one primary teacher for academics and no homework unless the student does not finish his or her work in class. Instructions are provided in shorter time increments with one more recess period to break up the day. The students are with the class whenever they travel to different areas in the building. Jacob's problems may have been less evident because he was not required to be as independent. It was recommended that Jacob receive a neurological assessment by a physician.

Case A-10 Mr. McMasters

Scott Johnson

Mr. McMasters was referred to occupational therapy by his neurosurgeon 5 days after the removal of a large malignant tumor of the left parietal and occipital lobes. He showed right hemiparesis, right-sided visual difficulty, and cognitive function deficits. He is a slightly overweight, middle-aged individual. His affect is somewhat flat and presents as depressed; however, he makes some attempt at socializing when family is present.

Mr. McMasters' chart information is as follows:

Employment History: Mr. McMasters is a 58-year-old former high-school social-studies teacher and coach who moved to Carmel Townsville from Beltsville, Wisconsin, a year ago to retire.

Social History: Mr. McMasters is accompanied by his wife Mildred of 35 years and their son, Jim, who lives out of state. The family has been present at the rehabilitation center daily since Mr. McMasters' admittance. Mr. McMasters's father died from lung cancer at age 82.

Habits: Patient's wife reports that Mr. McMasters occasionally drinks alcohol and smokes cigarettes.

Avocational Interests: Bicycling, hunting, fishing, gardening, swimming, dancing, music, playing cards, and volunteering for Meals-on-Wheels.

Allergies: Penicillin.

Past Medical History: History of polio as a child and a myocardial infarction 8 years ago.

Past Surgical History: Appendectomy 14 years ago, tonsillectomy as a child, and tumor excision as above.

History of Present Illness: Patient's wife reports that it dates back 2 months previous to Mr. McMasters's hospitalization, at which time he began to complain of very bad headaches. He also complained of having occasional vertigo and some uncoordination. The severity of the headaches increased, and shortly before Mr. McMasters was admitted to the hospital, he experienced a grand mal seizure while driving in Carmel Townsville. There was no vehicular accident reported; however, Mr. McMasters had bitten both sides of his tongue. Mrs. McMasters immediately took him to the local small-town doctor who referred him to a large, city hospital.

One week later, a magnetic resonance imaging scan revealed a large edematous mass over both the left parietal and occipital lobes of Mr. McMasters's brain. Surgery was performed the following day to remove the mass. Mr. McMasters was referred to occupational therapy to increase strength and cognitive awareness. No seizure activity is present postsurgery.

Occupational Therapy Assessment: Initial evaluation demonstrates areas of difficulty for Mr. McMasters in the following performance areas. Mr. McMasters is right-hand dominant.

Cognition: Mr. McMasters demonstrated difficulty with sequencing, two- and three-step commands, short-term memory, judgment, and attention. Mr. McMasters is oriented to date, time, and place. He has the ability to follow one-step commands and has intact long-term memory.

Perception: Mr. McMasters demonstrated impaired ability to identify two- and three-dimensional block designs, impaired figure ground perception, and difficulty with right and left discrimination.

Visual Motor: Mr. McMasters demonstrated an impaired right visual field with tracking. His left visual field is intact. Mr. McMasters is aware of his right visual difficulty.

Positioning: A lap board was issued to Mr. McMasters to assist with his right upper extremity placement.

Passive Range of Motion (PROM), Active Range of Motion (AROM), and Strength: PROM is within functional limits (WFL) both upper extremities. AROM: Left upper extremity is WFL.

Right upper extremity as follows:

Shoulder	Elbow
Flexion 35 degrees	Flexion 90 degrees
Extension not tested	Extension 90 degrees
Abduction 35 degrees	Pronation 45 degrees
Adduction 0 degrees	Supination 20 degrees
Horizontal abduction not tested	
Horizontal adduction not tested	
Internal rotation not tested	
External rotation not tested	

Wrist	Fingers
Flexion 30 degrees	WFL
Extension	30 degrees

Strength: Left upper extremity is WFL. Right upper extremity Manual Muscle Test (MMT) was not used due to limited AROM against gravity.

Grip Strength: Right 30 pounds. Left 70 pounds

Pinch Strength: Palmer – Right 5 pounds. Left 20 pounds

Lateral – Right 10 pounds. Left 22 pounds

Nine Hole Coordination Evaluation: Not tested

Box and Block Coordination Evaluation: Not tested

Sensation: Left upper extremity, intact except stereognosis; right upper extremity, impaired

Activities of Daily Living (ADL) Status:

Feeding: Independent with setup, requires maximum assistance to cut food

Grooming: Minimum assistance

In the areas of Toileting, Clothing Management, Bathing Tasks, Meal Preparation, and Homemaking, Mr. McMasters is dependent.

Mr. McMasters is able to communicate his needs; however, he is unable to write them.

Case A-11 Jeremiah

Jeffery Jones

Jeremiah is an 11-year-old boy, extremely sociable, with an unending smile. He wears wire-framed glasses with a relatively strong prescription. At an appropriate height for his chronological age, he is seated in a wheelchair, which is adapted to maintain eye contact at an age-appropriate level with peers.

Maximally dependent in his self-care activities; Jeremiah takes great pride in his limited abilities to feed himself. Mealtimes tend to become long and drawn out because of his socializing with others. His diagnoses include: cerebral palsy; structural deformities; difficulties with breathing, feeding, speech, and vision; increased overall tone; and decreased range of motion. Jeremiah uses an electric wheelchair equipped with a joystick to accommodate for limited upper-extremity mobility and has received therapy since birth at the same clinic. He enjoys outside activities (swimming, horseback riding, baseball, etc.) as well as verbal sparring and jokes with therapeutic personnel and peers. When out of his chair, he enjoys "roughhousing" with therapeutic personal during interventions.

Jeremiah's mother is employed at the Estherbrooke Children's Center, where he is treated on an outpatient basis. Since she is involved as a staff member she is acutely aware of Jeremiah's needs and continuing care requirements. Jeremiah lives with his mother and stepfather in federally subsidized housing that is not compliant with the Americans with Disabilities Act. Both parents utilize a staggered schedule to attend to his therapeutic needs and treatment. Schedules are staggered to assist in caring for and maintaining academic and therapeutic schedules. Jeremiah's mother is concerned with and involved in his daily care. His stepfather holds a lesser position in daily care. Accusations have been made by friends and therapeutic personnel toward the stepfather in regard to mental and physical abuse to Jeremiah.

Jeremiah receives therapy from both the Estherbrooke Children's Clinic and the Tri-State Elementary School at which he is mainstreamed. He receives occupational, physical, and speech therapies twice a week at both locations on alternating days. These sessions include both intensive individualized and combined interdisciplinary intervention.

Case A-12 Alice

Amy Kratz

Alice is an 87-year-old widow who suffered a left cerebrovascular accident resulting in right hemiparesis. Alice went through extensive physical, occupational, and speech therapy after her stroke. Not long after her stroke, her husband of 60 years passed away. Four months poststroke, Alice moved into the assisted-living portion of the continuing care retirement community where she was living, as she was unable to return home to care for herself. Alice was able to feed herself and get around using her wheelchair and walker with assistance. Alice still required assistance with basic activities of daily living, such as dressing.

Alice's retirement community provides its residents with a continuum of care that includes independent living, assisted living, nursing home, and Alzheimer's care. Residents have access to a weight room, indoor pool, library facilities, and walking paths. Prior to her stroke, Alice was involved in many groups utilizing these facilities.

Alice had been expressing a great desire to return to the pool at the facility. She had been an avid user while living in the independent-living apartments. To get an understanding of Alice, I chose to administer the Occupational Performance History Interview (Version 2.0) (OPHI-II) (Kielhofner et al., 1998). After a thorough interview, it became apparent that Alice has been swimming all her life. Alice stated, "There has never been a body of water that I haven't wanted to get in." She was upset that she was no longer able to engage in this valued occupation. Alice's goal was to be able to swim again and return to the weekly water aerobics class with her friends in the independent-living section of the retirement community.

Alice was able to use her right hand for functional tasks, but it was uncoordinated and weak. Alice participated in water-based occupational therapy in the pool three times per week for 3 months. Initial sessions focused on getting used to being in the water, gradually increasing to swimming with supportive devices, and concluding with swimming unsupported. We were also able to address Alice's ability to dress herself and practice using her right hand to dry herself after getting out of the pool.

Through this pool-based intervention, Alice was able to accomplish her goal and resume swimming. She recognized the importance of this occupation in her daily life both physically and emotionally and commented on how much stronger she felt because of it. Staff and family members commented on the change they saw in Alice from the aquatic interventions. Based on a thorough understanding of Alice's occupational history, the occupational therapist was able to create occupation-based intervention that had a broad impact on her health, quality of life, and daily functioning.

Kielhofner, G., Mallinson, T., Crawford, C., Nowak, M., Rigby, M., Henry, A., et al. (1998). A user's manual for the occupational performance history interview (Version 2.0). Chicago: Model of Human Occupation Clearinghouse, University of Illinois at Chicago.

Case A-13 John

Matthew J. Kraus

John is a 54-year-old married man who has been recently admitted to a state psychiatric hospital for suicidal ideation and major depression. His symptoms have manifested and increased in the last 9 months, since suffering from a cerebrovascular accident (CVA) 21 months ago.

Prior to his CVA, John was a boisterous and outgoing individual. He was at times considered uncouth because of his tendency toward tasteless jokes and lewd jocularity. In general, he was well-liked by his friends and peers.

John's prime source of income is as a welder. He began the welding trade after graduating from high school. He is self employed, working out of his garage, but primarily contracts out his skills to construction companies. Sometimes labeled a "handyman," he has above-average competence in mechanics, electrical wiring, carpentry, and home repair. He is a practical problem solver and his good "horse-sense" has given him a respectable reputation in the community.

John truly enjoys working with his hands. Welding provides his income, but he also enjoys creating things for fun such as furniture, handrails, and barbecue pits. One of John's favorite activities revolves around his classic car, a 1960 Corvette. He restored this car himself, and it is his pride and joy. He frequently takes his car cruising to the Friday night drive-ins where he meets up with friends who also have classic cars. He also enjoys seasonal fishing at

Pecan Valley Lake and hunting trips with friends. John's leisure pursuits usually involved consuming beer. He at times would drink heavily and his inebriation would further disinhibit his already outgoing personality.

John was married to his first wife Martha for 27 years and was divorced 10 years ago. He has no contact with her. They dated each other while in high school and got married shortly thereafter. Together, they raised two children. Both children are grown, married, and live with their respective families in different states. Contact with the children is through occasional phone calls, letters in the mail, or get-togethers during holidays like Thanksgiving, Christmas, or Easter. His relationship with his children is considered good and functional, although minimal.

John married his present wife, Tanya, 5 years ago. The couple has no children. Prior to this admission, his relationship with his present wife, although cycling through bouts of tension, was generally positive and functional. According to her, the subject of greatest tension in their relationship was his uncontrolled beer drinking.

John was taken to the county hospital 21 months ago by emergency medical service (EMS) complaining of a severe headache and a sudden loss of function in his right upper and lower extremities, after collapsing at his home. At the hospital, function on his right side as well as his ability to communicate deteriorated. A magnetic resonance imaging (MRI) test revealed an burst aneurysm in the middle cerebral artery in the left hemisphere.

After 3 months of rehabilitation, John was able to walk only a short distance with a quad cane, with moderate assistance from staff. In his weakened condition, he generally preferred, and at times insisted on, ambulating in a wheelchair. John's communication skills were greatly impaired by partial expressive and receptive aphasias. Initially, and shortly after the onset, John's motivation to recover and return to his previous vocation and lifestyle was good. As the months passed and his physical condition did not substantially improve, his morale began to deteriorate. After 3 months of rehabilitation, he plateaued at the level described and was discharged.

John's wife, Tanya, made few attempts to support him, either physically or psychologically. His impaired communication skills were frustrating to both of them. This challenging environment placed a maximal strain on the marriage. Tanya did not feel ready to dedicate the rest of her life to him as a caregiver. The relationship steadily deteriorated. Altercations between John and Tanya became frequent. John had difficulty communicating in their arguments due to his aphasia. Most attempts at communication became shouting matches. Despite his debilitated condition, Tanya was verbalizing fear that he would physically retaliate and hurt her. As a result of this mistrust, Tanya became very bitter toward John and wanted out of the marriage. Unbeknownst to John, she started selling off all their possessions. At a yard sale she conducted, she practically gave away all of his tools, books, and equipment, as well as his Corvette.

Reacting to the lack of control he had in correcting the downward spiral of his life, John became increasingly depressed. He also became increasingly intolerant of his wife's lack of attention and empathy for his situation. His frustrations were directed toward not only the actions of his wife but also his feelings of inadequacy and impotence in managing his own life.

During an explosive altercation in the home, Tanya called the police. When the police arrived at the house, they noted that John was sitting in a wheelchair weeping and shouting incoherent verbalizations to his wife. Tanya was sitting on the staircase, clinging to the banister and wielding a broomstick. She stated to the police that she was fearful for her life and he was going to attack her. The police reminded her that he was in a wheelchair and unable to climb the steps of their two-story house. Tanya stated that the wheelchair was a ploy and he could walk just fine.

Seeing that John was in physical distress, the police decided to call EMS to have him assessed. The EMS technician noted that John was very dehydrated and in a state of very poor hygiene. In treating John, the technician also heard between the incoherent gestures possible suicidal and homicidal ideations. With that, the police brought John to the state hospital for psychiatric testing.

Case A-14 Mr. Lowenstein

Curtis Quinn Marti

Mr. Lowenstein is a 33-year-old man of medium build. He is married and a father of a boy and girl, ages 5 and 9, respectively. He was involved in a single-car rollover and subsequent ejection of 40 feet. He initially had a Glasgow Coma Scale level of 4, and an alcohol level of 0.150. A CT scan reveals a right parenchymal and interparenchymal hemorrhage, a subdural arachnoid hemorrhage, and a C2 fracture. He also has a liver laceration and left pulmonary contusion. He was weaned off of the ventilator.

ADL/Home/Community Assessment: Mr. Lowenstein is independent with all of his self-care but requires verbal cues to comb his hair in the morning. He is able to independently feed himself. He is within functional limits (WFL) with clock and calendar use, but requires minimum verbal cues when counting money up to $20.00. When making change up to $10.00, Mr. Lowenstein requires moderate verbal cues. Minimum verbal cues are required for him to write a check accurately. He requires assistance with higher-level money management tasks. Mr. Lowenstein requires maximum verbal cues to find the emergency numbers in a phone book, but is able to locate numbers in the white and yellow pages with minimum to moderate verbal cues. He is able to dial a written phone number independently. When verbally responding to crisis situation questions, Mr. Lowenstein answers appropriately and completely 40 percent of the time.

Neuromuscular Assessment: Mr. Lowenstein's active range of motion (AROM) in the right upper extremity (RUE) was WFL, with the exception of the first digit's distal interphalangeal (DIP) joint. The client reports that skin was removed from his thumb and grafted onto his first digit, as a result of an injury with a saw. Consequently, the resultant scar tissue led to decreased AROM and passive range of motion (PROM) in the DIP joint. The joint's position at rest is minus 40 degrees from full extension. The joint cannot be passively moved because of complaints of pain. Manual Muscle Test (MMT) grades in the right UI are 5/5. AROM in the left UE is WFL, but he does complain of pain in the left shoulder upon movement. MMT grades in the left UE are 5/5, with the exception of shoulder flexion, which is 4/5.

Mr. Lowenstein's fine motor coordination, measured by the 9-Hole Peg Test, requires 24 seconds with the right hand and 32 seconds with the left. These scores indicate that the right hand is WFL and the left hand is slightly impaired. His grip strength, measured by the Jamar dynamometer on the #2 setting, is 70 pounds with the right hand and 55 with the left. These scores indicate that the right hand is moderately impaired and the left hand severely impaired for grip strength. His palmar pinch strength is 11 pounds with the right hand and 9 with the left. These scores indicate that palmar pinch strength is severely impaired bilaterally.

Upon admission, Mr. Lowenstein was wearing a cervical collar. He is not able to wear it at his own discretion. He reports that he wears the collar when his neck begins to feel weak. Active neck rotation is WFL. He ambulates independently without the aid of a device.

Perceptual Assessment: Sensation in Mr. Lowenstein's RUE is moderately impaired for sharp/dull (hand-forearm). Sensation in the LUE was moderately impaired for sharp/dull (forearm-hand). The accuracy of this sensory evaluation is decreased in light touch because he reports touches when no stimulus is present. Sensation will be re-tested when his cognitive level improves.

Mr. Lowenstein's combined score for the Motor-Free Visual Perceptual Test (MVPT) is 34/36. His errors occur in the visual closure section, which requires good attention/concentration as well as increased attention to detail. He demonstrates impulsivity and distractibility during the test.

Mr. Lowenstein's ability to visually track is WFL. However, he reports that his vision blurs during reading activities. Nystagmus is not observed during these visual tasks.

Cognitive Assessment: Upon initial evaluation, Mr. Lowenstein was oriented to person, date, situation, and place (not to the hospital's name). However, when he was asked the date on the following day, he was incorrect with the month and the day. He was able to repeat back a five-number sequence, which indicated that immediate recall is WFL. He demonstrated difficulty with short-term memory, as evidenced by his inability to recall his therapist's name or activities that he had participated in earlier. Mr. Lowenstein's long-term memory appears to be WFL. He was unable to count to 40 by threes and required maximum verbal cues with categorization skills. Moderate-maximum verbal cues were necessary when the client performed sequencing. He demonstrated impaired sequencing when he attempted to write out the alphabet. Mr. Lowenstein exhibits difficulty with reading and spelling. During verbal problem solving, he was WFL when identifying effects, but required minimum verbal cues when identifying causes. He demonstrates impulsivity that results in mistakes during activities, such as counting money. He also exhibited impaired attention/concentration and attention to detail during activities.

Behavioral and Psychosocial Assessment: Mr. Lowenstein responds appropriately and is willing to participate in therapy sessions. He displays a flat affect, except for occasional smiles during greetings. He participates during verbal exchanges, but does not seek out socialization with staff and other clients. He demonstrates poor insight into his deficit areas, as evidenced by his reporting that he needed to go home to care for his children and to return to work.

During dialogue with Mr. Lowenstein, he expressed that his top two priorities were to return to his job in a furniture-manufacturing plant and to resume his fathering duties. He expressed dissatisfaction with his present situation, by stating that he was "missing out on time spent with my kids."

Because of Mr. Lowenstein's strong background in constructing furniture, he expresses an interest in working with wood as a hobby. He feels that constructing wooden toys for his children would be a useful way to spend his time.

Mr. Lowenstein did not express that he had a serious alcohol problem, although he stated that he had made "bad decisions around the time of the car accident." Upon evaluation, he was already enrolled in a hospital-based drug- and alcohol-treatment program. Mr. Lowenstein appeared to be tentative when answering questions that were proposed and often asked for clarification. His locus of control was observed to be external, due to the number of questions that he asked therapists and department personnel prior to taking action on a task. The client's sense of personal causation appeared to be limited in view of the limited amount that he invested himself into a task. However, this may have developed secondary to his car accident.

Upon speaking with Mr. Lowenstein's family, they stated that he had basically the same personality characteristics as before the accident, only to a greater degree. His parents stated that he was "always a very dependent person who pretty much did what everyone around him was doing." Mr. Lowenstein's postdischarge aspirations were discussed with his family, and they were assured that they would be notified of any progress that he made in therapy. His family is very concerned about his alcohol problem and stated that it has been an ongoing issue since his teen years. They stated that he had been in and out of treatment programs over the years and none seemed to have a long-lasting effect.

During the family conference, both the stronger and the weaker performance areas of Mr. Lowenstein were discussed. Occupational therapy then collaborated with the family in regard to treatment interventions that would be beneficial to Mr. Lowenstein within the scope of occupational therapy.

Case A-15 Alta

Teddy R. Rudder

I was working as an occupational therapist in central Texas for a senior adult program when I met Alta. She had been referred to occupational therapy from a nursing home after a decline in ability to perform activities of daily living and symptoms of depression. I had already encountered the power of occupation-based treatment, but not like this case was about to reveal to me.

Alta was in her late seventies, a widow of 10 years with a diagnosis of diabetes mellitus and an above-knee amputation of the right leg secondary to complications from her diabetes. She had been living at the nursing home for 6 years. Her records painted a portrait of a lonely woman who spent most of her time alone in her room. She infrequently participated in facility activities and dined in her room for all meals. Nursing notes recorded her increasing desire to stay in bed and certified nursing assistants had reported increasing levels of assistance with activities of daily living. She had also declined from independent status with wheelchair management and mobility to moderate assistance.

I arrived at the local hospital where the senior adult program was based to find a prim and proper-looking woman sitting in her wheelchair. I had my clipboard in my hand as I walked up to her and introduced myself. She looked up and said, "I am not doing any exercise and I have been through this therapy before." I asked her about her previous experiences with occupational therapy and she said simply she had "been through it all before" and would be happy if she could go back to the nursing home and lie down. I set the clipboard aside and told her I would very much like to hear her story and promised her there would be no exercises. With that she began her story.

After her husband died Alta had been very depressed. Before he died, he had purchased her a Cadillac and it was her pride and joy. She spent her days running little errands in town and taking care of her birds. Her memory had began to fail shortly after her husband's death and got progressively worse. She began staying home more often, focusing on her birds. One day, on a trip to the local market, she ran a stop sign and struck another car. There was not much damage but it began her downward spiral. Her daughter-in-law came the following day to take her out to lunch. "Lunch" turned out to be the local nursing home and she had been there ever since. She was very bitter and angry as she told more. Her son had gained power-of-attorney over her and admitted her to the nursing home against her will. She missed her house and her birds. She began to cry.

The several years she had been at the nursing home involved many "escape" attempts, an infection that led to the above-knee amputation, and use of a wheelchair for mobility. She did not want to sit with the other residents during meals because "they made noises and were messy eaters." She just wanted to be left alone so she could "die in peace." I told her that I wanted to help and asked if she would give me a chance. She said that since I was the only one who ever let her talk that long without interrupting that she would return the next day but there would be no exercises. I agreed and we ended the session.

I obtained her charts and confirmed her story. In her evaluation I set goals to obtain a new wheelchair for her, to achieve independence with wheelchair mobility, to explore and develop leisure interests, to participate in a senior adult program peer discussion group, and to become independent in her abilities to perform activities of daily living. Occupational therapy would see her five times weekly at the senior adult program. I could only hope that she would return.

The next day found Alta in attendance and I took her to a private conference room to discuss her goals. I started with the new wheelchair and made an analogy to it as her new Cadillac. She liked this and immediately perked up. Together we chose the wheelchair and components and decided on a lightweight, hemi-height manual chair with a backpack for carrying items, wheel lock extensions, and a new honeycombed seat cushion. When she was able to choose the color (bright red), she was already referring to it as her new Cadillac. I told her that I would like for her to join the discussion group, which included other residents from the nursing home. She reluctantly agreed to "give it a try." I explained to her that the group would discuss leisure interests and dealing with life stressors. I also told her that each day the group did exercises but that she could choose to not participate. She agreed and asked what must have been a hundred times when she would get her new Cadillac. Luckily, I had a supplier that worked closely with me and went the extra mile so that I could tell her that the chair would be delivered in 2 weeks. She was like a child waiting for Christmas the whole time.

During the first discussion group, which I led, there was an obvious distance between Alta and some of the other group members. One big problem was that Alta had been married to a banker and the rest of the group members came from ranches. The group did not know that Alta had grown up on a ranch and she did not offer that information. The next day I presented a quiz game in which the group would look at a collection of western memorabilia and cowboy gear and then identify each item and its uses. The activity was a big hit and as the group discussed the answers, Alta scored highest. Her explanation that she had spent her youth on a large Texas ranch broke the ice and she was accepted into the group. She continued to show no interest in leisure activities, however.

During the fourth group discussion that Friday, Alta told us about her birds. When she had mentioned her birds before, I imagined a couple of parakeets. We learned that she had converted a school bus into an aviary and kept over 100 birds! I knew then that she had lost a cherished life role. Indeed, she had lost her reason to live when she lost her birds. I did not press to find out what had happened to them, but after confirming with the nursing home that it would be OK for her to have birds, I bought her a pair of baby parakeets. I cannot adequately describe how she beamed when I delivered the two birds on Saturday. She set her own goals at once: She would teach them to talk and to sit on her shoulder. I demonstrated to her how she could safely and independently rise from her seat to stand to reach the cage on top of her dresser. She practiced without one complaint. Before I left her room that day, she already exhibited an increased ability to transfer.

To make a long story short, I designed every exercise and activity-of-daily-living training session around those two birds. The wheelchair was delivered as promised and I do not think a real Cadillac would have made her any happier. Over the 4 weeks that I saw Alta, she met all her initial goals and new goals as well. Another woman in the senior adult program revealed that she also had a hard time eating in the dining room so she and Alta began taking turns eating in each other's rooms. I suggested to Alta that when her birds were trained to sit on her shoulder that she might enjoy sharing them with some of the nursing home residents who were confined to their beds most of the time. She and her birds became an attraction for all the residents.

I ended the occupational therapy treatment of Alta with her returning to independence with activities of daily living to include independent wheelchair mobility, her daily engagement in leisure interests (the birds), and a marked decline in symptoms of depression. On the day of discharge, I had to laugh to myself when Alta said she was so glad we had met and that she did not have to go through all the "old therapy" again! Ah, the power of occupational therapy.

Case A-16 Donald

Kris Seidner

Donald is an 18-year-old youth who resides in a public psychiatric facility for emotionally disturbed adolescents. His Axis I and II diagnoses are schizophrenia with borderline intelligence and schizoaffective personality. He has a refraction disorder resulting in a moderate visual impairment that corrects with his wearing glasses. Schizophrenia is a thought disorder that results in distorted reality during exacerbations of the illness. His schizoaffective personality is characterized by a tendency to withdraw from social situations and choose isolative activities. He is a shy young man, who appears unfriendly upon initial contact. He is hesitant to engage in interpersonal interactions and refuses to participate in any unfamiliar activities. The treatment team referred him for an occupational-therapy evaluation. The team's specific questions were related to his potential for living and working in the community.

Donald's social history provides a clearer image of this client. He was adopted at the age of 18 months by a white, middle-class couple, following a period of abuse and neglect beginning at birth. His adoptive mother is an administrative assistant in a law firm and his adoptive father is a hospital administrator in a nonprofit medical center. He has a sister who has completed college and is working as a computer analyst. Donald's family relationships with both parents and sister are strained. He was aloof with family members from the time of early childhood. He had developmental delays that became more obvious when he went to preschool. He didn't make friends with other children and related minimally with his teachers. When he was tested for kindergarten, he was placed in Special Education for emotional disturbance. His educational experiences were basically negative in terms of feedback received on academic performance and peer interactions. When he reached high school, it was difficult for his parents to get him to go to school. His behavior at home became more antisocial and he refused to comply with parental requests to assist in household tasks. His only interests seemed to be playing computer games, "surfing the net," and playing basketball. He usually kept his emotions hidden, but eventually they would build up. Emotional outbursts in which he was verbally abusive and threatening to family members were the result. He came to a point where he threatened suicide. At this time, his parents got him involved in counseling. After a 2-year period of counseling with few observable results, it was recommended that Donald be placed in a group home for adolescents.

Donald's adjustment to the group home setting was fair. He had difficulty forming meaningful relationships with peers and staff. However, he enjoyed playing basketball, which he had played consistently at home since he was a young child. After Donald was living in the group home for about a year, he threw a chair at another resident during an argument. His behavior was becoming increasingly more agitated with accompanying symptoms of paranoid ideation, loose associations, and insomnia. Donald was taken to a general hospital psychiatric unit where he was evaluated for appropriate placement. Upon admission, his affect was blunted, but he was friendly to the examiner, showing a sense of humor. Donald showed little spontaneity in conversation and lacked insight into his behaviors. When reciting the story of throwing the chair, he failed to take personal responsibility, but rather blamed the staff from the group home. Donald had poor long- and short-term memory and showed impoverishment of thought. The recommendation was admittance to an intermediate-term adolescent hospital for stabilization of emotions and behavior. The team felt Donald needed long-term rehabilitation for community living because he was almost 18. He was referred to a residential adolescent program in the community.

The residential program is for adolescents who need intermediate- to long-term treatment (4 to 12 months). Therapy groups, such as relationships, anger management, and self-esteem, are scheduled during the school day. Other group therapies are scheduled in the afternoon and evening, such as occupational therapy, therapeutic recreation, substance-abuse counseling, depression group, and Journeyman (a group for male issues). Individual-therapy sessions are scheduled with a social worker, licensed counselor, or psychiatrist a minimum of three times a week. The school program that the residents attend is from 8:30 AM until 1:30 PM Monday through Friday. The school is accredited and staffed with qualified special-education teachers. Classes include career planning, cooking skills, computer skills, and art as well as the traditional academic curriculum.

Donald was assigned to the school program but resists attending because "I have already graduated and should have my diploma." The school he last attended says he still has two credits to complete prior to graduation. Therefore, Donald has been assigned to attend school. He frequently refuses to go, which means he has to stay on the living unit and do paper and pencil tasks assigned by the staff as homework. On the living unit, Donald likes to watch television and seldom interacts with either peers or staff.

Donald's counselor and social worker are concerned because Donald says he wants to work, but he has a poor work history. He says he wants to live in the community, but again, he has had difficulty adjusting to his environment and lacks independent living skills. Donald reluctantly agreed to come for an evaluation in occupational therapy.

Donald was given the Adolescent Role Assessment (ARA), an interview that explores the relationship of childhood play to occupational choice and performance. He was also asked to complete the Perceptual Memory Task (PMT) to examine overall information processing, short- and intermediate-term memory, spatial relationships, and learning style. The ARA revealed that Donald had difficulty identifying childhood games and other childhood experiences. He said he played basketball in his neighborhood and learned to play computer games, but couldn't remember at what age these events occurred. He reported that it was difficult for him to make friends with the same or opposite sex and that he preferred to spend time by himself. Donald said he graduated from high school, but that the teachers at Eldon Center had not been able to get his diploma. He said it was upsetting to him to have to continue to attend school because he had graduated already. When asked about jobs, Donald reported that he had three different jobs, but was fired from each one after a few weeks. He spoke in detail about his last job at a buffet-style restaurant. He said that in his opinion he did a good job, but that his supervisors didn't appreciate him. He described his tasks as food preparation, washing dishes, cleaning, and vacuuming the floor. He wasn't sure why he got fired, but thought it was because his supervisors didn't like him. When Donald was asked to complete the PMT, he attempted three of the spatial designs. He had difficulty remembering the designs when the card was taken away and refused to do any more. He was scheduled to come on a second day for more testing.

The therapist's intent was for Donald to complete a standardized comprehensive vocational evaluation (McCarron-Dial Work Evaluation System) which was to evaluate verbal/spatial/cognitive, sensorimotor, and social/emotional functioning with a resultant predictive vocational level and independent living skill level. Donald completed the first subtest, the haptic test of sensory integration (of visual, tactile, and kinesthetic stimuli). His standard score overall was 67 (less than two standard deviations below the mean for the general population), with lowest scores on size and texture discrimination. When asked to do the Bender, a test of visual motor integration, Donald looked at the first card, which contained a circle and touching diamond which he was to draw while looking at the card. He stared at the examiner, refusing to do anything. When pushed for a response, he said, "I hate to draw." Then the examiner asked him to do a fine motor task of putting small beads from one box into another. Again he stared at the examiner, refusing to do the task or to talk about it. At this point, the examiner moved back from the table, as Donald appeared to be decompensating in his thoughts as evidenced by his facial expression and blank stare. When gently pushed again for a response, he said, "I have been tested by psychiatrists many times and I never do well." When asked what he wanted to do to make some vocational plans, he said he didn't know. When the examiner asked him if he would like to prepare some food and do a cleaning task, his face lit up. He said, "Could I show you what I know how to do?" When this was affirmed, he relaxed, smiled, and made a contract with the therapist. He agreed to make an omelet with onions, green peppers, and mushrooms, and some toast. He also agreed to vacuum the floor.

Donald came to the third session with a positive attitude. He appeared motivated to do the cooking task, as evidenced by his socially appropriate affect, movements, and interactions. The therapist oriented Donald to where his supplies were in the kitchen. He walked around the room aimlessly for about a minute. Then he turned on the stove burner, put the frying pan on it, and sprayed it with cooking oil. He did not check the pan again until he was ready to put in the eggs after the vegetables were cut. He tried to prepare his food, but had difficulty sequencing, planning, and organizing. He cut the vegetables in large chunks and had too many for the number of eggs. He hesitated when trying to figure out how to get the eggs in the pan and then how to mix in the vegetables. He had difficulty getting the toast out of the toaster and slightly burned his fingers on each of the four pieces. He dipped his fingers in the egg mixture while it was cooking. He had spills that he did not clean up or even seem to notice. Eventually he said the food didn't taste very good, but he had fun cooking it.

After cooking, Donald vacuumed a small office where he was told to move a chair and a wastebasket in order to vacuum the entire floor. He moved erratically, missing several places on the carpet. He left dirt, although he was redirected. He did not vacuum under things, nor move the chair and wastebasket. He said he did a good job.

Case A-17 Lou

Cheryl L. Stewart

Lou is 25 years old, blond with brown eyes, and a golden suntan. She is 5 feet 5 inches tall, with pretty, angular features. She has a history of hypoxia causing a massive seizure resulting in respiratory and cardiac arrest. Lou suffered significant brain damage. Lou's family reports that her seizure resulted from her spouse's attempt to suffocate her following a heated argument over custody of their 15-month-old daughter and pending divorce proceedings. Evidence of drugs was found in her blood on emergency room admission. There is suspicion she was drugged before the suffocation attempt. Because of legal technicalities, no charges have been filed in this case. Lou was admitted to an acute rehabilitation center following initial hospitalization and condition stabilization. Acute rehabilitation records indicate status plateau. Lou was recently admitted to On With Life at Glenwood because her family was unable to care for her at home. On With Life at Glenwood is a skilled-nursing facility specializing in the care of head-injured young adults.

Lou's family is very involved in her care and visit often. They seem pleased with her placement at Glenwood. They were very helpful in describing previous roles and favored occupations. Lou is the youngest of three girls. She had worked as an accountant for the local bank for several years. She is well liked in the community. She was active in local charitable organizations and enjoyed visiting with friends. She was a great seamstress and craftswoman. Lou had taken her crafts to multiple bazaars and shows. She enjoyed riding her bike and frequently set up 5- to 25-mile rides with friends and family. Lou was very active. Her family reports that she was always concerned about her weight, insisting she must stay active so she could eat. Lou was a "social butterfly" and every activity had to have just the right food.

Lou now presents as an alert nonverbal client with severe spastic quadriparesis. She seems to recognize family members and responds expressively with her eyes, facial expressions, and simple gestures. Her arms are held in the flexion synergy pattern. With inhibition techniques, increased time, muscle relaxation, and mobilization, she can achieve the following passive range of motion measurements:

- Functional shoulder range bilaterally.
- Right-elbow extension is within normal range.
- Left-elbow extension to minus 45 degrees.
- Supination results in pained response and a maximum of neutral bilaterally.
- Both wrists are contracted at minus 30 degrees flexion.
- If the wrist is allowed to drop to an at rest position, her hand passive-range-of-motion is within normal limits throughout bilaterally.
- If the wrists are passively extended, the fingers lose 15 to 20 degrees of extension. Her fingers seem to be extremely sensitive. She gives an expression of pain when the fingers are ranged into extension from the resting flexed pattern.
- Active movement is present in the mid-range of shoulder movements bilaterally and between 70 and 120 degrees of elbow flexion with gravity eliminated.
- Legs continue to move in an uncoordinated pattern, without weight-bearing.
- Head control is poor and tends to flex anteriorly and to the right.

The patient is unable to access the nurse's call light. Lou is very responsive when spoken to or when listening to others. She reportedly uses eye blinks for yes and no with 60 percent accuracy. Lou has very expressive facial features. She attempts to comply with simple one-step directions, requiring extra time to do so. Lou has difficulty relaxing to put her head back on a pillow or to use her headrest on her wheelchair.

She uses a Tilt'n Space wheel chair with an autobauch head support; "H" strap chest harness; bilateral swing-away lateral thoracic pads; lap tray (with elbow protective pads); seatbelt with auto-buckle; and 70-degree swing-away leg rests. Lou swings her leg over the outside of the leg rest and bed rails. Potential for injury to her legs while in her wheelchair or in bed is great. Additional padding is required. Within a few hours of admission, it was noticed that she has rubbed red sores on the lateral superior aspect of her feet, with the left worse than the right. Apparently, she has rubbed them along the bed-rail pads so much that it caused a friction burn.

Lou has high-topped tennis shoes to help prevent further foot drop bilaterally. She has bilateral anti-spastic ball splints that appear to be too big and spread the fingers too wide. Wrist-flexion contractures do not allow for placement of these splints.

Lou is totally tube fed, but has no significant drooling. She has not had any aspiration-type illnesses. She can, with effort, bring lips together on command, given significant time to do so. She requires at least 10 to 15 seconds to comply. She may require more time if distracted or otherwise stressed. She is very easily distracted. Her attention span is short—1 or 2 minutes without cues. Lou's records do not indicate that any swallow-study or oral-feeding programs have been tried.

Lou is dependent in all areas of self-care. She has been working with the previous placement staff to gain bladder control. She is continent up to 50 percent of the time, if toileted on 2-hour intervals for bladder, with occasional continent bowel movements

Lou's strengths include the following:

- Desire to comply with directives
- Beginning volitional movement in both upper extremities, movement of at least minimal control in the lower extremities
- Very expressive face and eyes
- Wheelchair meets her current needs
- Supportive family
- Good saliva control with imitation of oral movement patterns
- Possible potential for oral eating
- Appears alert and seems to be well oriented to at least one person
- In good general condition
- Possible potential for bowel and bladder control

Lou's weaknesses include the following:

- Moderate to severe spastic quadriparesis
- Contractures are beginning bilaterally at elbows, wrists, and hands, with painful fingers
- Beginning footdrop
- Nonverbal, without consistent communication of yes and no
- Cannot use nursing call light
- Non-oral feeder
- No appropriate splint program to decrease contractures
- Dependent in all self-care skills
- Poor head control
- Non—weight-bearing
- Poorly controlled lower extremities have strong injury potential
- Distractible with short attention span
- Difficulty relaxing—affects the success of her bowel and bladder training program

Case A-18 Tara

Christy Walloch

The members of a local early-intervention team referred Tara to occupational therapy because of her longstanding feeding problems. Tara was receiving weekly physical therapy and early-intervention educational services. Although an occupational therapist had worked with her when Tara was younger, her parents did not agree with the occupational therapist's approach to treating Tara. Therefore, her parents discontinued occupational therapy services approximately 6 months prior to this referral. Tara, a child of Hispanic descent, is 18 months old at the time of this evaluation. She lives with her parents, paternal grandparents, and older brother, all of whom accompanied Tara to her occupational-therapy evaluation. Her mother reports that Tara is the only girl in the last two generations born in her husband's family. Tara is very special to them.

At this time, Tara exhibits severe neurological dysfunction, uncontrolled seizures, and significant developmental delay. At the chronological age of 18 months, her motor and developmental skills are at the 4- to 5-month level. She displays quadriparesis with spastic and dyskinetic components. Her movements are impacted by the presence of residual primitive reflexes (bilateral asymmetrical tonic-neck reflex, symmetrical tonic-neck reflex, and tonic labyrinthine in both supine and prone positions). If held in a supported sitting position, she is able to swat at objects. She demonstrates a gross grasp and can hold toys for brief periods. Although she can bring her hands to midline while grasping a toy, she is unable to transfer it at midline. If placed on her stomach, she can roll to her back. However, she is unable to roll from her back to her stomach. She displays good eye contact and can follow objects with her eyes. Tara is interactive with her parents and the therapist.

Severe growth retardation and severe protein-energy malnutrition are exhibited (for example, weight for height, weight for age, and height for age parameters were less than 60 percent of ideal). Her parents report that Tara is very irritable, and suffers from frequent upper-respiratory infections. When queried about feedings, her parents report that feedings last up to $1\frac{1}{2}$ to 2 hours in duration. Tara is dependent for all feeding skills. Her parents state that Tara frequently coughs during meals. She is drinking liquids from bottle and sipper cup. Infant foods and mashed table foods are also given. Her parents express that Tara has to be held during eating, as she does not have the head and trunk control necessary to maintain a seated position in her highchair. When placed in a highchair, Tara extends and scoots out of the chair. She often falls to the side. Unsupported sitting in a highchair interferes with Tara's ability to volitionally open and close her mouth or move her tongue in a coordinated fashion because of her lack of stability. Evaluation of her swallowing shows that she has moderately to severely impaired oral and pharyngeal dysfunction. The oral dysfunction results in her inability to break down food and move it to the back of her mouth. She is unable to clear food from her mouth. Food and liquids are often lost from her mouth.

Videofluoroscopic exam of her swallow indicated mild aspiration. Some of the aspiration (food or liquid entering the trachea) during the evaluation occurred secondary to seizure activity during eating. Coughing is exhibited to help clear her airway after aspiration. Because of the poor timing of the pharyngeal phase of her swallow, Tara has to swallow three or four times to clear her throat. Feeding is a very arduous process for both her parents and herself. As she becomes increasingly irritable, her parents become increasingly tense and nervous.

Her parents reported that previous healthcare professionals who had evaluated Tara had recommended that oral feedings should be kept to a minimum and that a gastrostomy (tube feeding) was necessary. Her parents expressed that they were opposed to that recommendation. It is important to her parents that Tara be able to join them during mealtime. Her mother related that it is a social time for family and Tara needs to be part of it. Her parents also hold a number of underlying fears and anxieties, such as the following:

- Instituting gastrostomy feedings is a sign that they have given up on their daughter.
- They are abandoning the one thing that Tara is able to do that is normal.
- Gastrostomy feedings are just one more thing to emphasize their daughter's problems.
- Family and friends will view them as failures because they are not able to feed their daughter.
- No one will assist with childcare if Tara has a gastrostomy.
- People will not interact with her because she is technology dependent.
- Tara might not tolerate the gastrostomy surgery and could possibly die.

It is very clear after talking with her parents that tube feedings are not an option they care to explore. They have come here "to learn how to feed their daughter."

The immediate goal is to improve Tara's nutritional status. Therefore, a high-density calorie formula that is thickened to a nectar texture is recommended. Drinking nectar-textured liquids appears to be the safest and most efficient way Tara can eat orally. Since Tara is unable to consume sufficient calories through foods, foods are to be kept to minimum, as they only serve to lengthen the mealtime and tire her out. Her caloric requirements will be met by the formula. A regime of pulmonary percussion before mealtimes and at bedtime is introduced to help keep her airway clear. An adaptive seating insert is fabricated to assist Tara in maintaining a stable well-aligned skeletal system while seated in her highchair. This increased stability helps to optimize her oral motor skills during eating. Her parents are trained in how to perform the pulmonary percussion, prepare her formula, and feed her. These measures will help improve her nutrition for the current time.

Case A-19 Barb

Mary Way

Barb is an 85-year-old black woman who is currently admitted to the hospital with a diagnosis of a right hip fracture. The secondary diagnoses are: diabetes mellitus (DM), Parkinson's disease, coronary artery disease (CAD), and arthritis.

Barb is a rather shy woman who is one of five children who grew up in a small town in Georgia. She finished high school and also went on to complete 2 years of college. Barb earned a degree in education, which enabled her to teach in a local school district in Georgia. She continued to teach until she met her husband, Robert. After their marriage, she discontinued her role as a teacher and began to pursue a new role as a wife and homemaker. She was primarily responsible for the cooking, cleaning, shopping, and laundry tasks. She reported her husband used to help her "when he could."

Throughout the years of their marriage, Barb gave birth to five children: three boys and two girls. Unfortunately, her second boy, John, was killed in an automobile accident when he was 15. This was a very difficult emotional crisis for Barb and required years of therapy and counseling. However, despite the unfortunate circumstances, she remained a strong and stable force in the lives of her other four children. She participated in many parent organizations and organized a variety of charity and benefit events for the clubs and sports in which her children were involved. She took great pleasure in watching them grow up and continues to be proud of their accomplishments. She also currently enjoys her twelve grandchildren and eight great-grandchildren.

Barb currently lives alone in a two-bedroom apartment. She has lived there since the death of her husband 1 year ago. She comments that she is still adjusting to the loss of her husband and has not fully "gotten used to being alone." Her children, some of whom still live in Georgia, have asked her to come and live with them. However, Barb wants to remain independent and prefers to stay on her own for as long as she is able. Twelve steps lead to the entrance to her apartment. However, the apartment itself is all on one level.

Her past hobbies have included reading, embroidery, sewing, gardening, writing letters, and participating in church discussion groups. Because of her current impaired eyesight and the arthritis in her hands, she does not participate in the fine motor tasks as frequently as she previously did. Besides maintaining her apartment with help from her children, she usually engages in listening to the radio, listening to mystery books on tape, watching television, and praying. Prior to admission she was independent in self-care and meal preparation. However she did require extra time to complete all tasks.

Barb's overall physical condition is poor due to general debilitation. Her physical deficits include: weakness in her upper extremities (UE) (with more severe weakness in her right UE) and lower extremities, and arthritis in her neck, spine, hands, and knees.

Barb is alert and oriented times three and is able to recall past and present events and information. Perceptual skills are within normal functional limits, but were not directly assessed. Some visual perceptual deficits may exist due to her impaired eyesight.

Her strengths include:

- Pleasant disposition
- Good motivation
- Cooperation
- Good cognitive/perceptual abilities
- Good family support

Barb's weaknesses include:

- Lack of muscle strength
- Severe arthritis
- Lives alone

- Overall general debilitation
- Right hip fracture (pain, limited range of motion, and limited functional abilities)
- Parkinson's disease (slow movements, resting tremors, memory loss, and postural instability)

Barb wants desperately to return home as soon as possible. She is worried how she will be able to care for herself at home with her fracture. She wants to be independent in all of the activities she needs to function at home. However, she realized that her eyesight and arthritis are becoming more of a problem. She wants to know about different ways she can become independent, so as not to be a problem for her children.

Recommended Narratives of Disability

Narratives of disability are listed here for your use in combination with the Power Builders at the ends of the chapters. This list includes four very recent narratives of living with disability reviewed by Bennett, Cunningham, Pierce, and Tuminski (2002). They also recommended seven other classic narratives as useful to practitioners in developing their understanding of the life stories and occupational patterns of persons with disabilities. Effective practice requires such a depth of insight. The narratives are also fascinating to read. I warn you, they can also provoke some strong feelings as you put yourself in the place of someone living with a disability.

Reference

Bennett, O., Cunningham, A., Pierce, D., & Tuminski, K. (2002). Reflections on disability: Ethnography, cultural biography, and essay. *American Journal of Occupational Therapy, 56,* 595–597.

Bibliography

Bauby, J. (1998). *The diving bell and the butterfly: A memoir of life in death.* New York: Holt.

Beisser, A. R. (1989). *Flying without wings: Personal reflections on being disabled.* New York: Doubleday.

Clare, E. (1999). *Exile and pride: Disability, queerness, and liberation.* Cambridge, MA: South End Press.

Fadiman, A. (1997). *The spirit catches you and you fall down.* New York: Farrar, Strauss, and Giroux.

Frank, G. (2000). *Venus on wheels: Two decades of dialogue on disability, biography, and being female in America.* Berkeley, CA: University of California Press.

Hockenberry, J. (1995). *Moving violations: War zones, wheelchairs, and declarations of independence.* New York: Hyperion.

Keller, H. (1903). *The story of my life.* New York: Doubleday.

Klein, B. S. (1997). *Slow dance: A story of stroke, love, and disability.* Berkeley, CA: Page Mill Press. (Also published in Canada By Alfred A. Knopf under the title *Out of the blue.*)

Murphy, R. (1987). *The body silent.* New York: Henry Holt.

Price, R. (1994). *A whole new life: An illness and a healing.* New York: Atheneum.

Zola, I. (1982). *Missing pieces: A chronicle of living with a disability.* Philadelphia: Temple University Press.

Recommended Narratives of Occupational Experience

The following list provides a variety of descriptions of occupational experience from the perspectives of very different people. They are provided here for your use in combination with Power Builders at the ends of the chapters. You may just find them enjoyable to read too. Many of them are written for the popular press. If you are looking for a bit more conceptual growth, the books by DeVault, Lancy, and Scott would probably fit the bill. Perhaps you have read other narratives of occupational experience? To me, a strong narrative of occupational experience tells about doing from the perspective of the person, describes it at a fairly detailed level, and includes the contextual dimensions of occupation.

Bibliography

Bateson, M. C. (1990). *Composing a life*. New York: The Penguin Group.

Baxandall, R., & Gordon, L. (1995). *America's working women: A documentary history 1600 to the present*. New York: W. W. Norton & Company.

Bird, C. (1995). *Lives of our own: Secrets of salty old women*. New York: Houghton Mifflin Company.

DeVault, M. L. (1991). *Feeding the family: The social organization of caring as gendered work*. Chicago, IL: University of Chicago Press.

Dillard, A. (1989). *The writing life*. New York: HarperCollins.

Ehrenreich, B. (2001). *Nickel and dimed*. New York: Henry Holt and Company.

Foley, M. (1999). *Mankind: Have a nice day! A tale of blood and sweatsocks*. New York: Regan Books.

Lancy, D. (1996). *Playing on the motherground: Cultural routines for children's development*. New York: Guilford Press.

Lydon, S. G. (1997). *The knitting sutra: Craft as a spiritual practice*. New York: HarperCollins.

Myerhoff, B. (1980). *Number our days*. New York: Simon & Schuster.

Sarton, M. (1973). *Journal of a solitude*. New York: W.W. Norton & Company.

Scott, S. (1995). *Two sides to everything: The cultural construction of class consciousness in Harlan County, Kentucky*. Albany, NY: State University of New York Press.

... *Index*

Page numbers followed by a "t" indicate tables.